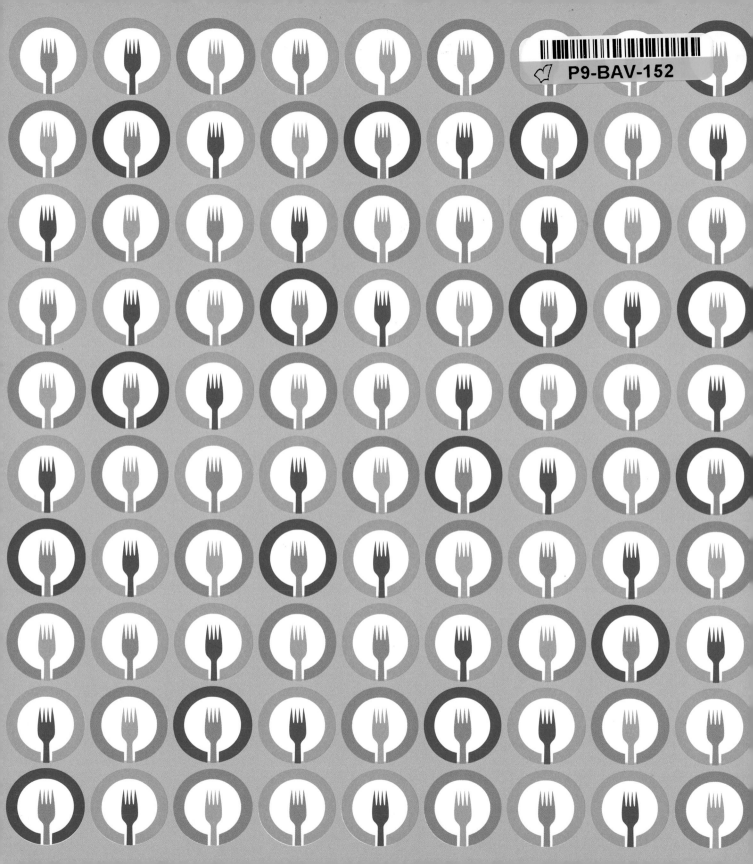

THE WHOLE30

FAST & EASY

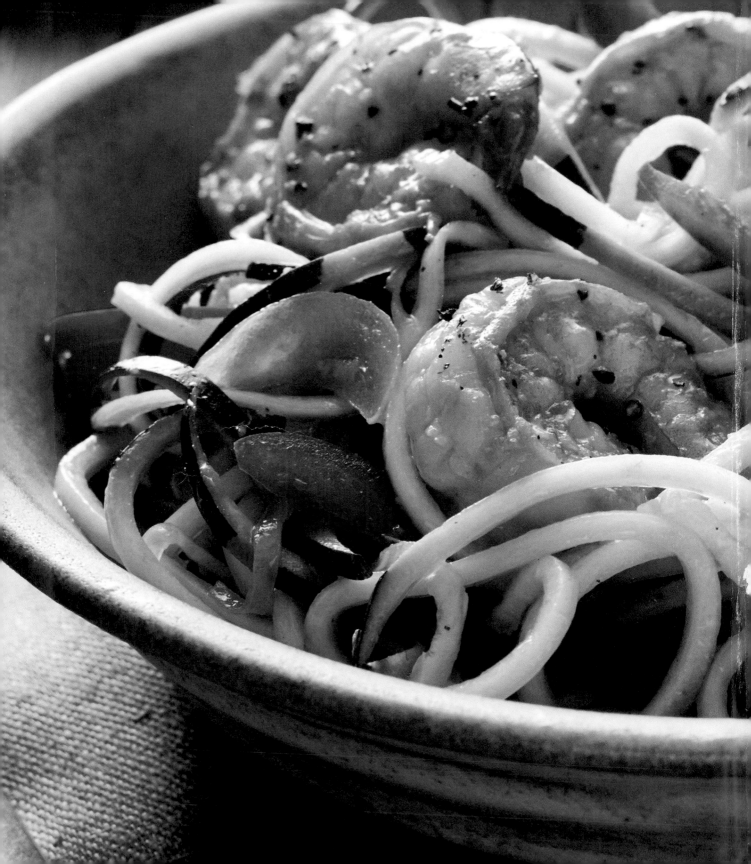

THE WHOLE30® FAST&EASY

150 Simply Delicious Everyday Recipes for Your Whole30

MELISSA HARTWIG

Co-author of the *New York Times* best-selling *The Whole30*

Photography by Ghazalle Badiozamani

Houghton Mifflin Harcourt
BOSTON   NEW YORK

For you, my faithful Whole30ers

For information about permission to reproduce selections from this book, write
to trade.permissions@hmhco.com or to Permissions, Houghton Mifflin Harcourt
Publishing Company, 3 Park Avenue, 19th Floor, New York, New York 10016.

hmhco.com

Library of Congress Cataloging-in-Publication Data is available.

ISBN 978-1-328-83920-6 (hbk)

ISBN 978-1-328-83939-8 (ebk)

Book design by Vertigo Design NYC

Printed in the United States of America

DOC 10 9 8 7 6 5

4500697373

CONTENTS

ACKNOWLEDGMENTS vi

PREFACE vii

WHAT IS THE WHOLE30? viii

THE WHOLE30 RULES x

GETTING STARTED WITH THE WHOLE30 xiii

WHOLE30 KITCHEN ESSENTIALS xv

Main Dish Salads and Wraps 1

Skillet Meals, Stir-Fries, and Sautés 45

Sheet Pan Suppers 113

Soups, Stews, and Noodle Bowls 157

Stir-and-Go Slow Cooker Recipes 211

Simple Sides 257

Sauces and Dressings 273

Basics 279

WHOLE30 RESOURCES 285

WHOLE30 APPROVED 290

WHOLE30 SUPPORT 293

COOKING CONVERSIONS 294

INDEX 295

ACKNOWLEDGMENTS

To Justin Schwartz, my editor at Houghton Mifflin Harcourt, writing and editing with you continues to be a joy. I like you more and more with every book we work on together—and we have worked on a lot of books.

To Bruce Nichols, Ellen Archer, Marina Padakis, Deb Brody, Claire Safran, Jessica Gilo, Rebecca Liss, and the entire Houghton Mifflin Harcourt team, you give so much to me and to the Whole30 community. I am so happy you are my people.

To Andrea Magyar and Trish Bunnett at Penguin Canada, you continue to encourage, support, and motivate me to better serve our Canadian Whole30ers. Thank you for your continued faith in this program and our mission.

To Christy Fletcher, you are my advocate, my sounding board, and my sympathetic ear when the writing gets hard. Thank you for being on my team.

To Grainne Fox, Melissa Chinchillo, Erin McFadden, Sylvie Greenberg, Sarah Fuentes, and the Fletcher and Company team, thank you for your tireless efforts to support my books and my engagements. I love working with all of you.

To Ghazalle Badiozamani, your talents were so well-suited to this book. Thank you for supporting our vision so beautifully.

To Paola Andrea and Monica Pierini, you took our ingredients and turned them into meals that will inspire hundreds of thousands of budding cooks. Thank you for sharing your passion with our readers.

To our talented guest contributors: Dana Monsees, Anya Kaats, Scott Gooding, Jessica Beacom, Stacie Hassing, Kelly Smith, ChihYu Smith, Brian Kavanagh, Laura Miner, and Ronny Joseph. Thank you for everything you do for our community, and for sharing your creative, healthy dishes here with us.

To Sarah Steffens, our Whole30 in-house recipe creative, bringing you on board was one of the best ideas I've ever had. Thank you for all of your hard work reviewing these recipes to make sure they're as fast, easy, and delicious as possible, and contributing your own favorite dishes to the project.

To my Whole30 team: Kristen Crandall, Shanna Keller, Jen Kendall, Karyn Scott, and Tawni Schall; thank you for giving so much of yourselves to our mission, vision, and community. You are Whole30.

To my family and friends, thank you for your love, support, and encouragement. And don't ever let me write two books at the same time again. I mean it. Where were you people in December?

To Dallas, thank you for your contributions to the Whole30 program and this community. I will always be grateful.

For my son, you are my whole world.

Finally, to YOU, my Whole30ers. I will always do as much as I can to make you healthy, happy, and successful in the Whole30 and your food freedom. You give more to me than I could ever give to you. Thank you.

PREFACE

There are so many good things to say about the Whole30. It has the power to radically transform your health in just 30 days. It's incredibly effective at breaking undesirable food-related habits. It fosters a comfortable, healthy, secure relationship with food. It can be one of the most life-changing, empowering experiences of your life.

But the dishes. Oh, the dishes.

And the grocery shopping. And the label-reading. And the prepping. And the cooking. Did we mention the chopping? *So much chopping.* Making the switch from grab-and-go, processed, convenience, or take-out foods to home-cooked whole food meals can have a bit of a learning curve, especially if you'd describe yourself as "kitchen challenged." But if there's one thing I've learned in my own Whole30 and food freedom journey, it's not to overthink this part.

Your Whole30 meals don't have to be complicated, time-consuming, or use obscure ingredients to be incredibly satisfying, totally delicious, and make you feel like a kitchen rock star. You can get an impressive Whole30 dinner on the table in under 20 minutes. You can buy "normal" foods from any old grocery store and use simple techniques to transform them into delicious, hearty, nourishing meals. You can throw five things into a slow cooker, walk away, and come back to an incredible, ready-to-serve feast. And thanks to modern conveniences like packaged "veggie noodles," precut produce, and minced garlic in a jar, if you *really* don't want to chop, you probably don't have to.

Truth is, all you need to succeed with the Whole30 are whole-food ingredients and some helpful instructions to help you prep, cook, and serve them in a way that's fast, easy, *and* tasty. In fact, this is an entire book full of recipes that do just that—

plus the tips, tricks, and hacks I've cultivated in my own Whole30 kitchen. We've created more than 150 recipes using few ingredients, simple preparation instructions, short start-to-finish times, and/or little hands-on time. The end goal? Delicious, creative, satisfying Whole30 meals that won't keep you chained to your cutting board, stovetop, or oven.

Along the way, I'll also share my favorite Whole30 shortcuts: pre-packaged whole foods that help you prep faster, Whole30 Approved grab-and-go condiments to add flavor and keep things fresh, and kitchen tools that make almost any job easier and more fun.

Even chopping.

Finally, keeping in the spirit of "fast and easy," I'll offer this last piece of Whole30 advice: Let good enough be good enough. Not every Whole30 meal has to be a from-scratch, candlelit, religious experience. Some days, you might be in the car with left-over One-Pan Meatballs (page 147), or eating your Warm Salmon and Potato Salad (page 16) stone-cold out of the glass storage container, or topping your Steamed Cod with compliant jarred tomato sauce instead of the Spicy Roasted Tomato-Fennel Sauce (page 214).

This is all *totally okay.*

Did you stick to the Whole30 rules? Yes. Did you feed yourself a satisfying, nutrient-dense meal? Yes. Should we let good enough be good enough here, given our modern lives, busy schedules, and emotional capacity for picking thyme leaves off the stem one by one? HELL YES.

And with that, I'll leave you to it . . . but first, a quick refresher on the Whole30 program.*

Best in health,
MELISSA HARTWIG

*For a detailed planning and preparation guide, including an extensive FAQ and reintroduction schedule, refer to *The Whole30: The 30-Day Guide to Total Health and Food Freedom.*

WHAT IS THE WHOLE30?

Think of the Whole30 like pushing the reset button with your health, your habits, and your relationship with food.

The premise is simple: Certain food groups (like sugar, grains, dairy, and legumes) could be having a negative impact on your body composition, health, and quality of life without you even realizing it. Are your energy levels inconsistent or nonexistent? Do you have aches and pains that can't be explained by over-use or injury? Are you having a hard time losing weight no matter how hard you try? Do you have some sort of condition (like skin issues, digestive ailments, seasonal allergies, or chronic fatigue) that medication hasn't helped? These symptoms may be directly related to the foods you eat—even the "healthy" stuff.

So how do you know if (and how) these foods are affecting you? Eliminate them from your diet completely. Cut out all the psychologically unhealthy, hormone-unbalancing, gut-disrupting, inflammatory food groups for a full 30 days. Let your body heal and recover from whatever effects those foods may be causing. Push the reset button on your metabolism, systemic inflammation, and the downstream physical and psychological effects of the food choices you've been making. Learn how the foods you've been eating are actually affecting your day-to-day life, long-term health, body composition, and relationship with food.

these foods for a set period of time, experiencing what life is like without these commonly problematic triggers while paying careful attention to improvements in energy, sleep, digestion, mood, attention span, self-confidence, cravings, chronic pain or fatigue, athletic performance and recovery, and any number of symptoms or medical conditions. This elimination period will give you a new "normal"— a healthy baseline where, in all likelihood, you will look, feel, and live better than you ever imagined you could.

At the end of the 30 days, you'll then carefully and systematically reintroduce those foods you've been missing, again paying attention to any changes in your experience. Do your two p.m. energy slumps return? Does your stomach bloat? Does your face break out, your joints swell, your pain return? Does your Sugar Dragon rear his ugly head? The reintroduction period teaches you how specific foods are having a negative impact on *you*, and exactly how these foods are making you look and feel less than your best.

Put it all together, and for the first time in your life, you'll be able to make educated decisions about when, how often, and in what amount you can include these "less healthy" foods in your daily diet in a way that feels balanced and sustainable, but still keeps you looking feeling as awesome as you now *know* you can look and feel.

How It Works

For a full 30 days, you'll completely eliminate the foods that scientific literature and my clinical experience have shown to be the most commonly problematic in one of four areas—your cravings, metabolism, digestion, and immune system. During the elimination period, you'll completely eliminate

The Results

I cannot possibly put enough emphasis on this simple fact—the next 30 days will change your life. They will change the way you think about food, they will change your tastes, they will change your habits and your cravings. It will restore a healthy emotional relationship with food, and with your body. It has the potential to change the way you eat for the rest of your life. I know this because I did it, and millions of thousands of people have done it since, and it changed my lives (and their lives) in a dramatic and permanent fashion.

The physical benefits of the Whole30 are profound. A full 96 percent of participants lose weight and improve their body composition without counting or restricting calories. Also commonly reported? Consistently high energy levels, better sleep, improved focus and mental clarity, a return to healthy digestive function, improved athletic performance, and a sunnier disposition. (Yes, many Whole30 graduates say they felt "strangely happy" during and after their program.)

The psychological benefits of the Whole30 may be even more dramatic. Through the program, participants report effectively changing long-standing, unhealthy habits related to food, developing a healthier body image, and dramatically reducing or eliminating cravings, particularly for sugar and carbohydrates. The words so many Whole30 participants use to describe this place?

"Food freedom."

Finally, testimonials from thousands of Whole30 participants document the improvement or "curing" of any number of lifestyle-related diseases and conditions.

• high blood pressure • high cholesterol • type 1 diabetes • type 2 diabetes • asthma • allergies • sinus infections • hives • skin conditions • endometriosis • PCOS • infertility • migraines • depression • bipolar disorder • heartburn • GERD • arthritis • joint pain • ADHD • thyroid dysfunction • Lyme disease • fibromyalgia • chronic fatigue • lupus • leaky gut syndrome • Crohn's • IBS • celiac disease • diverticulitis • ulcerative colitis

THE WHOLE30 RULES

For the next 30 days, you'll be eating meat, seafood, and eggs; lots of vegetables and fruit; natural, healthy fats; and herbs, spices, and seasonings—with no slips, cheats, or special occasions. Eat foods with very few ingredients, all pronounceable ingredients, or better yet, no ingredients listed at all because they're whole and unprocessed. Below are the program rules. (Please refer to *The Whole30: The 30-Day Guide to Total Health and Food Freedom* for a complete list of rules, and use that book to prepare for and succeed with your program.)

DO NOT CONSUME ADDED SUGAR OF ANY KIND, REAL OR ARTIFICIAL. No maple syrup, honey, agave nectar, coconut sugar, date syrup, stevia, Splenda, Equal, Nutrasweet, xylitol, etc. Read your labels, because companies sneak sugar into products in ways you might not recognize.

DO NOT CONSUME ALCOHOL IN ANY FORM. No wine, beer, champagne, vodka, rum, whiskey, tequila, etc., whether consumed on its own or used as an ingredient—not even for cooking.

DO NOT EAT GRAINS. This includes wheat, rye, barley, oats, corn, rice, millet, bulgur, sorghum, sprouted grains, and all gluten-free pseudo-cereals like amaranth, buckwheat, or quinoa. This also includes all the ways we add wheat, corn, and rice into our foods in the form of bran, germ, starch, and so on. Again, read your labels.

DO NOT EAT LEGUMES. This includes beans of all kinds (black, red, pinto, navy, white, kidney, lima, fava, etc.), peas, chickpeas, lentils, and peanuts. This also includes all forms of soy—soy sauce, miso, tofu, tempeh, edamame, and all the ways we sneak soy into foods (like soybean oil or soy lecithin). No peanut butter, either. The only exceptions are green beans and snow/snap peas.

DO NOT EAT DAIRY. This includes cow's-, goat's-, or sheep's-milk products such as milk, cream, cheese, kefir, yogurt, sour cream, ice cream, and frozen yogurt. The only exceptions are clarified butter or ghee.

DO NOT CONSUME CARRAGEENAN, MSG, OR ADDED SULFITES. If these ingredients appear in any form in the ingredient list of your processed food or beverage, it's out for the Whole30.

DO NOT RE-CREATE BAKED GOODS, "TREATS," OR JUNK FOODS WITH APPROVED INGREDIENTS. Re-creating or buying sweets, treats, and foods-with-no-brakes (even if the ingredients are technically compliant) is totally missing the point of the Whole30, and will compromise your life-changing results. These are the same foods that got you into health trouble in the first place—and a pancake is still a pancake, even if it is made with coconut flour.

Some specific foods that fall under this rule include: pancakes, waffles, bread, tortillas, wraps, biscuits, muffins, cupcakes, cookies, brownies, pizza crust, cereal, or ice cream. No commercially prepared chips (potato, tortilla, plantain, etc.) or French fries either. However, this list is not limited strictly to these items—there may be other foods that you find are not psychologically healthy for your Whole30. Use your best judgment with those foods that aren't on this list, but that you suspect are not helping you change your habits or break those cravings. Our mantra: When in doubt, leave it out. It's only 30 days. (See page 95 in *The Whole30* for further guidance.)

DO NOT STEP ON THE SCALE OR TAKE MEASUREMENTS. The Whole30 is about so much more than just loss, and to focus only on body composition means you'll overlook all of the other dramatic and lifelong benefits this plan has to offer. So no weighing yourself, analyzing body fat, or breaking out the tape measure *during* your Whole30. (We do encourage you to weigh yourself *before* and *after*, so you can see one of the more tangible results of your efforts when your program is over.)

The Fine Print

These foods are exceptions to the rule and are allowed during your Whole30.

CLARIFIED BUTTER OR GHEE. Clarified butter (page 283) and ghee are the only sources of dairy allowed during your Whole30, as they've had their milk solids rendered out. Plain old butter is *not* allowed, as its milk proteins could impact the results of your program.

FRUIT JUICE AS A SWEETENER. Some products or recipes will include fruit juice as a stand-alone ingredient or natural sweetener, which is fine for the purposes of the Whole30. (We have to draw the line somewhere.)

GREEN BEANS AND SNOW/SNAP PEAS. While these are technically legumes, they are far more "pod" than "bean," and green plant matter is generally good for you.

VINEGAR. Most forms of vinegar, including distilled white, balsamic, apple cider, red wine, white wine, champagne, and rice, are allowed during your Whole30 program. The only exceptions are flavored vinegars with added sugar, or malt vinegar, which is thought to contain gluten.

COCONUT AMINOS. All brands of coconut aminos (a brewed and naturally fermented soy sauce substitute) are acceptable, even if you see the word "coconut nectar" in the ingredient list.

IODIZED SALT. All iodized salt contains a tiny amount of dextrose (sugar) as a stabilizer, but ruling out table salt would be unreasonable. This exception will not impact your Whole30 results in any way.

It's for Your Own Good

Here comes the tough love, heavy on the *love*—perhaps the most famous part of the Whole30. This is for those of you who are considering taking on this life-changing month, but aren't sure you can actually pull it off, cheat-free, for a full 30 days. This is for people who have tried to make lifestyle changes but "slipped" or "fell off the wagon" or "just *had* to eat [fill in food here] because of this [fill in event here]."

IT IS NOT HARD. Don't you dare tell me this is hard. Beating cancer is hard. Birthing a baby is hard. Losing a parent is hard. Drinking your coffee black is. not. hard. You've done harder things than this, and you have no excuse not to complete the program as written. It's only 30 days, and it's for the most important health cause on earth: the only physical body you will ever have in this lifetime.

DON'T EVEN CONSIDER THE POSSIBILITY OF A "SLIP." Unless you physically trip and your face lands in a box of doughnuts, there is no "slip." You make a choice to eat something unhealthy. It is always a choice, so do not phrase it as if you had an accident. Commit to the program 100 percent for the full 30 days. Don't give yourself an excuse to fail before you've even started.

YOU NEVER, EVER, EVER HAVE TO EAT ANYTHING YOU DON'T WANT TO EAT. You're all big boys and girls. Toughen up. Learn to say no (or make your mom proud and say, "No, thank you"). Learn to stick up for yourself. Just because it's your sister's birthday, or your best friend's wedding, or your company picnic does not mean you have to eat anything. It's always a choice, and we would hope that you stopped succumbing to peer pressure in seventh grade.

THIS DOES REQUIRE A BIT OF EFFORT. Grocery shopping, meal planning, dining out, explaining the program to friends and family, and dealing with stress will all prove challenging at some point during your program. We've given you all the tools, guidelines, and resources you'll need in our books and on our website, but you also have to take responsibility for your own plan. Improved health, fitness, and quality of life don't happen automatically just because you're now taking a pass on bread.

YOU CAN DO THIS. You've come too far to back out now. You want to do this. You need to do this. And I know that you *can* do this. So stop thinking about it, and start doing it. Right now, this very minute, commit to the Whole30.

I want you to be a part of our community. I want you to take this seriously, and see amazing results in unexpected areas. I want you to look, feel, and live better than you have in years—or maybe ever. I want you to find lasting food freedom. Even if you don't believe this will actually change your life, if you're willing to give it 30 short days, DO IT. It is that important. I believe in it that much. It changed my life, and I want it to change yours too.

Welcome to the Whole30.

GETTING STARTED WITH THE WHOLE30

Planning and preparation are the key to success on the Whole30. Here are some basic steps for getting your home and your head Whole30-ready. For a more detailed step-by-step plan for getting started with the program, see pages 17 to 31 in *The Whole30*.

Step 1: Choose Your Start Date

Start *as soon as you possibly can*, but plan carefully. If you've got a once-in-a-lifetime vacation, a new baby due any day now, or a wedding (especially your own!) in your immediate future, consider starting the Whole30 after those events. It's also important not to have your Whole30 end the day before a vacation, holiday, or special event. The reintroduction phase is just as critical as the 30-day elimination. Ideally, you'll allow at least 10 days after your Whole30 is done to go through your Fast Track or Slow reintroduction, *then* enjoy your special event. (See page 42 in *The Whole30* for reintroduction guidance.)

Finally, take a look at your calendar during the proposed 30-day period and see what business or personal commitments you have in place. If you've got a family dinner, a business lunch, or a bridal shower in your imminent future, excellent! Consider it an opportunity to take your Whole30 skills out on the town, and create a plan for how to handle it (see Step 4). You'll have to deal with lots of new situations during your program, so *don't* let them push your Whole30 off.

In summary, there will never be a "perfect" time to do the Whole30, so think about what you have coming up, choose a date, and circle it on your calendar in permanent marker. (Really—write it down. Habit research shows that putting your commitment on paper makes you more likely to succeed.)

Step 2: Build Your Support Team

Finding the right support network will be critical to keeping you motivated, inspired, and accountable during your program. The first step is sharing a bit about the program, leading with the things you *will* be eating. Say something like, "For thirty days, I'll eat lots of whole, fresh, nutritious foods—no calorie counting at all! Breakfast could be a vegetable frittata, fresh fruit, and avocado; lunch is a spinach salad with grilled chicken, apples, pecans, and a raspberry-walnut vinaigrette; and dinner is pulled pork carnitas with roasted sweet potato and a cabbage slaw."

You should also share with those you care about *why* you are choosing to embark upon this journey. Make it personal. Share your current struggles, your goals, and all the ways you believe the program will make you healthier and happier. Try something like, "Every day at three p.m., I feel like I need a nap. I'm hoping the Whole30 will help me keep my energy up without my usual afternoon soda and candy bar."

Finally, don't forget to *ask* for their support. Saying very directly, "Can I count on you to support me for the next thirty days?" lets them know how important these efforts are to you and how much you'd value their encouragement and help.

Still, despite all your best efforts, family and friends may be less than supportive of your Whole30 plan. If you're having a hard time talking to friends and family about the Whole30 or are dealing with pushback during your conversations, read the Friends, Family, and Food section in *Food Freedom Forever* for guidance.

Step 3: Get Your House Ready

First, get all the stuff you won't be eating out of the house. It's time to clean out the pantry—be thorough; throw out the foods you won't be eating, give them to a neighbor for safekeeping, or (if you feel right about this) donate them to a local food bank.

If you're the only one at home doing the Whole30, dedicate one drawer in your fridge and one out-of-the-way cabinet for your family's off-plan items, so you don't have to reach around the Oreos every time you need a can of coconut milk.

Even if you're not the planning type, make a plan for what you'll eat for breakfast, lunch, and dinner for the first three to seven days of your Whole30. Then, go grocery shopping and buy everything you need for your first set of meals, plus Whole30 pantry staples. (See whole30.com/pdf-downloads for a detailed Shopping List.)

Step 4: Plan for Success

Think about the next 30 days, and write down every potentially stressful, difficult, or complicated situation you may encounter during your Whole30. These may include business lunches, family dinners, travel plans, a long day at work, birthday parties, holiday celebrations, office gatherings, family stress, job stress, financial stress... anything you think might derail your Whole30 train. Then, make a plan for how you'll handle it. Use if/then statements when crafting plans. Some examples might include:

BUSINESS LUNCH: If my coworkers pressure me to have a drink, then I'll say, "I'm doing this food experiment to see if I can improve my allergies, so no alcohol right now—I'll just have a mineral water, please."

FAMILY DINNER: If Mom invites me out for dinner, then I'll either choose a Whole30-friendly restaurant or ask if we can cook together instead.

TRAVEL DAY: If I get to the airport and my flight is delayed, then I'll snack on the meat stick, apples, baby carrots, and small packet of almond butter I brought in my carry-on.

Finally, find three quick and easy "go-to" recipes in this cookbook; meals you can make in 20 minutes or less with foods you always have on hand. Write your list down and pin it to your fridge so you'll always have a plan for nights when things just get crazy.

Step 5: Toss That Scale

This is your last and final step in preparing for the Whole30—for the next 30 days, get rid of your scale. Put it in the garage, give it to a friend to "hold," or better yet, take it out back and introduce it to your sledgehammer in a nice little pre-Whole30 ritual.

We don't want you to ignore your body for the next 30 days—keep an eye on how your clothes are fitting, whether your stomach is flatter, your rings are looser, or your skin is clearer. You can also take before and after measurements; weigh yourself, take body measurements, and/or a photograph on Day 0, and then again on Day 31.

Ready, Set, Whole30!

And with that (and perhaps a quick refresher of the program details, FAQs, and Whole30 Timeline in *The Whole30*), it's time for your Whole30 journey to begin! But before we jump straight into the food, let's talk about some planning and preparation tips to make the most of your *Whole30 Fast and Easy* recipes.

WHOLE30 KITCHEN ESSENTIALS

Fast & Easy Kitchen Tools

If you want to keep your Whole30 truly fast and easy, you'll want to invest in a few kitchen tools to help you do the job. (Because ain't nobody got time for mincing garlic by hand at 7 p.m. on a Wednesday night.) The good news is that most of these are pretty inexpensive and offer major time-saving bang for the buck.

We'll also suggest some "bonus" gadgets here, based on what Melissa uses in her own kitchen. These are more expensive non-essentials, but you'll be happy you made the investment the first time you realize you can have mashed sweet potatoes on the table in just 15 minutes.

Knives and Sharpener

We know you have knives, but do you have Whole30-worthy knives? With all the chopping you'll be doing, a good knife (or three) will save you time and energy.

Start with a paring knife for small cuts like dicing, an 8-inch chef's knife designed for chopping, and a long, thin slicing knife for carving. If you often have kitchen helpers, double up on the paring and chef's knives, so no one is waiting for a slow chopper.

Look for knives that are all one piece (not a blade and handle joined together), and spend some money here. Trust us, this is one investment that will pay you back every single time you cook. (And don't forget the sharpener! A good knife is only good when it's sharp.)

Kitchen Shears

You might think these are duplicative (wait, I have knives?) but a good set of shears lets you "chop" whole tomatoes still in the can, cut fresh herbs right over the dish, chop bacon into bits, and crack poultry bones with ease. We had you at "bacon," didn't we?

Multiple Measuring Cups

A set of measuring cups are pretty cheap, and how often do you waste precious time looking for the ½ tablespoon? (Hint: it's in the sink.) Doubling up on measuring cups also lets your kitchen helpers join in the fun, getting dinner on the table that much faster.

Multiple Cutting Boards

We already mentioned all the chopping, so make sure you have enough surfaces to work on—especially if raw meat is in the mix. Multiple boards let you chop your chicken separate from the veggies, reducing the trips to the sink to wash and rinse. Buy a few different sizes, including one really big one. Throw a flexible cutting board into the mix to take your ingredients straight to the pot, and consider wood fiber composite boards from Epicurean—they're durable, non-porous, and dry *really* fast.

Small Bowls

One trick to cooking faster is *mise-en-place*, the French term for "everything in its place." That means reading the whole recipe through and prepping and measuring every ingredient before you start to cook. It may sound counter-intuitive (isn't it faster to cook as I go?) but trust—having all of your ingredients measured and ready to go exactly when you need it will save you from overcooked meat while you search for the paprika. For mise-en-place to work, you'll want a variety of small bowls to hold measured spices, minced garlic, diced vegetables, and cooking oils. (And use the tricks on page xix to reduce the number of bowls you'll need to wash later.)

Big Sheet Pans

Roasting a bunch of vegetables at once is one of the fastest and tastiest ways to batch-prep for the week. Crowding your roasting tray, however, means your veggies will steam instead of roast, leaving you with soggy potatoes instead of brown, crisp, caramelized cubes. Buying two big sheet pans (with very low sides) will let you make the most of your oven and keep your vegetables, salmon cakes, or meatballs brown and toasty instead of pale and soggy. (Look for a "three-quarter sheet pan"; a full sheet pan is too big for most home ovens.)

Parchment Paper

Want to make clean-up a snap? (Duh.) Line baking sheets with parchment paper lightly coated with cooking fat before you roast. The surface will help keep vegetables and meat from sticking, and when you're done, just toss the paper and put the tray away. (Or copy Melissa and reuse it once or twice . . . all that leftover ghee or duck fat still on the paper shouldn't go to waste.)

Garlic Peeler and Press

This one could have come first, for the simplicity of the gadgets and the time they will save you. A garlic peeler is just a little silicone tube—insert your clove, rub it briskly between your hands, and the peel is removed in three seconds flat. Then, insert the clove into your press and *voilà*! Minced garlic *and* clean hands. Seriously. Buy these.

Citrus Juicer

This is another simple gadget that seems redundant, but saves you time in the squeezing and gets every last drop from those lemons or limes without the forearm cramps or messy hands.

Microplane

This handy mini-grater is perfect for making citrus zest or grating fresh ginger, two very simple ingredients that will add major punch to your fast-and-easy Whole30 meals. Just watch your knuckles; we know this from experience.

Vegetable Chopper

These handy tools come in a variety of styles, but are designed to do just one thing—take your onions/bell peppers/mushrooms/zucchini and chop them in one fell swoop. You may not want to bust this out just to dice up half an apple, but for making salsa, gazpacho, or a vegetable frittata, a chopper can easily cut your prep time by 72%. It's science.

Spiral Slicer

A spiral slicer does *way* more than turn hunks of vegetables and fruit into cool-looking noodles. Spiral-slicing your sweet potato, butternut squash, or other dense vegetables dramatically reduces the baking or roasting time, and can take the place of time-consuming grating (like for breakfast hash). Splurge a little here and buy a big one with a handle to crank (like the Paderno)—small spiralizers aren't tough enough for root vegetables, and can be a pain.

Food Processor

Blenders are great, but only if your dish has enough liquid. For effortlessly making cauliflower rice (page 75), Egg-Free Mayonnaise (page 281), or Cauliflower-Cashew Alfredo Sauce (page 276), you'll want a food processor. You *can* buy inexpensive small-capacity processors, but adding hearty portions one small batch at a time is more trouble than it's worth. Get a big one (at least 8 cups), and save smaller jobs for the immersion blender.

Immersion Blender

This powerful hand mixer is perfect for smaller jobs, where you don't want to put together (and clean) the food processor. Use it for Mayonnaise (page 281), Apple Butternut Squash Soup (page 168), or to blend your homemade salad dressing.

Slow Cooker

There is no easier meal than something you add to the slow cooker in the morning and pull out to serve as soon as you get home. We've got a lot of slow cooker meals featured here, and this is one investment that will pay you back in time and weeknight stress over and over again. Buy a big one (at least six quarts) for cooking large pieces of meat, make sure it has a timer and "keep warm" setting, and if you want to be extra-fancy, look for one with a built-in "sear" function to brown meat effortlessly.

Alternative: Instant Pot

An Instant Pot is like an all-in-one pressure cooker, slow cooker, and steamer (and includes some features you won't need on your Whole30 but might come in handy later, like a rice-cooker setting). It cuts your cooking time tremendously (spaghetti squash in 10 minutes, a whole sweet potato in under 15 minutes, and bone broth just 2 hours), and takes the place of your slow cooker—one less gadget to store. It also means you can start dinner when you get home from the office, instead of scrambling in the morning to get the slow-cooker loaded. It comes with a bit of a learning curve, but once you have it down, you'll never again wait eight hours for that beef stew to be done. (Bonus; it makes *perfect* soft-boiled eggs that peel like a dream!)

Fast & Easy Kitchen Hacks

There's a saying in the project management world: you can have it fast, you can have it cheap, you can have it right . . . pick two. Here in the world of Whole30 recipes, this basic premise holds, but we've adapted it to suit our context. When it comes to your Whole30 meals:

You can have it fast, you can have it cheap, you can have it mouth-wateringly delicious . . . pick two.

Now, you don't *really* have to pick two. (Whew.) This book is full of meals that are fast, easy, AND mouth-wateringly delicious. But if you want it on the table really fast without breaking the bank, you may have to compromise on taste. If you want to spend less money and still end up with something totally delicious, it might take you a little longer. And if you want it super-fast but it has to taste incredible, you'll probably spend a little more.

Here are some ideas to help you succeed in all three areas.

If you want it fast . . .

These tips will all have the food in your belly faster, but you'll either spend a little more, compromise the flavor a bit, or both.

- Buy pre-cut or spiral-sliced vegetables.
- Buy Whole30 Approved condiments (like mayo or salsa) instead of making your own.
- Buy Whole30 Approved bone broth instead of making your own.
- Buy a compliant rotisserie chicken instead of roasting your own.
- Buy Whole30 Approved emergency food (see page 290) instead of prepping your own.
- Use dried herbs instead of fresh.
- Use minced garlic or ginger from a jar.
- Use pre-packaged lemon or lime juice, and skip the zest.

- Buy Whole30 Approved spice mixtures that are close enough to the spices used in the recipe (e.g., the recipe calls for paprika, cayenne, salt, and black pepper; sub with your favorite compliant Mexican blend).
- Skip browning the meat in slow-cooker meals.
- Make double and freeze for a later meal.
- Invest in an Instant Pot.
- Reheat leftovers in the microwave.

TIP *It may be tempting to buy the pre-made salmon patties, Mexi-burgers, or barbecue chicken thighs from the grocery store, but read your labels! Most of these pre-seasoned or prepared meats won't be Whole30 compliant, because of bread crumbs, added sugar, cheese, or other off-plan ingredients.*

If you want it mouth-wateringly delicious . . .

These steps may take a little more time or dig into your budget a bit, but the flavor payoff is totally worth it.

- Make your own mayonnaise, bone broth, and dressings (tailored to your palate).
- Roast your own chicken (like on page 236).
- Use fresh herbs as often as possible.
- Mince your own ginger and grate your own garlic.
- Squeeze your own lemon or lime juice—and *never* skip the zest!
- Buy *all* the specialty spices called for in a recipe—even the unusual ones.
- Invest in an Instant Pot (makes even cheap cuts of meat taste incredible).
- Brown your meat before tossing it into the slow-cooker or Instant Pot.
- Reheat leftovers in a frying pan or pot.

TIP *This last bullet point is my favorite for maximizing the flavor of your Whole30 recipe replays. In a microwave, foods are re-warmed inconsistently, leaving unpleasant "cold pockets." Plus, it tends to make salmon cakes, roasted sweet potato, or bacon soggy . . . and reheating liquids can leave a mess when they splatter all over the inside—not exactly "fast and easy" to clean. Take a little extra time and reheat your leftovers on the stove, in fresh cooking oil where appropriate, adding fresh ingredients or spices to mix things up. Your taste buds will thank you, and you'll probably waste less food, too.*

If you want it cheap . . .

These tips will help you pinch your Whole30 pennies, but you'll need to spend a little more time, or (perhaps) sacrifice on flavor.

- Chop your own everything.
- Make your own everything (almost—see Tip).
- Prep your own portable or on-the-go emergency food.
- Buy spices in bulk.
- Buy frozen meat, seafood, vegetables, or fruit.
- Skip optional toppings like chopped nuts or seeds or bacon bits.
- Shop at multiple grocery stores, based on advertised sales.
- Invest in a freezer (for buying meat in bulk and storing leftovers).
- Invest in a Thrive Market membership, saving up to 50% off retail on Whole30 staples (see page 290).

TIP *In a Whole30 cost comparison of "convenience" versus "homemade," the homemade version (ghee, emergency food, salad dressings, mayonnaise, or flavored water) always came out on top, with one* *exception . . . beef jerky or "meat sticks." These are tricky to make at home, so if you want emergency meat on hand, either allocate a portion of your budget to buying some (see page 290), or find other protein sources that work on-the-go (like canned tuna or hard-cooked eggs).*

If you want it clean . . .

Finally, kitchen hacks aren't just related to cooking. On the Whole30, you'll soon find the dishes (and measuring spoons, and cutting boards . . .) tend to pile up, leaving you feel chained to the kitchen in an endless cycle of prep/cook/clean. It doesn't have to be like that. Here are our best tips for making clean-up fast and easy, too.

- During mise-en-place, combine ingredients or spices that go into the pot or pan at the same time in the same prep bowl.

- Use one cutting board for all your veggies, moving them from the board to the prep bowl to make room for the next. (Give raw meat its own cutting board, though.)

- Keep a plastic bag handy for scraps, instead of running back and forth to the garbage can a dozen times.

- Use the same pan for the whole meal wherever possible. When making hash and eggs, cook your hash, transfer into a serving dish, then add a little more oil and cook the egg in the same hot pan.

- When presentation isn't important, save yourself some dishes and store, reheat, and eat out of the same glass storage container. (Don't use plastic in the microwave, please.)

- Clean as you go. No, really, you should do this. If you've added garlic to your pan and it needs 2 minutes to soften, that's four dishes you could wash or a counter you could wipe. (Because you've mise-en-place'd, you don't have meal prep taking up time here!)

- Reuse the parchment paper on sheet pans after you've pulled your veggies out of the oven—no need to toss the paper and wash the pan before using again.

- Speaking of roasting, skip the step where you add the veggies and oil to a bowl and toss to coat—just place the raw vegetables on the parchment paper-lined baking sheet, drizzle the oil, and mix it up good with your hands; one less bowl to wash.

- Two words: Paper plates. Sometimes, you have to let good enough be good enough.

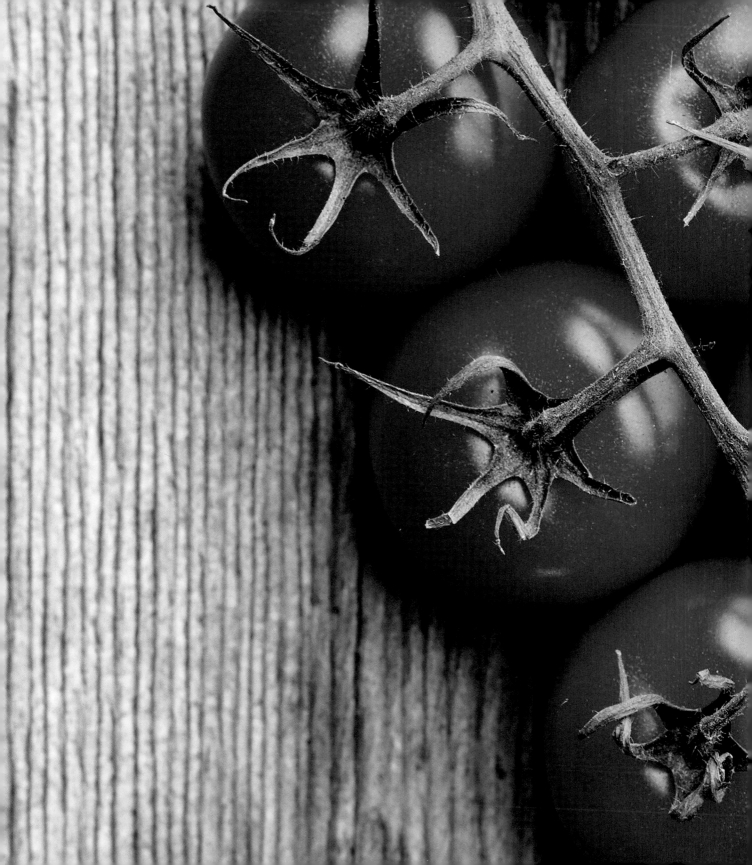

CHAPTER 1

MAIN DISH SALADS AND WRAPS

Banh Mi Pork Salad

SERVES 2

This colorful salad delivers all of the flavors and elements of the popular Vietnamese sandwiches called *banh mi*—without the bread. The quick-pickled vegetables add tremendous flavor and crunch to the salad—and you won't believe how easy they are to make!

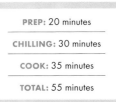

PREP: 20 minutes	
CHILLING: 30 minutes	
COOK: 35 minutes	
TOTAL: 55 minutes	

FOR THE QUICK-PICKLED VEGETABLES

½ cup thinly sliced unpeeled English cucumber

½ cup packaged shredded carrots, or 1 medium carrot, shredded

½ teaspoon coarse salt

3 cloves garlic, peeled and smashed

1 piece (1 inch) fresh ginger, thinly sliced

1 teaspoon whole black peppercorns

1 cup rice vinegar

½ cup unsweetened pineapple juice

FOR THE CABBAGE AND PORK

1 small head green cabbage (about 1½ pounds), core intact, cut into 4 wedges

2 tablespoons extra-virgin olive oil

Coarse salt and black pepper

2 boneless center-cut pork chops (5 ounces each)

FOR THE DRESSING

⅓ cup Whole30-compliant mayonnaise or Basic Mayonnaise (page 281)

2 to 3 teaspoons Whole30 Sriracha (page 274) or Whole30-compliant hot sauce

1 jalapeño, seeded and thinly sliced

½ cup loosely packed fresh cilantro

MAKE THE QUICK-PICKLED VEGETABLES: In a medium bowl, combine the cucumber, carrots, and salt. Place the garlic, ginger, and peppercorns in a 4 x 4-inch piece of cheesecloth; tie closed with cotton kitchen string, and place in the bowl. In a small saucepan, combine the vinegar and pineapple juice. Bring to a boil over medium heat; pour over the cucumber mixture. Place the bowl in the freezer to cool the vegetables while preparing the cabbage and pork.

MAKE THE CABBAGE: Meanwhile, heat a cast-iron grill pan or cast-iron skillet over medium heat. Brush the cabbage wedges with 1 tablespoon of the olive oil and lightly season with salt and black pepper. Cook the cabbage, turning frequently, until charred all over, about 15 minutes. Let the cabbage cool slightly, then remove the cores and coarsely chop.

MAKE THE PORK: In the same grill pan or skillet, heat the remaining 1 tablespoon olive oil over medium-high heat. Lightly season the pork chops with salt and black pepper. Cook the chops until golden brown and the internal temperature is 145°F, 5 to 6 minutes per side. Let rest for 5 minutes. Thinly slice the chops.

MAKE THE DRESSING: While the pork is resting, in a small bowl, whisk together the mayonnaise and Sriracha.

DRAIN the pickled vegetables in a colander and discard the cheesecloth packet. Place the chopped cabbage on a large platter. Arrange sliced pork, pickled vegetables, sliced jalapeño, and cilantro on top. Drizzle with the dressing and serve.

TIPS *The Whole30 Sriracha can be made ahead and stored in an airtight container in the refrigerator for up to 1 week.*

The Quick-Pickled Vegetables can be made up to 8 hours ahead and stored, drained, in an airtight container in the refrigerator.

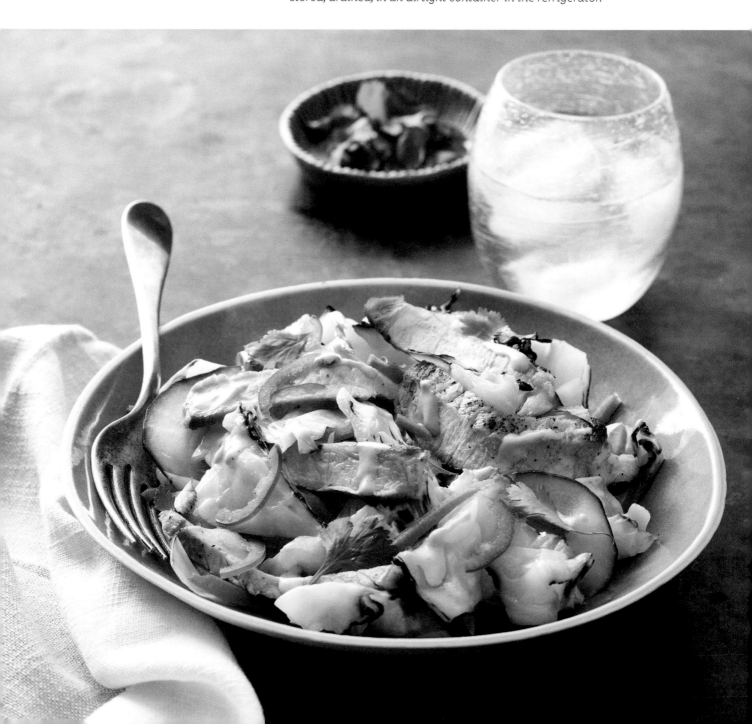

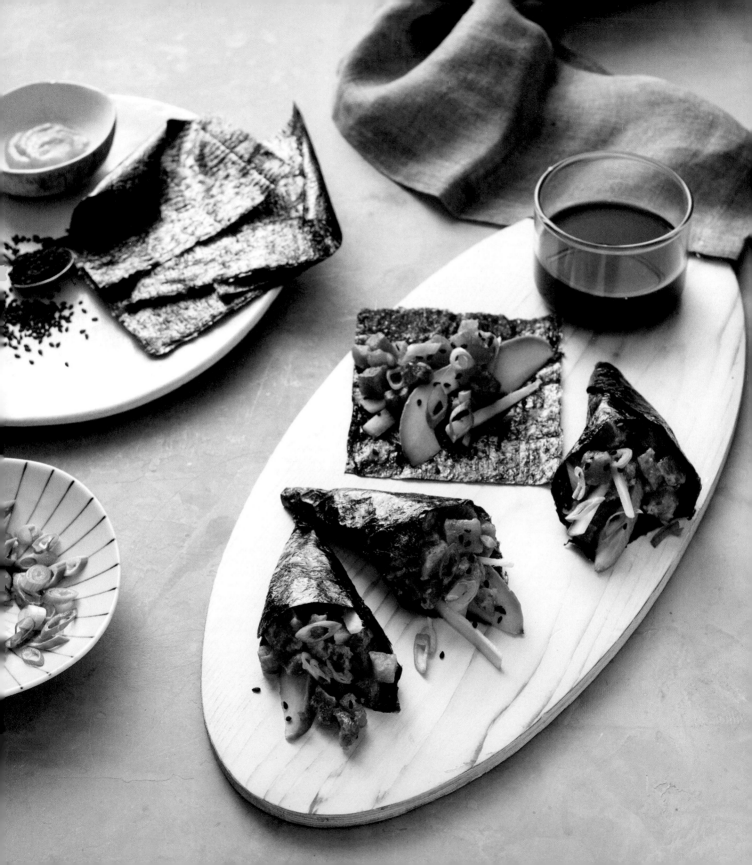

No-Rice Spicy Tuna Rolls

SERVES 2

FROM *Anya Kaats of Anya's Eats*

Who said you can't have sushi on Whole30? These rolls are not only Whole30-compliant, but they're so satisfying and delicious that you won't even notice there isn't any rice. With just a few simple ingredients, you can create restaurant-quality sushi right in your own kitchen!

PREP: 35 minutes

TOTAL: 35 minutes

½ pound sushi-grade tuna, diced

1 tablespoon Whole30-compliant mayonnaise or Basic Mayonnaise (page 281)

1 tablespoon Whole30 Sriracha (page 274)

4 nori sheets

½ unpeeled English cucumber, cut into matchsticks (1 cup)

1 piece (3 inches) fresh ginger, peeled and cut into matchsticks

1 avocado, halved, pitted, peeled, and cut into 16 slices

¼ cup thinly sliced green onions

1 tablespoon black sesame seeds

Whole30-compliant wasabi

Coconut aminos

IN a large bowl, combine the tuna, mayonnaise, and Sriracha.

FOLD each nori sheet lengthwise and crosswise until it breaks easily into 4 pieces to create 16 squares.

FOR each roll, place about 2 cucumber matchsticks, 2 ginger matchsticks, 1 slice avocado, 2 slices green onion, and 1 rounded tablespoon of tuna mixture diagonally at the bottom left corner of a nori square. Sprinkle with some of the sesame seeds. Gently roll into a cone and tuck the pointed end under; use your fingers to wet the edge of the nori square with water to seal.

SERVE the rolls with wasabi and coconut aminos for dipping.

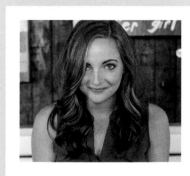

Anya Kaats

Anya Kaats is the San Diego-based blogger behind Anya's Eats. She's also a health coach and a professional marketer for natural-products brands. From sharing delicious, whole-foods recipes on her blog and social channels to helping small natural-products brands thrive, Anya is honored to be a part of the ripple effect that's inspiring people to prioritize their health and the health of our planet through real food and sustainability.

Hot Beef and Broccoli Salad

SERVES 4

The vegetables in this salad are cooked just enough so the first bite is slightly tender, but the rest is satisfyingly crunchy.

PREP: 15 minutes

COOK: 5 minutes

TOTAL: 20 minutes

1 pound boneless beef sirloin steak or stir-fry meat

½ teaspoon salt

¼ teaspoon black pepper

2 teaspoons grated lemon zest

6 tablespoons Whole30-compliant lemon-garlic dressing

3 cups broccoli florets

1 large orange or red bell pepper, seeded and thinly sliced

1 package (9 ounces) spring mix/baby spinach

¼ cup snipped fresh chives

THINLY slice the meat across the grain into bite-size pieces and season both sides with the salt, pepper, and lemon zest. In a medium bowl, toss the meat with 2 tablespoons of the dressing.

IN a large bowl, combine the broccoli, bell pepper, and 3 tablespoons of the dressing. Toss to coat.

IN a large skillet, cook the broccoli and bell pepper over medium-high heat, stirring, for 3 minutes. Return the vegetables to the large bowl. Add the meat to the hot skillet and cook, stirring, until slightly pink in center, 1 to 2 minutes. Add the vegetables to the skillet and stir to combine with the meat.

IN a large bowl, toss the greens with the remaining 1 tablespoon dressing. Serve the meat and vegetables over the greens. Sprinkle the salad with the snipped chives.

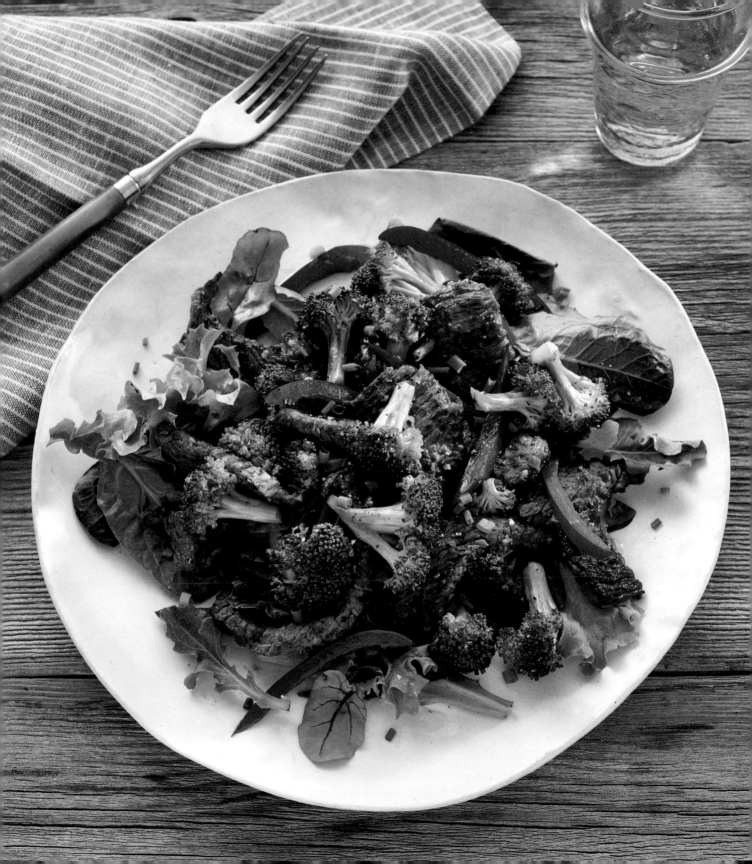

Cashew-Crusted Chicken and Wilted Kale Salad

SERVES 2

While the chicken bakes to crisp-crusted deliciousness in the oven, you quickly wilt the kale and onion in bacon drippings in a skillet—then toss it with raw shredded carrot and grape tomatoes. The contrast of temperatures and textures is a nice change of pace from a traditional salad.

PREP: 15 minutes
COOK: 15 minutes
TOTAL: 30 minutes

FOR THE CHICKEN
Extra-virgin olive oil

1 large egg

½ cup almond flour

⅓ cup finely chopped raw cashews

½ teaspoon salt

½ teaspoon black pepper

6 boneless, skinless chicken breast tenderloins (about 12 ounces total)

FOR THE SALAD
3 slices Whole30-compliant bacon, chopped

4 cups torn fresh kale

1 small red onion, slivered

½ cup packaged shredded carrot

½ cup grape tomatoes, halved

¼ cup raw cashews, toasted (see Tip) and chopped

MAKE THE CHICKEN: Preheat the oven to 425°F. Lightly brush olive oil on a medium baking sheet.

WHISK together the egg and 1 tablespoon olive oil in a shallow dish. In another shallow dish, stir together the flour, cashews, salt, and pepper. Dip each tenderloin into the egg, turning to coat. Allow the excess to drip off, then dip into the cashew mixture, turning to coat. Place on the prepared pan.

BAKE the chicken, turning once halfway through cooking, until the internal temperature is 165°F and the chicken is no longer pink, 15 to 18 minutes.

MAKE THE SALAD: Meanwhile, in a large skillet, cook the bacon, stirring, until browned and crisp. Using a slotted spoon, transfer the bacon to a plate lined with paper towels, reserving the bacon fat in the skillet. Add the kale and onion to the skillet with the bacon fat. Cook, tossing frequently with tongs, until the kale is wilted and tender, 2 to 3 minutes.

REMOVE the skillet from the heat. Stir in the cooked bacon, carrot, and tomatoes. Serve the chicken on top of the kale salad. Sprinkle with the cashews.

TIP *To toast cashews, heat in a dry skillet over medium heat, stirring, until fragrant and lightly browned, about 2 minutes.*

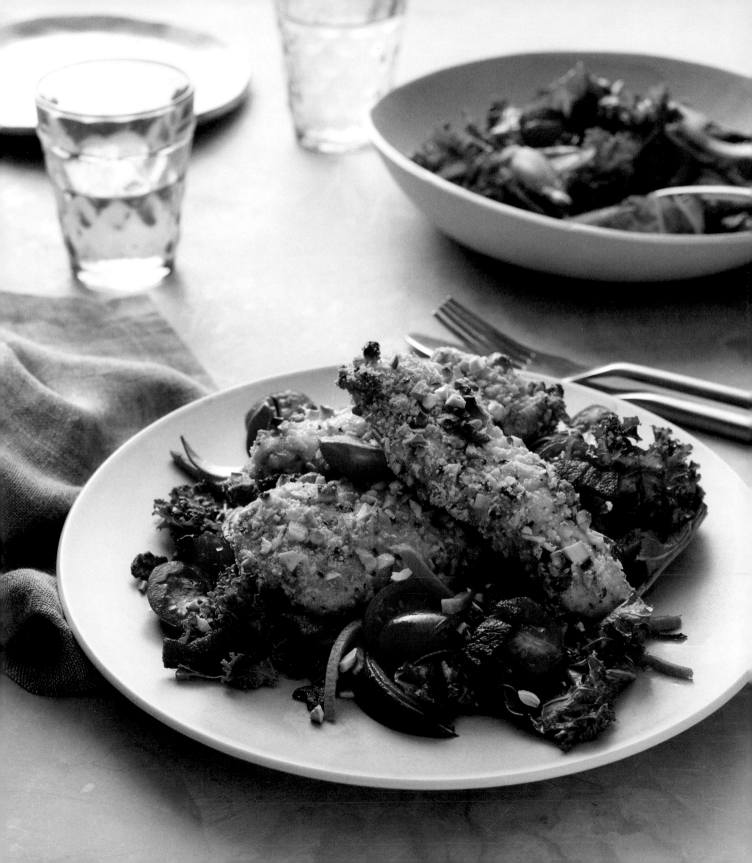

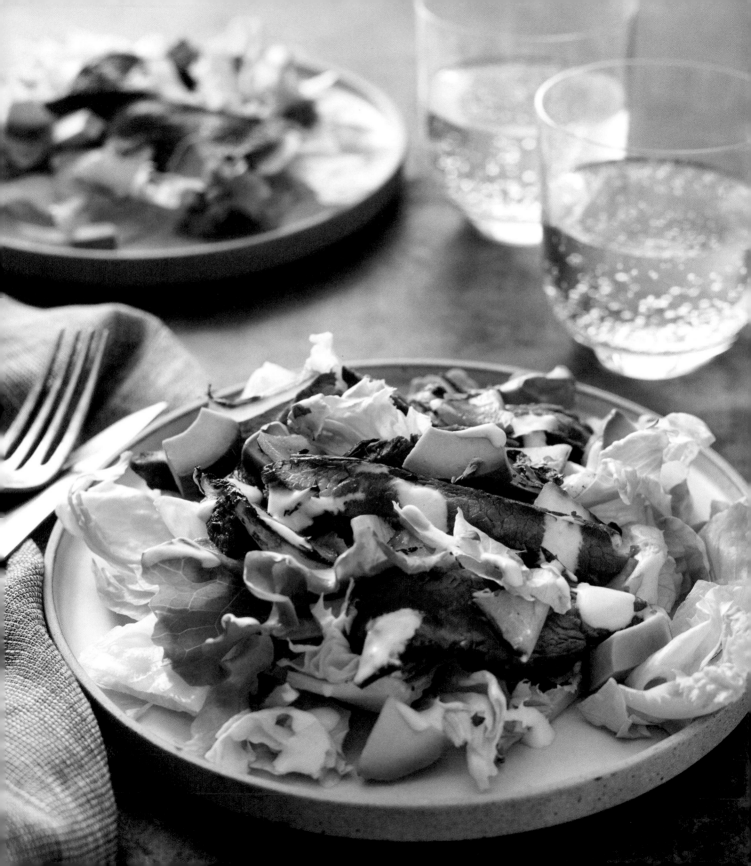

Grilled Steak and Charred Onion Salad

SERVES 4

The creamy dressing for this salad has just three ingredients—mayo, lime juice and zest, and hot sauce—but it tastes like there's much more going on. It's a perfect accompaniment to the cumin-spiced steak.

PREP:	15 minutes
GRILL:	20 minutes
TOTAL:	35 minutes

FOR THE STEAK AND ONIONS

1 flank steak or skirt steak (16 to 20 ounces)

1 tablespoon cumin seeds, lightly crushed

1 teaspoon salt

1 teaspoon black pepper

1 large onion

2 tablespoons extra-virgin olive oil

FOR THE DRESSING

¾ cup Whole30-compliant mayonnaise or Basic Mayonnaise (page 281)

Grated zest and juice of 1 lime

2 teaspoons Whole30-compliant hot sauce

8 cups chopped butterhead or iceberg lettuce

2 avocadoes, halved, pitted, peeled, and diced

Chopped fresh cilantro

PREHEAT a grill to medium-high heat (375°F) or a grill pan over medium-high heat.

GRILL THE STEAK AND ONIONS: Season the steak with the cumin seeds, salt, and pepper. Cut the onion into ½-inch-thick slices. Drizzle the steak and onions with the olive oil.

GRILL the steak and onion slices over direct heat, turning once, until the onion is lightly charred, 5 to 6 minutes, and the steak is cooked to desired doneness, 15 to 20 minutes for medium (160°F). Remove the steak and onion and let rest for 5 minutes.

MAKE THE DRESSING: Meanwhile, in a small bowl, combine the mayonnaise, lime zest and juice, and hot sauce.

THINLY slice the steak against the grain and coarsely chop the onions. Place the lettuce in a serving bowl and top with the steak and onions. Drizzle the dressing over the salad. Top with the avocado and cilantro.

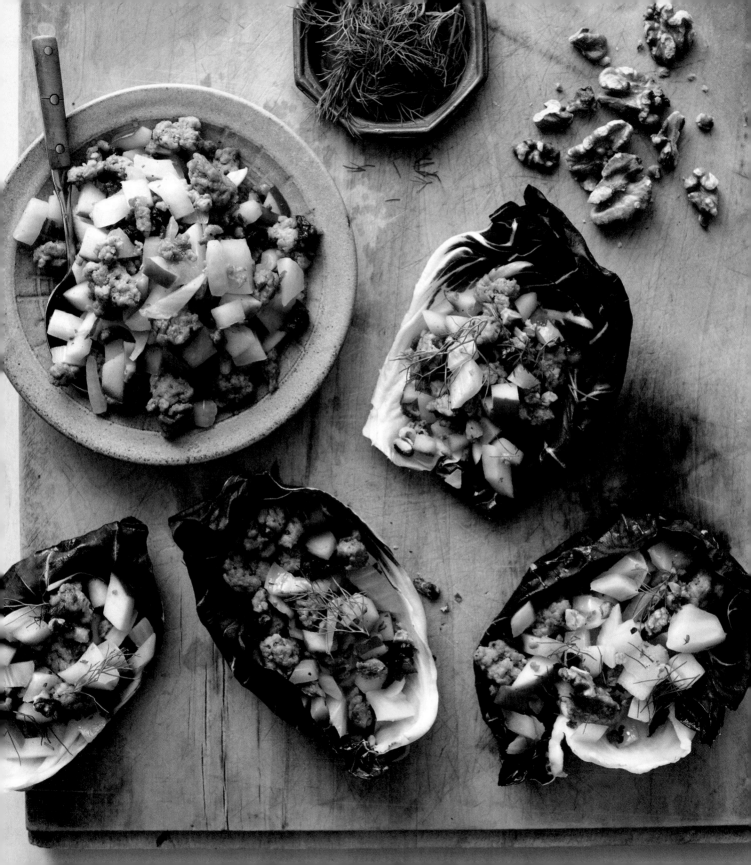

Apple, Fennel, and Pork Radicchio Wraps

SERVES 2

Lots of people like the pleasantly bitter flavor of radicchio. If you're not one of them, opt for cabbage, butterhead, or Bibb leaves instead.

PREP:	15 minutes
COOK:	10 minutes
TOTAL:	25 minutes

1 small fennel bulb

1 tablespoon extra-virgin olive oil

8 ounces ground pork

1 small cooking apple (such as Granny Smith or McIntosh), cored and diced

1 teaspoon dried sage, crushed

¼ teaspoon salt

2 tablespoons finely chopped unsulfured dried apricots

2 tablespoons Whole30-compliant mayonnaise or Basic Mayonnaise (page 281)

1 tablespoon cider vinegar

8 medium radicchio, cabbage, butterhead lettuce, or Bibb lettuce leaves

¼ cup chopped walnuts, toasted (see Tip)

TRIM the fennel bulb, reserving the feathery tops (fronds). Remove the core and then coarsely chop the bulb. Heat the olive oil in a medium skillet over medium heat. Add the chopped fennel and the pork and cook, stirring, until the pork is almost cooked through, 3 to 4 minutes.

ADD the apple, sage, and salt. Cook, stirring, until the pork is no longer pink and the apple is crisp-tender, 2 to 3 minutes. Stir in the apricots. Remove from the heat. In a small bowl, whisk together the mayonnaise and vinegar. Add to the pork mixture and stir until combined.

PLACE the radicchio leaves on a large serving plate. Spoon the pork filling into the center of the leaves. Sprinkle with the walnuts. Chop some of the reserved fennel fronds and sprinkle over the walnuts.

TIP *To toast walnuts, heat in a skillet over medium heat, stirring, until fragrant and lightly browned, about 2 minutes.*

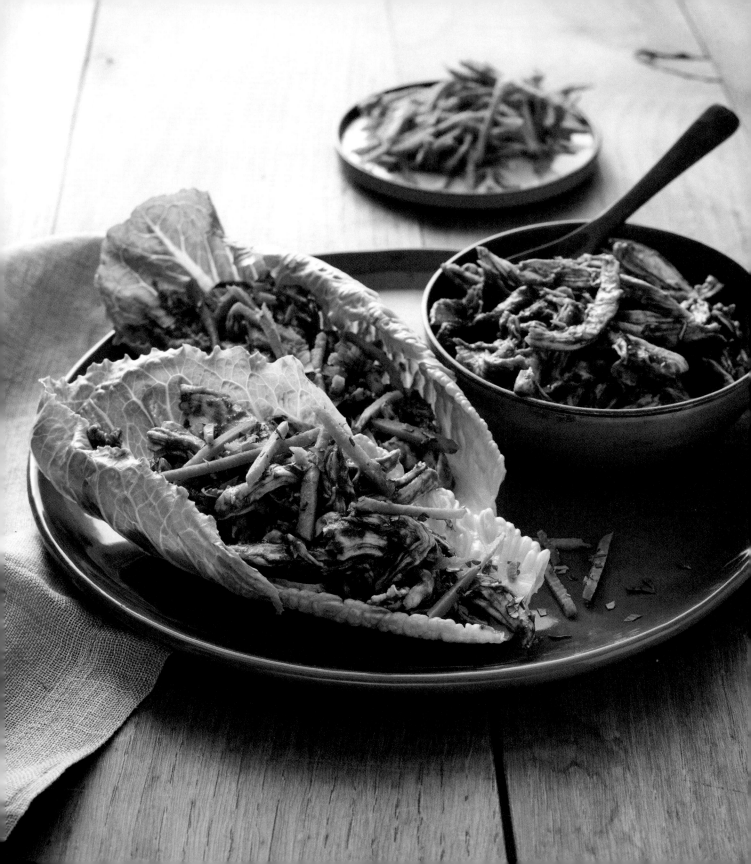

BBQ-Pulled-Chicken Lettuce Wraps

SERVES 4

These speedy wraps fly in the face of the "low and slow" barbecue mantra. Using chicken instead of a tough cut of pork means you get that same satisfying sweet and tangy flavor and fork-tender texture in minutes instead of hours.

PREP:	10 minutes
COOK:	25 minutes
TOTAL:	35 minutes

1 pound boneless, skinless chicken breasts or boneless, skinless chicken thighs

½ to ¾ cup Whole30-compliant barbecue sauce

1 cup packaged shredded carrots or 2 medium carrots, shredded

2 tablespoon chopped fresh cilantro

2 tablespoons fresh lime juice

8 Bibb or romaine lettuce leaves

PLACE the chicken in a medium saucepan and add enough water to cover. Bring to a boil. Reduce the heat to low, cover, and simmer until the chicken is cooked through, 15 to 20 minutes.

TRANSFER the chicken to a cutting board and let cool slightly. Discard the water in the pan and wipe dry with paper towels. Use two forks to shred the chicken. Return the chicken to the pan and stir in the barbecue sauce. Cook over medium heat until heated through, about 2 minutes.

IN a small bowl, combine the carrots, cilantro, and lime juice. Serve the BBQ chicken and some of the shredded carrot mixture in the lettuce leaves.

Warm Salmon and Potato Salad

SERVES 4

FROM *Brian Kavanaugh of The Sophisticated Caveman*

Baby potatoes are tossed in a simple Dijon vinaigrette and served warm. The addition of arugula and salmon makes this a hearty side or even a quick lunch.

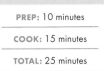

PREP: 10 minutes

COOK: 15 minutes

TOTAL: 25 minutes

1 ½ pounds baby yellow potatoes, halved

⅓ cup avocado oil

1 tablespoon Whole30-compliant Dijon mustard

1 tablespoon fresh lemon juice

½ teaspoon salt

½ teaspoon black pepper

1 can (6 ounces) salmon, drained

2 cups arugula

3 green onions, sliced

2 tablespoons snipped fresh chives

1 tablespoon minced fresh parsley

PLACE the potatoes in a medium pot and add enough cold water to cover. Bring to a low boil and cook until tender, about 15 minutes. Drain.

IN a large bowl, whisk together the avocado oil, mustard, lemon juice, salt, and pepper. Add the potatoes, salmon, arugula, green onions, chives, and parsley. Gently toss until the potatoes are coated. Serve warm.

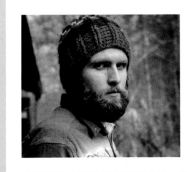

Brian Kavanagh

Brian Kavanagh, otherwise known as The Sophisticated Caveman, is an outdoor enthusiast with a special place in his heart for food. After struggling for years with weight loss, he recently discovered that he could satisfy his passion for cooking delicious meals while also using clean, healthy ingredients. He enjoys creating and sharing simple recipes that involve real food with an added "touch of class."

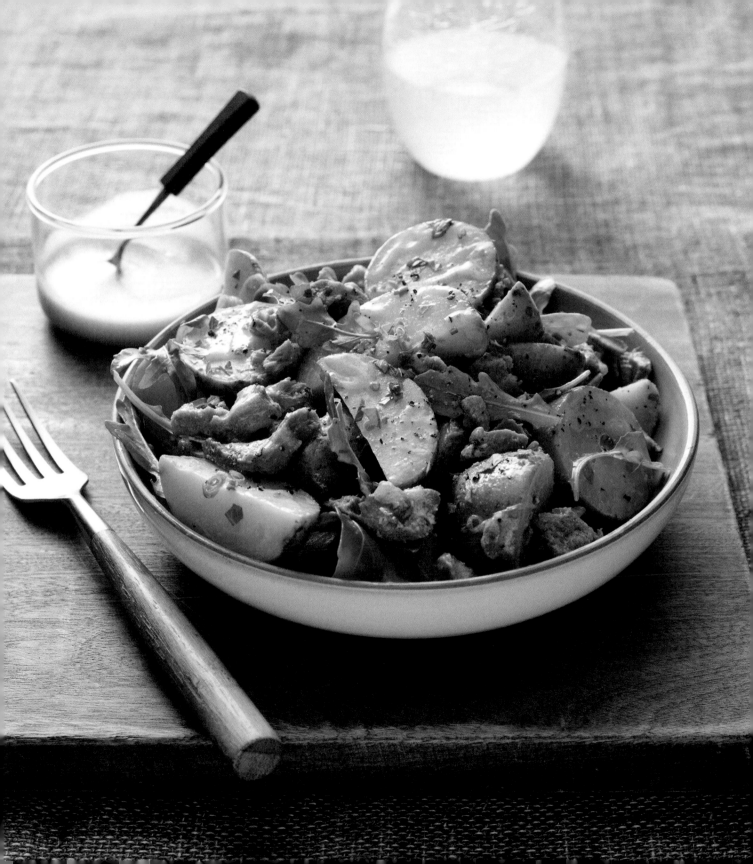

Curry Chicken Salad

SERVES 3 TO 4

FROM *Jessica Beacom and Stacie Hassing of The Real Food Dietitians*

Cool and creamy chicken salad gets a little exotic with the addition of antioxidant-rich curry powder, crisp vegetables, and crunchy cashews. This recipe is great for using up leftover chicken or turkey and makes for a great lunch when tucked inside a lettuce leaf, or served on a bed of greens or cucumber slices.

PREP: 15 minutes

TOTAL: 15 minutes

½ cup Whole30-compliant mayonnaise or Basic Mayonnaise (page 281)

1 tablespoon fresh lime juice

2 tablespoons fresh cilantro

2 teaspoons Whole30-compliant curry powder

¼ teaspoon salt

2 cups diced cooked chicken

½ medium apple, diced

1 celery stalk, finely diced

3 tablespoons finely diced red onion

¼ cup roughly chopped Whole30-compliant dry-roasted cashews

Sliced green onions, shredded cabbage, shredded carrots, and/or chopped cashews (optional)

IN a medium bowl, stir together the mayonnaise, lime juice, cilantro, curry powder, and salt. Add the chicken, apple, celery, and onion and toss to coat. Fold in the cashews. If desired, top the salad with green onions, cabbage, carrots, and/or additional cashews.

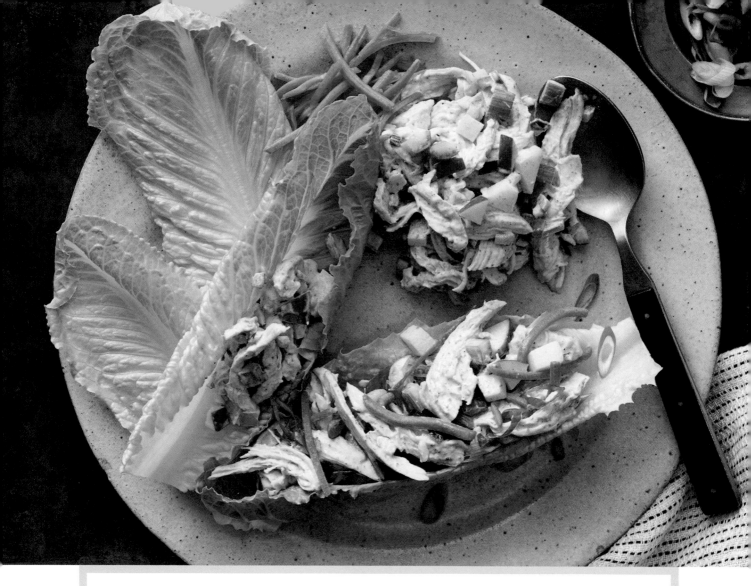

Jessica Beacom and Stacie Hassing

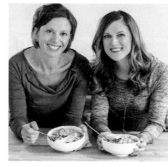

Jessica Beacom and Stacie Hassing are the Registered Dietitian Nutritionists (RDN) and Whole30 Certified Coaches behind The Real Food Dietitians website and blog. They create gluten-free and Whole30-friendly recipes designed to be big on taste and short on ingredients, so you can spend less time in the kitchen and more time doing the things you love. Together they provide expert guidance, meal plans, and a supportive online space for those completing a Whole30.

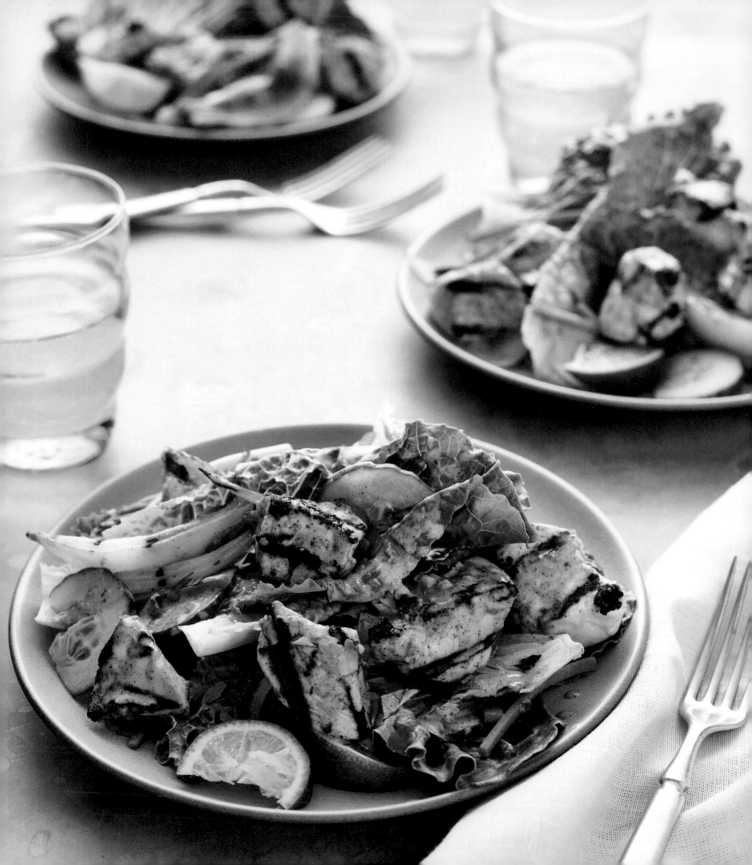

Grilled Chicken Satay Salad

SERVES 4

The yummy Almond Satay Sauce—flavored with lime, ginger, garlic, and coconut aminos—does double duty in this recipe as both a marinade for the chicken and a dressing for the salad.

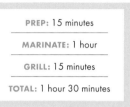

PREP: 15 minutes

MARINATE: 1 hour

GRILL: 15 minutes

TOTAL: 1 hour 30 minutes

FOR THE KABOBS

1 pound boneless, skinless chicken breasts, cut into 1-inch pieces

1 cup Almond Satay Sauce (page 278)

1 large onion, halved and cut into 16 wedges

FOR THE SALAD

½ cup Almond Satay Sauce (page 278)

2 teaspoons Whole30-compliant coconut milk

1 bag (9 ounces) hearts of romaine

2 medium cucumbers, sliced (2 cups)

3 medium carrots, peeled and cut into matchsticks (2 cups)

¼ cup chopped fresh cilantro

Lime wedges (optional)

MAKE THE KABOBS: Place the chicken in a resealable plastic bag. Add the satay sauce to cover the chicken. Seal the bag and marinate the chicken in the refrigerator for 1 to 8 hours. Remove the chicken from the refrigerator about 30 minutes before grilling.

PREHEAT the grill to medium heat (350° to 375°F). Remove the chicken from the marinade and discard the marinade. Alternate threading the chicken and onion on 8 skewers (see Tip), leaving a ¼-inch space between each piece.

GRILL the kabobs over direct heat, turning once or twice, until the internal temperature of the chicken is 165°F, 12 to 15 minutes.

MAKE THE SALAD: In a small bowl, stir together the satay sauce and coconut milk.

ARRANGE the romaine, cucumber, and carrots on serving plates. Sprinkle with the cilantro. Top each salad with the chicken and onions from two of the kabobs and drizzle with some of the sauce. Serve with lime wedges, if desired.

TIP *If using wooden skewers, soak them in water for at least 30 minutes to prevent burning.*

Six-Ingredient Chicken Salad

SERVES 2 GENEROUSLY

Using a compliant ranch dressing, cooked chicken, and a package of precooked beets means this gorgeous salad comes together in less than 15 minutes.

PREP: 10 minutes

COOK: 5 minutes

TOTAL: 15 minutes

8 ounces fresh green beans, trimmed

½ cup Whole30-compliant ranch dressing or Whole30 Ranch Dressing (page 282)

1 teaspoon finely chopped fresh tarragon or basil

2 cups chopped cooked chicken

1 cup yellow grape tomatoes, halved

1 package (8 ounces) steamed and peeled beets, diced

IN a large pot of boiling water, cook the green beans just until crisp-tender, about 2 minutes. Drain and immediately place in a large bowl of ice water until completely cool, about 1 minute. Drain and pat dry with paper towels.

IN a small bowl, stir together the ranch dressing and tarragon. Arrange the green beans, chicken, tomatoes, and beets in rows on serving plates. Drizzle the salads with some of the dressing and serve.

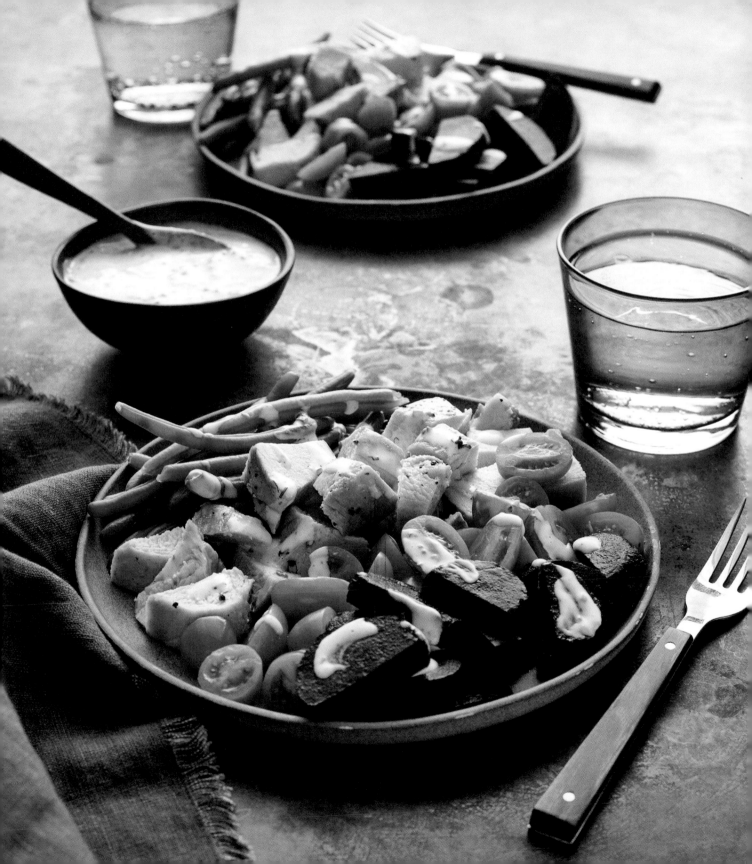

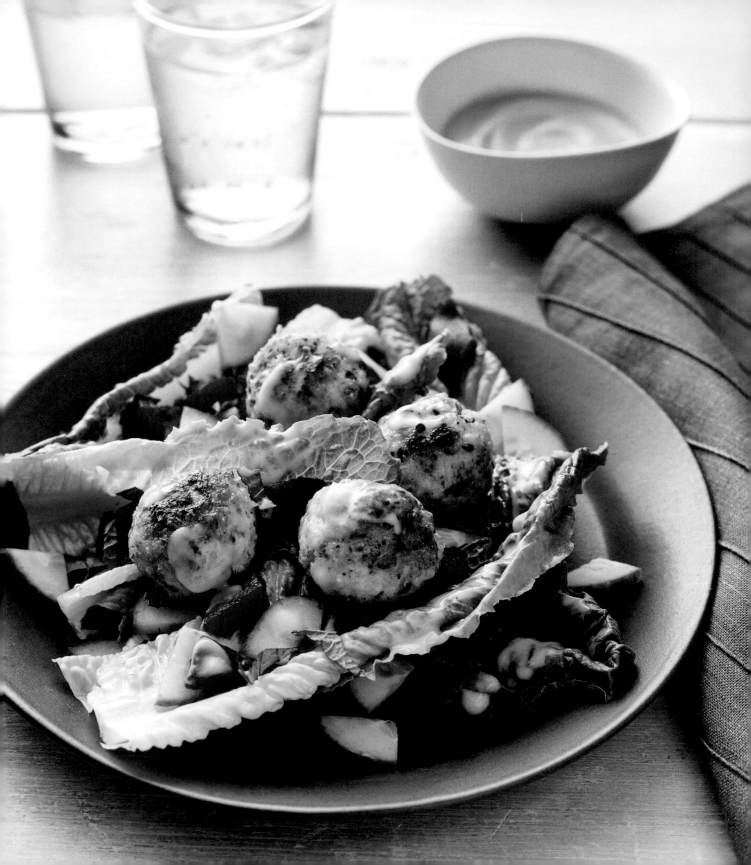

Greek-Style Meatball Salad

SERVES 2

The turkey meatballs—flavored with garlic and oregano—are wonderful on this crunchy and colorful salad, but they would be equally good on a pile of zucchini noodles and topped with a compliant marinara sauce.

PREP: 15 minutes

BAKE: 20 minutes

TOTAL: 35 minutes

FOR THE MEATBALLS

1 large egg

¼ cup almond flour

3 cloves garlic, minced

1 teaspoon dried oregano, crushed

½ teaspoon salt

¼ teaspoon black pepper

8 ounces ground turkey

FOR THE LEMON-AVOCADO SALAD

½ small avocado, pitted and peeled

¼ cup unsweetened flax milk or Whole30-compliant coconut milk

1 to 2 tablespoons fresh lemon juice

1 clove garlic, minced

¼ teaspoon salt

⅛ teaspoon black pepper

2 tablespoons chopped fresh mint

1 bag (9 ounces) hearts of romaine

½ English cucumber, sliced, slices quartered

⅔ cup drained roasted red pepper, patted dry and chopped

MAKE THE MEATBALLS: Preheat the oven to 400°F. Line a baking pan with parchment paper.

IN a medium bowl, whisk the egg until lightly beaten. Stir in the almond flour, garlic, oregano, salt, and black pepper. Add the ground turkey and gently mix to combine. Shape the mixture into 8 meatballs and place on the pan. Bake for 18 to 20 minutes, until the internal temperature is 165°F.

MAKE THE LEMON-AVOCADO SALAD: Meanwhile, in a blender combine the avocado, flax milk, lemon juice, garlic, salt, and black pepper. Cover and blend until smooth. Transfer the dressing to a small bowl and stir in the mint.

ARRANGE the romaine on serving plates. Top with the cucumber, roasted pepper, and meatballs. Drizzle with the dressing and serve.

Fruity Chicken Chopped Salad

SERVES 2

The pomegranate arils, or seeds, add juicy little bursts of flavor and crunchy texture to this salad. Look for small containers of the arils in the refrigerated case in the produce section of your grocery store.

PREP: 10 minutes

TOTAL: 10 minutes

FOR THE DRESSING

2 tablespoons fresh orange juice

1 tablespoon white wine vinegar

¼ cup extra-virgin olive oil

⅛ teaspoon salt

⅛ teaspoon black pepper

FOR THE SALAD

1 medium orange, peeled and white pith removed (see Tip)

6 cups chopped romaine lettuce

1½ cups coarsely chopped cooked chicken

¼ cup pomegranate seeds

¼ cup coarsely chopped roasted cashews

2 green onions, sliced

MAKE THE DRESSING: In a small bowl, whisk together the orange juice, vinegar, olive oil, salt, and pepper.

MAKE THE SALAD: Divide the orange into segments. Arrange the lettuce in serving bowls. Top with the orange segments, chicken, pomegranate seeds, cashews, and green onions. Drizzle with the dressing and serve.

TIP *If you have a few extra minutes, you can supreme the orange (remove the membrane from the orange so it can easily be served in slices): With a sharp knife, trim the fruit's ends. Set one end on a cutting board and slice off the peel and pith in sections. Set the fruit on its side. Cut toward the center, along a membrane. Then slice along the adjacent membrane until the cuts meet, releasing the segment. Repeat with the remaining segments.*

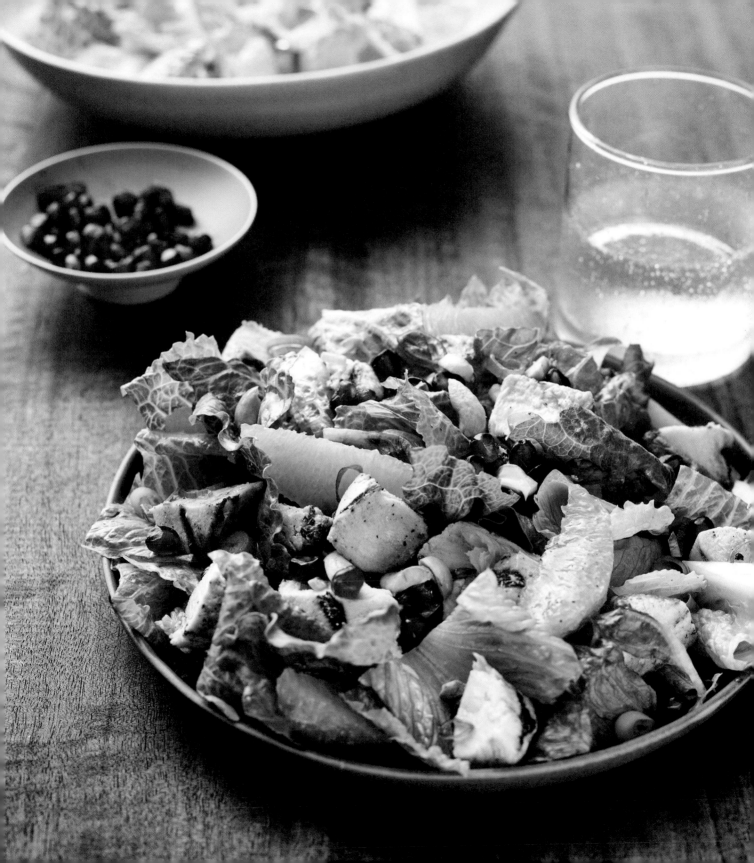

Mango and Ahi Tuna Poke Salad

SERVES 4

Hawaiian *poke* (pronounced POH-kay) is becoming super-popular across the mainland. A bit like deconstructed sushi, it's essentially seasoned cubes of raw fish tossed with fresh fruits and vegetables. Sometimes it's served over rice—but not this Whole30 version!

PREP: 20 minutes

TOTAL: 20 minutes

FOR THE DRESSING

3 tablespoons coconut aminos

1 tablespoon rice vinegar

1 teaspoon sesame oil

1 teaspoon grated fresh ginger

¼ teaspoon salt

⅛ teaspoon black pepper

FOR THE SALAD

1½ pounds sushi-grade ahi tuna, cut into bite-sized pieces

1 package (5 ounces) baby spinach

1 ripe avocado, halved, pitted, peeled, and chopped

1 ripe mango, pitted, peeled, and chopped

1 small unpeeled cucumber, sliced

1 cup packaged shredded carrots, or 2 medium carrots, shredded

Black sesame seeds (optional)

Sliced green onions (optional)

MAKE THE DRESSING: In a small bowl, stir together the dressing ingredients.

MAKE THE SALAD: In a medium bowl, gently toss the tuna with 2 tablespoons of the dressing to coat. Let stand and marinate while you assemble the salads.

DIVIDE the spinach among four plates. Arrange the avocado, mango, cucumber, and carrots on the spinach. Top with the marinated tuna and drizzle the salads with the remaining dressing. Top with black sesame seeds and sliced green onions, if desired, and serve.

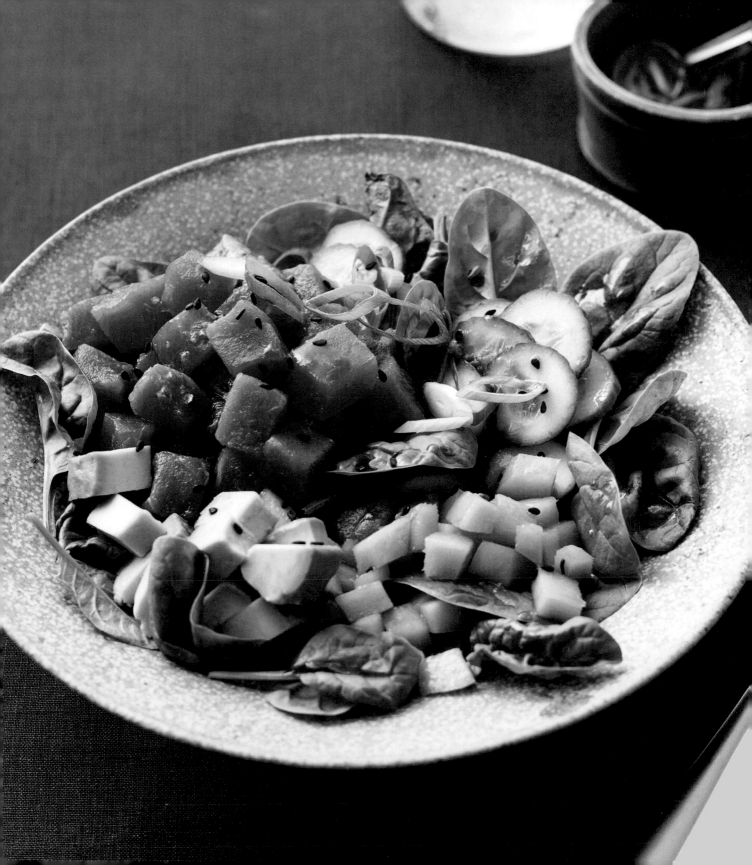

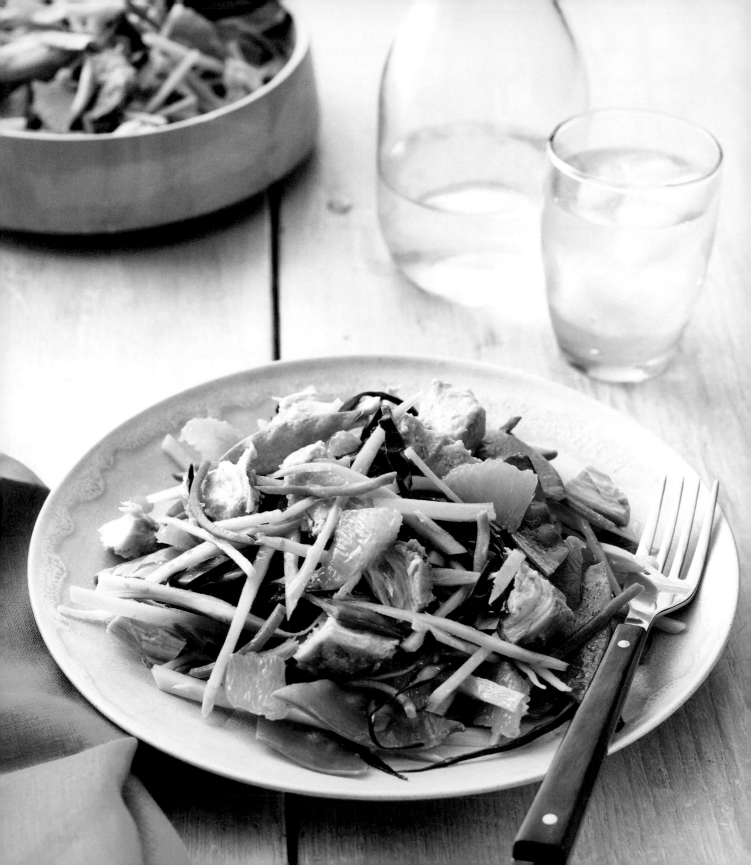

Asian Tuna, Snow Pea, and Broccoli Salad with Sesame Dressing

SERVES 4

Solid white albacore tuna has a meatier texture and richer flavor than chunk light tuna. Look for a brand that is troll- or pole-and-line caught, methods of fishing that are better for both the fish and the environment.

PREP: 10 minutes

TOTAL: 10 minutes

FOR THE DRESSING

1 teaspoon grated orange zest

3 tablespoons extra-virgin olive oil

3 tablespoons rice vinegar

1 tablespoon toasted sesame oil

FOR THE SALAD

1 orange, peeled and cut into bite-size pieces

1 bag (12 ounces) broccoli slaw

1 package (8 ounces) fresh snow peas, trimmed and halved diagonally

2 cans (5 ounces each) water-packed wild albacore tuna, drained and broken into chunks

MAKE THE DRESSING: In a small bowl, combine the orange zest, olive oil, vinegar, and sesame oil.

MAKE THE SALAD: In a large bowl, combine the orange pieces with the broccoli slaw, snow peas, and tuna. Drizzle with the dressing and gently toss.

Shrimp and Mango Salad

SERVES 2

To prep the mango for this salad, stand it upright on a cutting board and cut down along each side of the large pit. Place each mango half skin-side down on the cutting board and cut a crosshatch pattern in the flesh down to the skin. Run the knife closely against the inside of the skin to pop the flesh out and create diced fruit.

| PREP: 15 minutes |
| COOK: 5 minutes |
| TOTAL: 20 minutes |

FOR THE DRESSING

½ teaspoon grated lime zest

2 tablespoons fresh lime juice

¼ cup extra-virgin olive oil

1 tablespoon chopped fresh cilantro

2 teaspoons finely chopped seeded jalapeño

⅛ teaspoon salt

FOR THE SALAD

1 tablespoon extra-virgin olive oil

8 ounces peeled and deveined large shrimp (see Tip)

1 teaspoon chili powder

⅛ teaspoon salt

6 cups torn Bibb lettuce leaves

1 medium ripe mango, peeled, pitted, and diced

1 medium ripe avocado, halved, pitted, peeled, and diced

MAKE THE DRESSING: In a small bowl, combine the lime zest and juice. While whisking, drizzle in the olive oil until combined. Stir in the cilantro, jalapeño, and salt.

MAKE THE SALAD: In a large skillet, heat the olive oil over medium-high heat. Add the shrimp, chili powder, and salt. Cook, stirring, until the shrimp are opaque, about 5 minutes.

ARRANGE the lettuce on serving plates. Top with the mango, avocado, and shrimp. Drizzle the salads with the dressing and serve.

TIP *To make this recipe even faster, use cooked shrimp in place of the fresh shrimp. Cook shrimp with the chili powder and salt for just 1 to 2 minutes or until heated through.*

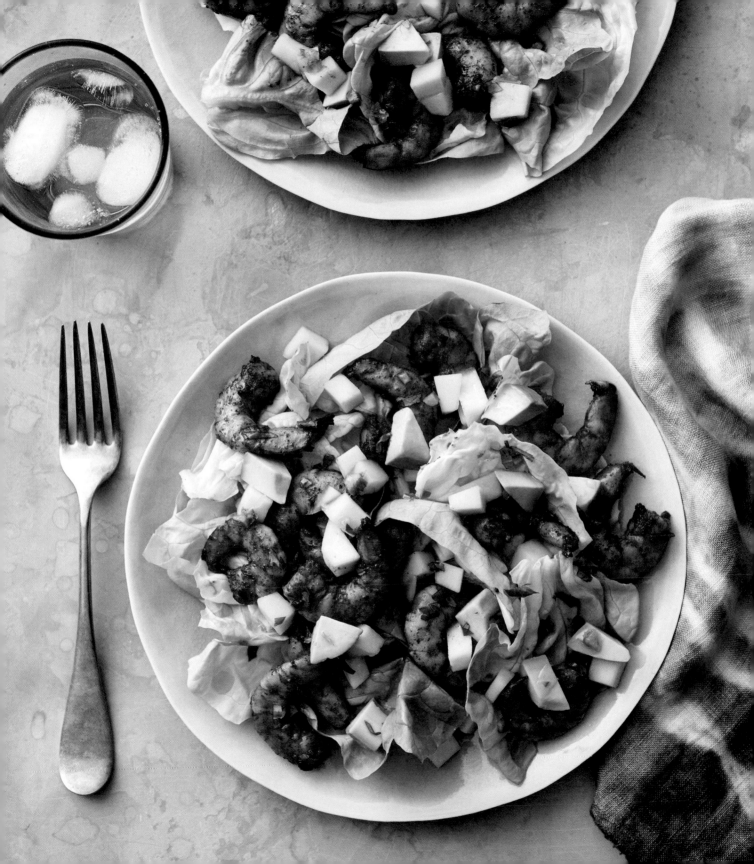

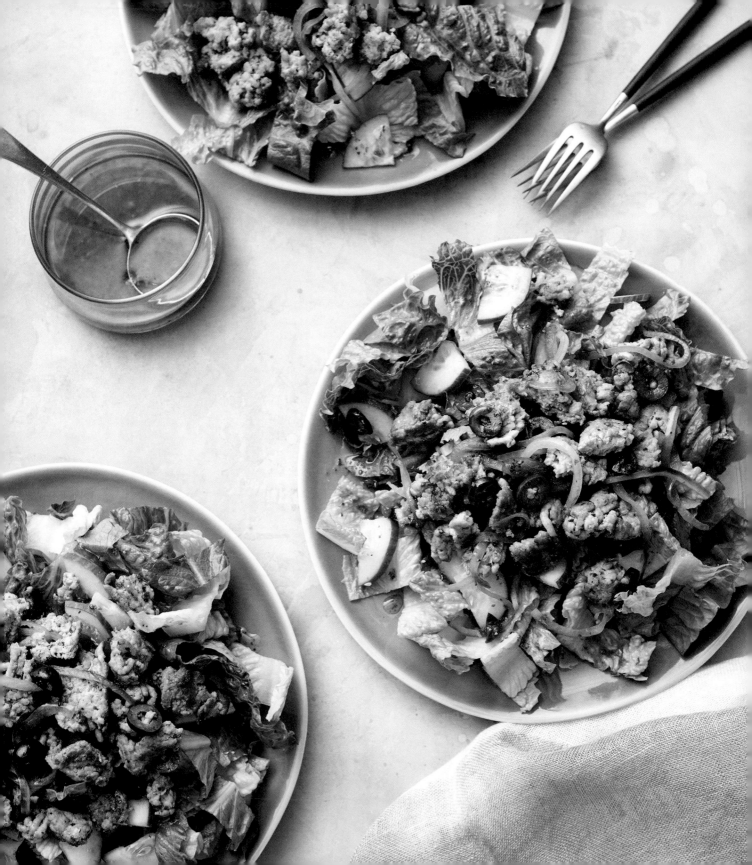

Sizzling Pork Greek Salad

SERVES 4

The "sizzle" in this salad comes from seasoned pork cooked in a skillet until browned and crispy, stirred together with briny Kalamata olives and red onion and served over crunchy romaine and cucumbers drizzled with a red wine vinaigrette.

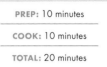

PREP: 10 minutes

COOK: 10 minutes

TOTAL: 20 minutes

FOR THE PORK

1 pound ground pork

1 teaspoon Greek seasoning (see Tip)

½ cup thinly sliced red onion

½ cup sliced pitted Kalamata olives

FOR THE SALAD

3 tablespoons red wine vinegar

1 or 2 cloves garlic, minced

1 teaspoon Greek seasoning

¼ cup extra-virgin olive oil

8 cups chopped romaine lettuce

1 medium cucumber, chopped

COOK THE PORK: In a large nonstick skillet, cook the pork and Greek seasoning over medium-high heat, stirring occasionally, until browned and crispy, 6 to 8 minutes. Turn off the heat. Stir in the red onion and olives. Let stand for 2 minutes to soften the onion.

MAKE THE SALAD: Meanwhile, in a small bowl, combine the vinegar, garlic, and Greek seasoning. Whisk in the olive oil until well combined.

LAYER the lettuce, cucumber, and pork in bowls. Drizzle with the dressing and serve.

TIP *If your store doesn't have Greek seasoning, it's easy to make your own. In a small bowl, stir together 1 tablespoon dried oregano, 1 teaspoon dried basil, ½ teaspoon dried mint, ½ teaspoon dried minced onion, and ½ teaspoon dried minced garlic. Makes about 2½ tablespoons. Store in an airtight container.*

Veggie Wraps with Lemon-Zucchini Dressing

SERVES 2

Use any leftover meat, poultry, or shrimp you have on hand to provide the protein in these veggie-packed wraps. A sprinkle of fresh dill is a terrific complement to the creamy sauce flavored with lemon and garlic.

PREP: 15 minutes

TOTAL: 15 minutes

FOR THE DRESSING

1 medium unpeeled zucchini, chopped

¼ cup almond butter

3 tablespoons fresh lemon juice

1 tablespoon extra-virgin olive oil

1 clove garlic, minced

½ teaspoon salt

2 cups assorted thinly sliced vegetables, such as cucumbers, carrots, bell peppers, radishes, and/ or green onions

10 ounces cooked chicken, beef, or shrimp, chopped or sliced

12 Bibb lettuce leaves

2 tablespoons chopped fresh dill

MAKE THE DRESSING: In a food processor, combine the zucchini, almond butter, lemon juice, olive oil, garlic, and salt. Process until smooth.

ARRANGE the lettuce leaves on two plates. Divide the vegetables and the chicken, beef, or shrimp among the leaves. Drizzle with some of the dressing, sprinkle with fresh dill, and serve.

TIP *Store any leftover dressing in an airtight container in the refrigerator for up to 2 days. Use as a dip for vegetables or as a sauce for zucchini noodles.*

Hearty Chopped Salad

SERVES 2

To ensure that you get the most perfect, ripe, and beautiful avocados, buy them when they are still quite firm to the touch so they don't get bruised in transit from the store. Let them ripen on your counter for a couple of days until they give just slightly when you press on them.

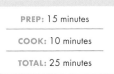

PREP: 15 minutes

COOK: 10 minutes

TOTAL: 25 minutes

4 slices Whole30-compliant bacon

4 cups chopped romaine lettuce

1 cup chopped cooked chicken

2 large hard-cooked eggs, quartered

1 ripe avocado, halved, pitted, peeled, and chopped

1 small unpeeled cucumber, chopped

1 cup grape tomatoes, halved

Whole30-compliant ranch salad dressing or Whole30 Ranch Dressing (page 282)

¼ teaspoon salt

¼ teaspoon black pepper

COOK the bacon in a large skillet over medium heat until crisp, about 10 minutes. Remove with a slotted spoon and place on paper towels to drain. Crumble the bacon when cool enough to handle.

ARRANGE the lettuce on two plates. Top with the chicken, bacon, eggs, avocado, cucumber, and tomatoes. Drizzle the dressing over the salads and season with the salt and pepper. Toss to combine and serve.

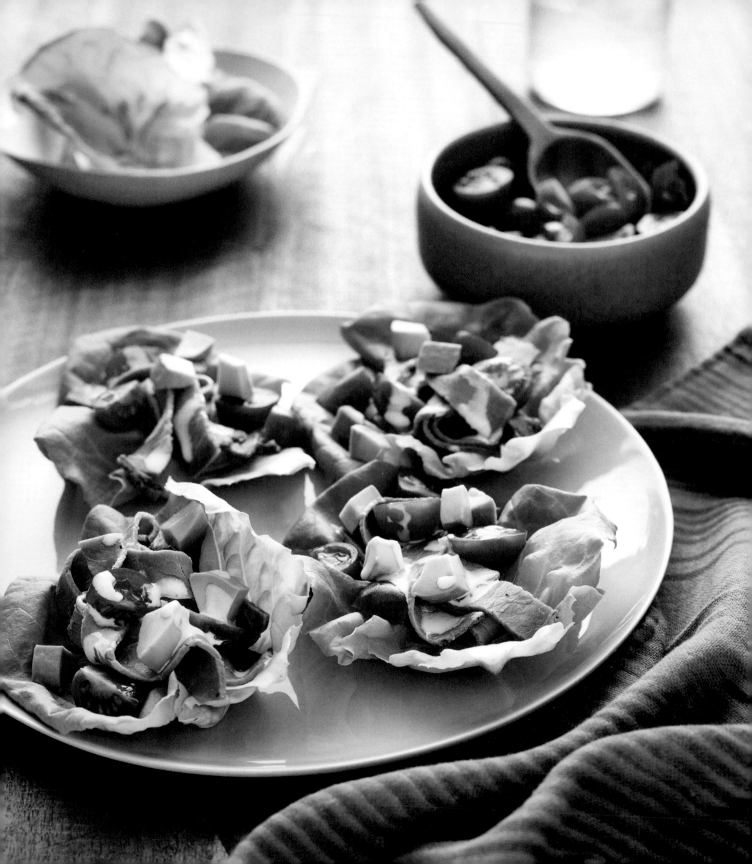

Easy Beef Salad Wraps

SERVES 2

"Easy" is an overstatement! A quick garlic-basil mayo provides the flavor for these wraps that come together in a flash—10 minutes or less. They're so simple and quick, you can make them in the morning before work and enjoy them for lunch.

PREP: 10 minutes

TOTAL: 10 minutes

FOR THE DRESSING

¼ cup Whole30-compliant mayonnaise or Basic Mayonnaise (page 281)

1 clove garlic, minced

1 tablespoon chopped fresh basil

½ teaspoon grated lemon zest

1 teaspoon fresh lemon juice

12 large Bibb lettuce leaves

8 ounces Whole30-compliant sliced roast beef, cut into ½-inch strips

1 medium avocado, halved, pitted, peeled, and diced

1 cup quartered or halved cherry tomatoes

MAKE THE DRESSING: In a small bowl, stir together the mayonnaise, garlic, basil, and lemon zest and juice.

ARRANGE the lettuce leaves on two serving plates. Divide the roast beef strips, avocado, and tomatoes among the leaves. Drizzle with the dressing and serve.

Shrimp-Prosciutto Red Cabbage Cups

SERVES 4

Delicate bits of crisp-cooked prosciutto are the magic in these shrimp-stuffed cabbage cups. They provide hits of both flavor and texture.

PREP:	15 minutes
COOK:	10 minutes
TOTAL:	25 minutes

2 tablespoons extra-virgin olive oil

2 ounces sliced prosciutto, chopped

1 pound peeled and deveined large shrimp (see Tip)

1 red bell pepper, chopped

3 cloves garlic, chopped

2 teaspoons Italian seasoning

½ teaspoon salt

½ teaspoon black pepper

½ cup chopped fresh basil

1 tablespoon white wine vinegar

1 small head red cabbage or Bibb lettuce (see Tip)

HEAT the olive oil in a large skillet over medium heat. Add the prosciutto and cook, stirring, until crisp, 2 to 3 minutes. Transfer the prosciutto with a slotted spoon to paper towels to drain.

INCREASE the heat to medium-high. Add the shrimp and bell pepper and cook, stirring occasionally, until the shrimp are almost opaque and the pepper is softened, about 2 minutes. Add the garlic, Italian seasoning, salt, and black pepper. Cook, stirring, until the shrimp are opaque, 2 to 3 minutes longer. Remove from the heat. Stir in the basil and vinegar.

SEPARATE the leaves from the cabbage and arrange on a platter. Spoon the shrimp filling into the leaves, top with the prosciutto, and serve.

TIPS *To use cooked shrimp instead of fresh, add them with the garlic, and reduce the cook time to 1 to 2 minutes or until heated through.*

Instead of in the cabbage cups, the filling can be served over lightly sautéed zucchini noodles.

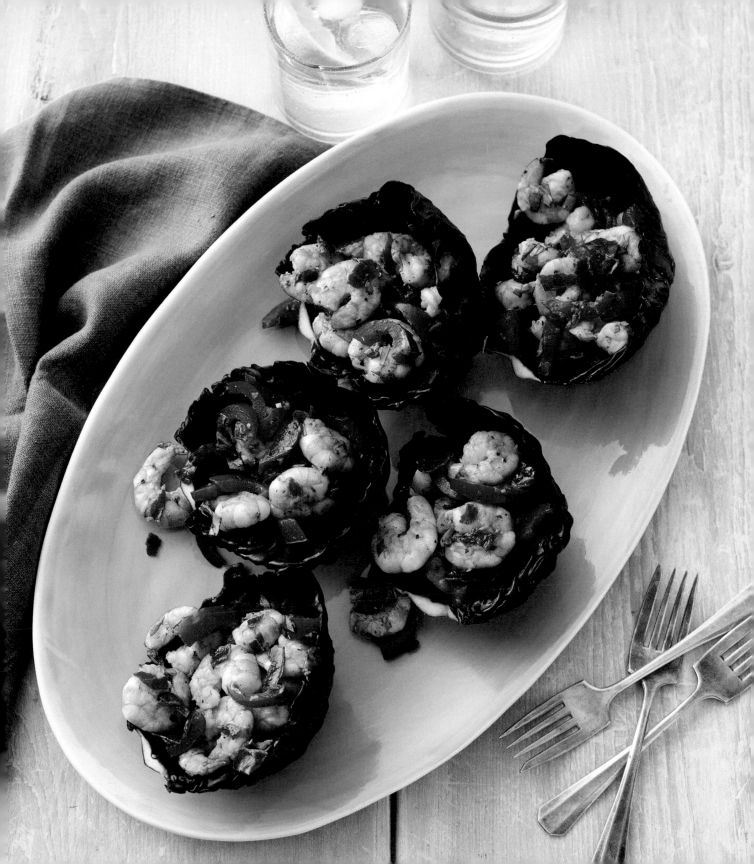

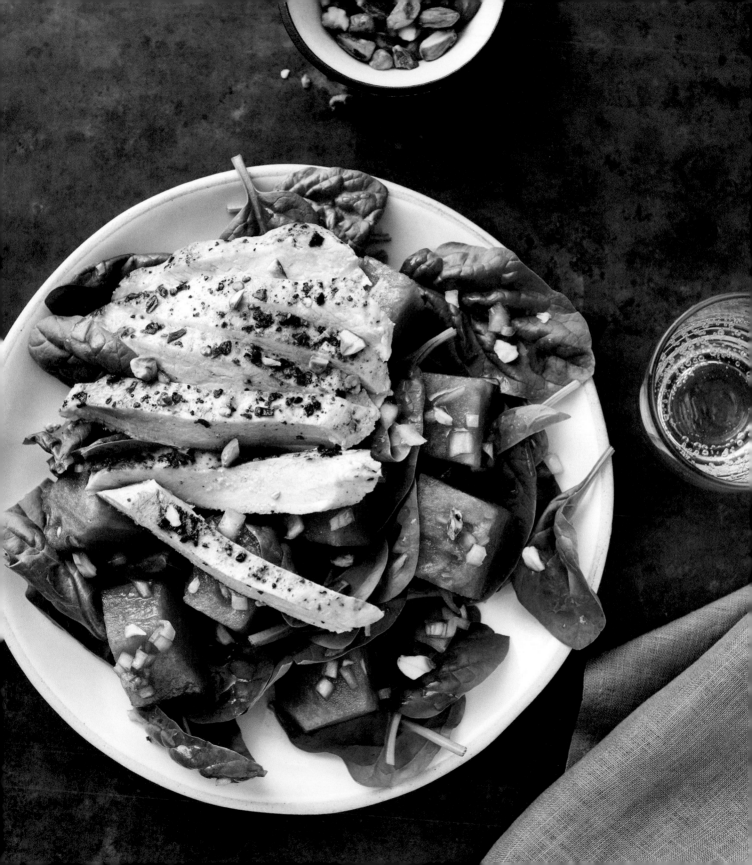

Spicy Seared Chicken with Watermelon-Spinach Salad

SERVES 2

This salad is a riot of temperatures, textures, and flavors that work really well together. The cool, slightly sweet salad balances the spicy, warm chicken in the most delicious way! A sprinkling of chopped roasted pistachios adds a buttery, salty crunch.

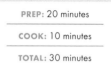

PREP: 20 minutes

COOK: 10 minutes

TOTAL: 30 minutes

FOR THE CHICKEN

2 boneless, skinless chicken breasts (about 6 ounces each)

1 teaspoon red pepper flakes

½ teaspoon garlic powder

½ teaspoon salt

½ teaspoon black pepper

2 tablespoons extra-virgin olive oil

FOR THE SALAD

4 cups baby spinach

2 cups chopped seedless watermelon

¼ cup finely chopped shallot

3 tablespoons extra-virgin olive oil

2 tablespoons red wine vinegar

½ teaspoon salt

½ teaspoon black pepper

⅓ cup roasted salted pistachios, chopped

MAKE THE CHICKEN: Place the chicken breasts between two pieces of plastic wrap and use the flat side of a meat mallet to flatten to a ¼-inch thickness. (You can ask your butcher to do this for you.) Combine the pepper flakes, garlic powder, salt, and pepper in a small bowl. Sprinkle the seasoning over the chicken.

HEAT the olive oil in a large skillet over medium-high heat. Add the chicken and cook, turning once, until browned and cooked through, about 8 minutes. Place the chicken on a cutting board and let rest for 5 minutes. Thinly slice the chicken.

MAKE THE SALAD: Combine the spinach, watermelon, and shallot in a large bowl. Drizzle with the olive oil and vinegar. Sprinkle with the salt and black pepper. Toss the salad to coat with the dressing.

ARRANGE the salad on two serving plates. Top with the sliced chicken, sprinkle with the pistachios, and serve.

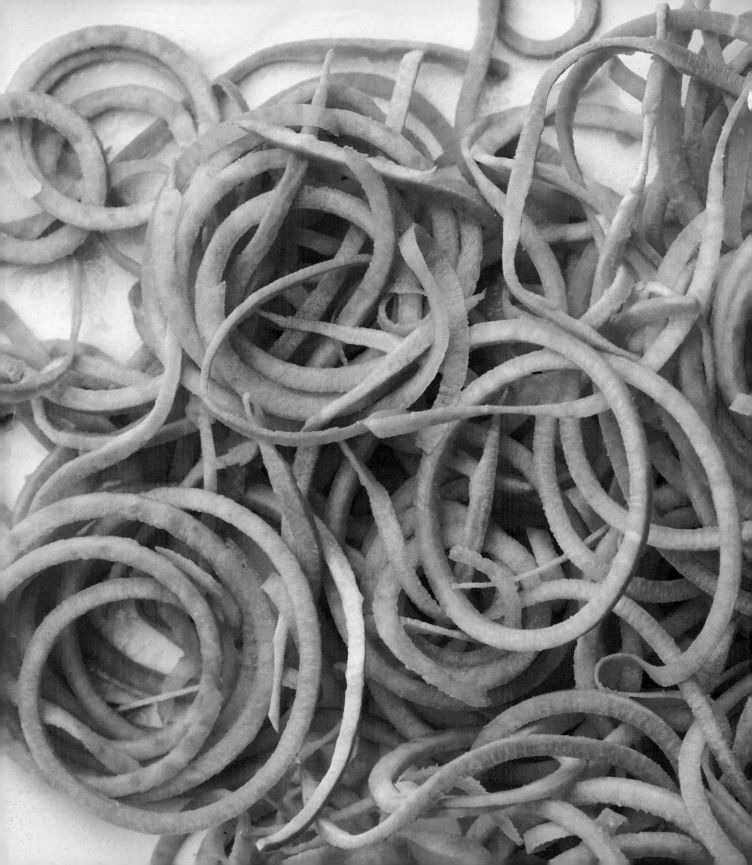

CHAPTER 2

SKILLET MEALS, STIR-FRIES, AND SAUTÉS

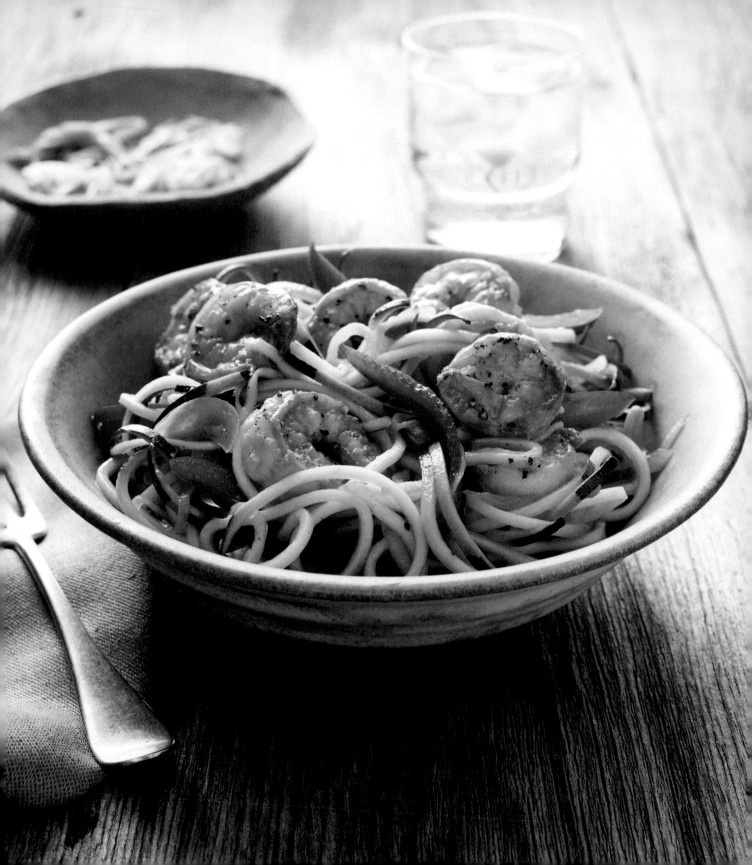

Ginger Shrimp and Zucchini-Noodle Stir-Fry

SERVES 4

Keeping a couple of 1-pound bags of peeled and deveined shrimp in your freezer means that with just a couple of fresh ingredients, dinner is a cinch to get on the table. And frozen shrimp thaw very quickly—just place them in cool water for 15 minutes or so, and change the water once.

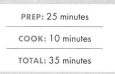

PREP: 25 minutes

COOK: 10 minutes

TOTAL: 35 minutes

¼ cup rice vinegar

3 tablespoons coconut aminos

3 cloves garlic, minced

1 tablespoon minced fresh ginger (see Tip)

¼ teaspoon salt

1½ tablespoons sesame oil

1 large yellow onion, slivered

1½ pounds peeled and deveined medium shrimp (see Tip)

3 medium red and/or green bell peppers, cut into matchsticks

2 packages (10.7 ounces each) zucchini noodles; or 3 medium zucchini, spiralized, long noodles snipped if desired

3 green onions, sliced

IN a small bowl, mix together the vinegar, coconut aminos, garlic, ginger, and salt.

HEAT the sesame oil in an extra-large skillet or wok over medium-high heat. Add the onion and cook, stirring, until it just starts to become tender, about 2 minutes. Stir in the vinegar mixture and cook until slightly reduced, about 1 minute. Add the shrimp, bell pepper, and zucchini noodles. Cook, stirring, until the shrimp are opaque and the vegetables are crisp-tender, 5 to 8 minutes. Top with the green onions and serve.

TIPS *Steer clear of store-bought jars of minced ginger, as they almost always contain added sugar and/or soybean oil.*

To make this recipe even faster, use cooked shrimp in place of the raw shrimp. Add after the vegetables are crisp-tender and continue to cook, stirring, until the shrimp are heated through, 1 to 2 minutes.

Turkey Tenderloins with Cherry Tomato–Serrano Peperonata

SERVES 4

Peperonata is an Italian relish of sweet peppers sautéed in olive oil that be served warm or cold. It can be flavored with all kinds of additional ingredients, such as tomatoes, onions, garlic, herbs, capers, olives, and vinegar. This version incorporates a serrano pepper for a little kick!

PREP:	15 minutes
COOK:	35 minutes
REST:	5 minutes
TOTAL:	55 minutes

1 ½ pounds turkey tenderloins

½ teaspoon salt

½ teaspoon black pepper

2 tablespoons extra-virgin olive oil

4 cups sliced sweet mini peppers

1 serrano chile pepper, halved, seeded, and thinly sliced

1 medium onion, sliced

3 cloves garlic, minced

1 pint cherry or grape tomatoes

¼ cup balsamic vinegar

2 tablespoons torn fresh basil

PREHEAT the oven to 425°F.

SEASON the turkey with the salt and black pepper. Heat the oil in an oven-proof skillet over medium-high heat. Add the turkey and cook until browned, 2 to 3 minutes per side.

REMOVE the turkey from the skillet. Add the bell peppers, chile, onion, and garlic to the skillet and cook, stirring occasionally, until just softened, 3 to 5 minutes. Stir in the tomatoes and vinegar.

RETURN the turkey to the skillet and transfer to the oven. Roast until the turkey is cooked through, 25 to 30 minutes. Let the turkey rest 5 minutes then cut into slices. Top with the basil and serve.

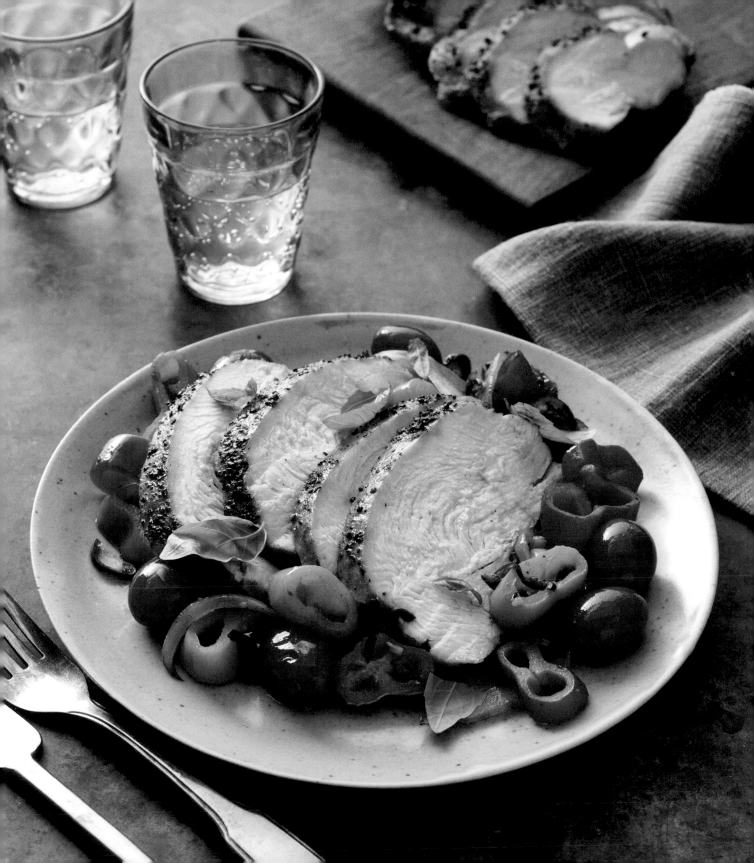

Thai Chicken and Brussels Sprout Skillet

SERVES 4

Pre-shredded Brussels sprouts make super-quick work of this one-pan meal. If you have the time to shred your own sprouts (see Tip), they will taste a little fresher.

PREP: 10 minutes
COOK: 10 minutes
TOTAL: 20 minutes

4 tablespoons extra-virgin olive oil or coconut oil

1 pound boneless skinless chicken thighs, thinly sliced (see Tip)

½ teaspoon salt

2 bags (9 to 10 ounces each) shaved Brussels sprouts

1 cup packaged shredded carrots, or 2 medium carrots, shredded

2 tablespoons chopped shallots

½ cup Asian Citrus Dressing (page 277)

Whole30 Sriracha (page 274)

IN an extra-large skillet, heat 2 tablespoons of the olive oil over medium heat. Add the chicken and cook, stirring occasionally, for 3 minutes. Sprinkle the chicken with the salt. Add the remaining 2 tablespoons olive oil to the skillet, then the Brussels sprouts, carrots, and shallots. Cook, stirring occasionally, until the sprouts are tender and lightly browned, 5 to 8 minutes. Add the dressing and heat through, about 1 minute. Serve with the Sriracha.

TIPS *To make this recipe even faster, use 3 cups chopped leftover cooked chicken.*

To shave your own Brussels sprouts, use a food processor to shave about 1¼ pounds trimmed Brussels sprouts. You should have about 10 cups shaved Brussels sprouts.

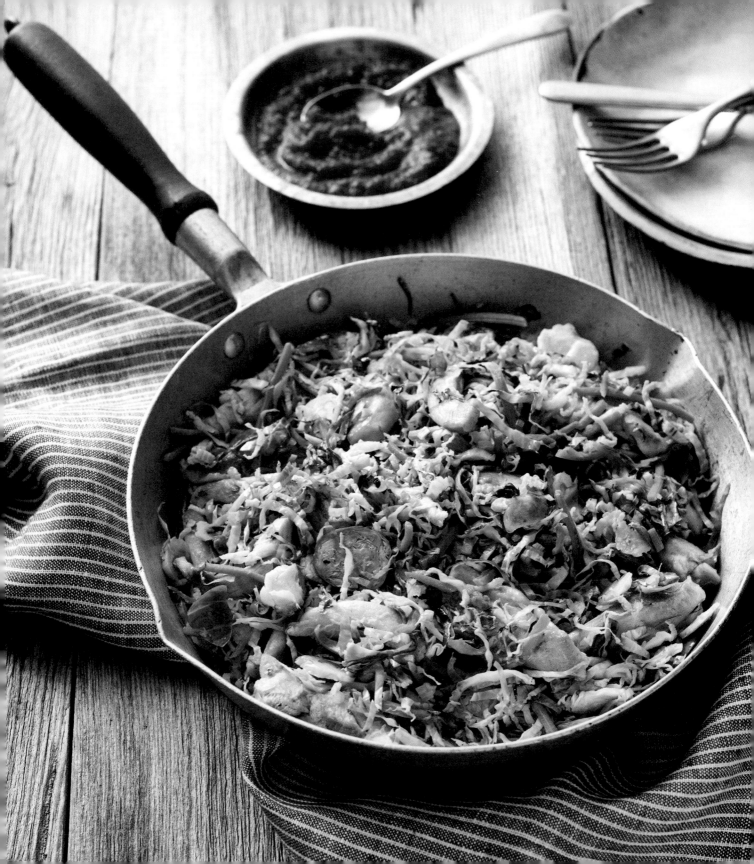

Pan-Seared Steaks with Chimichurri Brussels Slaw

SERVES 2

Chimichurri is an Argentinean condiment that is typically served with that country's famous grilled steak. It's garlicky, vinegary, a little spicy, and fresh—from a generous dose of herbs.

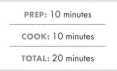

PREP: 10 minutes

COOK: 10 minutes

TOTAL: 20 minutes

FOR THE CHIMICHURRI

¼ cup red wine vinegar

½ cup packed fresh parsley

1 tablespoon fresh oregano leaves, or 1 teaspoon dried oregano

2 cloves garlic, chopped

½ teaspoon red pepper flakes

½ teaspoon salt

½ teaspoon black pepper

½ cup extra-virgin olive oil

FOR THE STEAKS

2 flat iron, strip, or sirloin steaks (6 to 8 ounces each)

¼ teaspoon salt

¼ teaspoon black pepper

1 tablespoon Clarified Butter (page 283) or ghee

1 bag (9 to 10 ounces) shaved Brussels sprouts (see Tip)

MAKE THE CHIMICHURRI: Combine the vinegar, parsley, oregano, garlic, pepper flakes, salt, and black pepper in a blender. Cover and blend until almost smooth. With the blender running, add the olive oil in a thin stream until combined. Set aside.

COOK THE STEAKS: Season the steaks with the salt and black pepper. Heat the butter over medium-high heat in a large skillet. Cook the steaks, turning once, until medium-well, 5 to 6 minutes. Remove the steaks from the skillet and let rest.

MEANWHILE, add the Brussels sprouts to the skillet. Cook over medium heat, stirring, until crisp-tender, 4 to 5 minutes. Stir in ¼ cup of the chimichurri. Serve the steaks with the Brussels sprouts and remaining chimichurri.

TIP *To shave your own Brussels sprouts, use a food processor to shave about 10 ounces Brussels sprouts, trimmed. You should have about 5 cups shaved Brussels sprouts.*

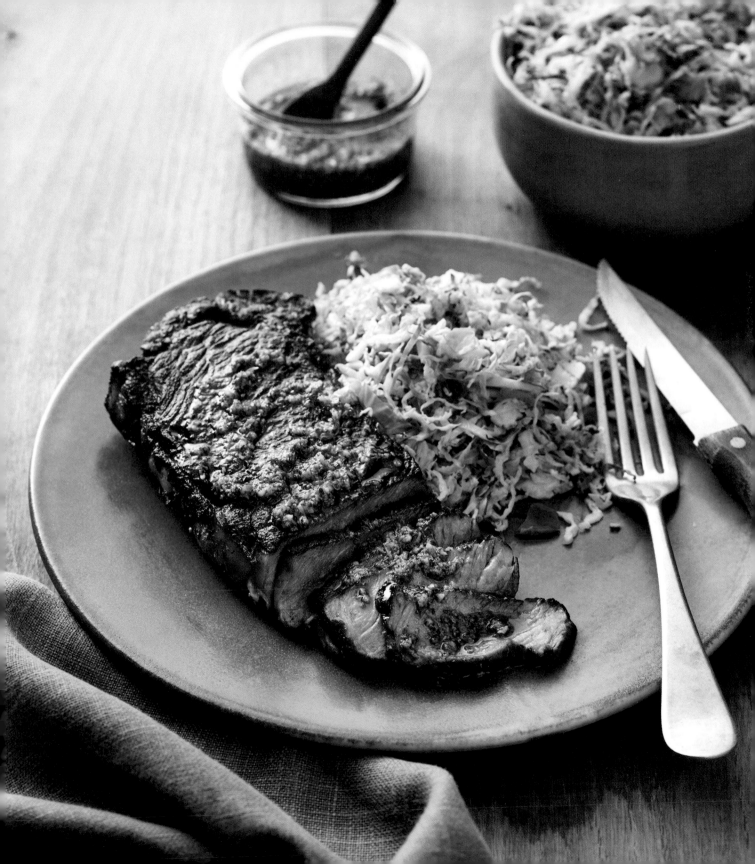

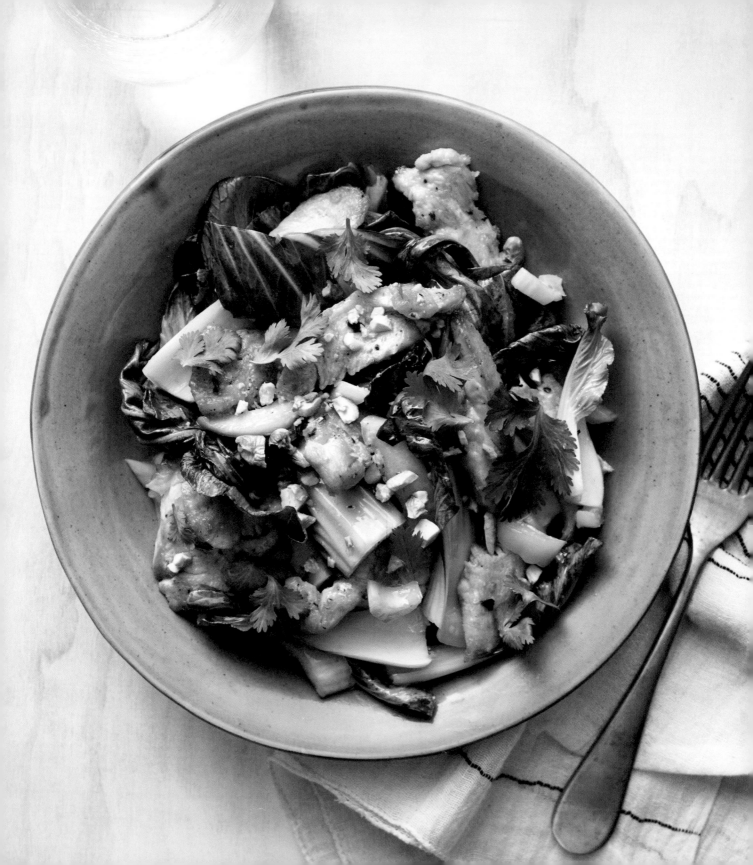

Spicy Lemongrass Chicken and Bok Choy Stir-Fry

SERVES 4

Lemongrass gives this stir-fry bright, fresh flavor. To prepare the lemongrass, trim off the root end of the stalk. Peel away the tough outer layers to get to the pale core. Use only the bottom 4 or 5 inches of the stalk, which is the most tender, and chop finely.

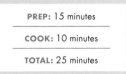

PREP: 15 minutes

COOK: 10 minutes

TOTAL: 25 minutes

1 pound chicken breast stir-fry strips

¼ teaspoon salt

¼ teaspoon black pepper

2 tablespoons extra-virgin olive oil

1 tablespoon finely chopped fresh lemongrass

1 tablespoon minced fresh ginger

4 cloves garlic, minced

½ teaspoon red pepper flakes

4 heads baby bok choy, coarsely chopped

¼ cup roasted salted cashews, finely chopped

¼ cup chopped fresh cilantro

SEASON the chicken with the salt and black pepper. Heat 1 tablespoon of the olive oil in a large skillet over medium-high heat. Add the chicken and cook, stirring occasionally, until the chicken is almost cooked through, about 5 minutes.

ADD the lemongrass, ginger, garlic, and pepper flakes to the skillet. Cook, stirring, for 1 minute. Add the remaining 1 tablespoon olive oil. Add the bok choy and cook, stirring, until beginning to soften but still crisp, 2 to 3 minutes. Remove the skillet from the heat. Top with the cashews and cilantro and serve.

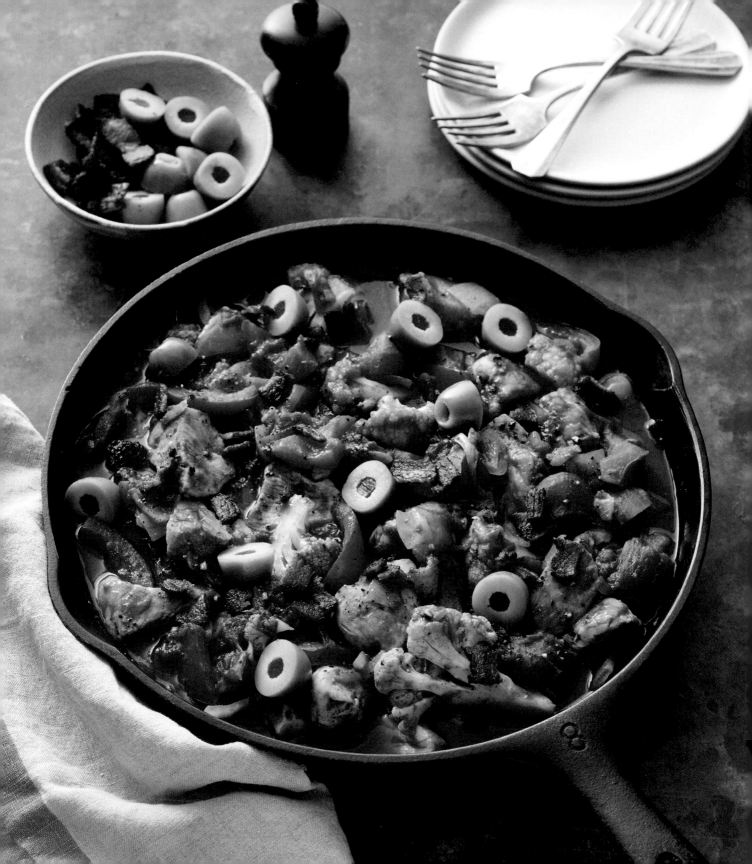

Spanish Chicken and Cauliflower Skillet

SERVES 4

Cooking the chicken and vegetables in a little bit of rendered bacon fat does amazing things for the flavor of this dish.

PREP: 20 minutes

COOK: 20 minutes

TOTAL: 40 minutes

4 slices Whole30-compliant bacon, chopped

1 pound boneless, skinless chicken breasts or thighs, diced

1 medium onion, chopped

1 red bell pepper, chopped

4 cloves garlic, minced

1 can (28 ounces) Whole30-compliant diced tomatoes

½ teaspoon black pepper

¼ teaspoon cayenne pepper

¼ teaspoon salt

4 cups cauliflower florets

½ cup pimento-stuffed Spanish olives, halved

IN a large skillet, cook the bacon over medium-high heat until crisp, about 5 minutes. Transfer with a slotted spoon to paper towels to drain, leaving the bacon fat in the skillet.

ADD the chicken to the skillet and cook, stirring, until opaque, 2 to 3 minutes. Stir in the onion, bell pepper, and garlic. Cook, stirring until the onions are softened, about 4 minutes. Add the tomatoes, black pepper, cayenne pepper, and salt. Bring to a boil and add the cauliflower. Cover and simmer until the cauliflower is just tender, about 5 minutes. Top with the bacon and olives and serve.

Spaghetti Squash with Sausage Arrabbiata Sauce

SERVES 4

The word *arrabbiata* means "angry" in Italian, in reference to the spiciness provided by a healthy dose of red pepper flakes in the sauce. Cut the pepper flakes to ¼ teaspoon if you don't like things quite so hot.

PREP: 20 minutes
COOK: 25 minutes
TOTAL: 45 minutes

1 spaghetti squash (about 2 pounds)

1 pound ground pork

3 ounces pancetta, chopped

1 medium onion, chopped

3 cups coarsely chopped seeded Roma (plum) tomatoes (see Tip)

½ cup drained Whole30-compliant roasted red peppers, chopped

4 cloves garlic, minced

2 teaspoons dried Italian seasoning

½ teaspoon salt

½ teaspoon red pepper flakes

½ teaspoon fennel seeds, finely crushed (optional)

¼ cup chopped fresh basil

1 tablespoon extra-virgin olive oil

CUT the squash lengthwise in half. Scrape out the seeds and strings. Place the squash halves, cut sides down, in a 2-quart rectangular microwave-safe baking dish. Add ½ cup water to the dish. Microwave, uncovered, on high until the squash is tender, 14 to 16 minutes. Let the squash stand until cool enough to handle.

MEANWHILE, in a large skillet, cook the ground pork, pancetta, and onion over medium-high heat, stirring, until the pork is no longer pink. Drain off the fat. Add the tomatoes, roasted peppers, garlic, Italian seasoning, salt, crushed pepper, and fennel seeds (if using). Cover and cook over medium heat, stirring occasionally, until the tomatoes are softened, 4 to 5 minutes. Uncover and continue to cook, stirring and mashing with a spatula, until the mixture is saucy and well combined, 3 to 4 minutes more. Remove from the heat. Stir in the basil.

USE a fork to scrape the squash flesh into a medium bowl. Drizzle with the olive oil and season lightly with salt. Toss gently to coat. Spoon the arrabbiata sauce over the squash and serve.

TIP *If fresh tomatoes are not in season, substitute 1 can (28 ounces) Whole30-compliant no-salt-added diced tomatoes.*

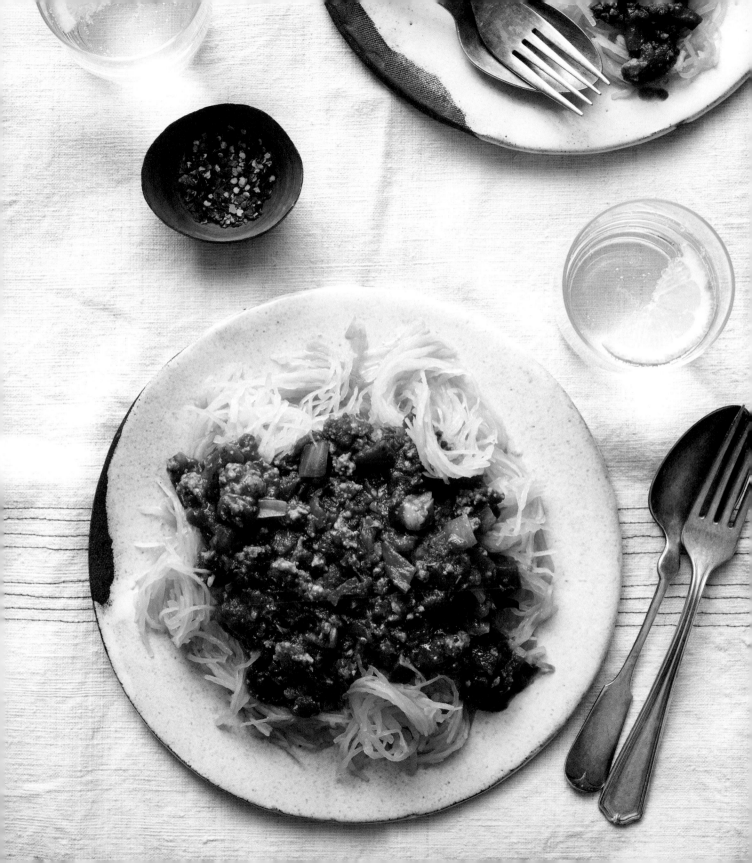

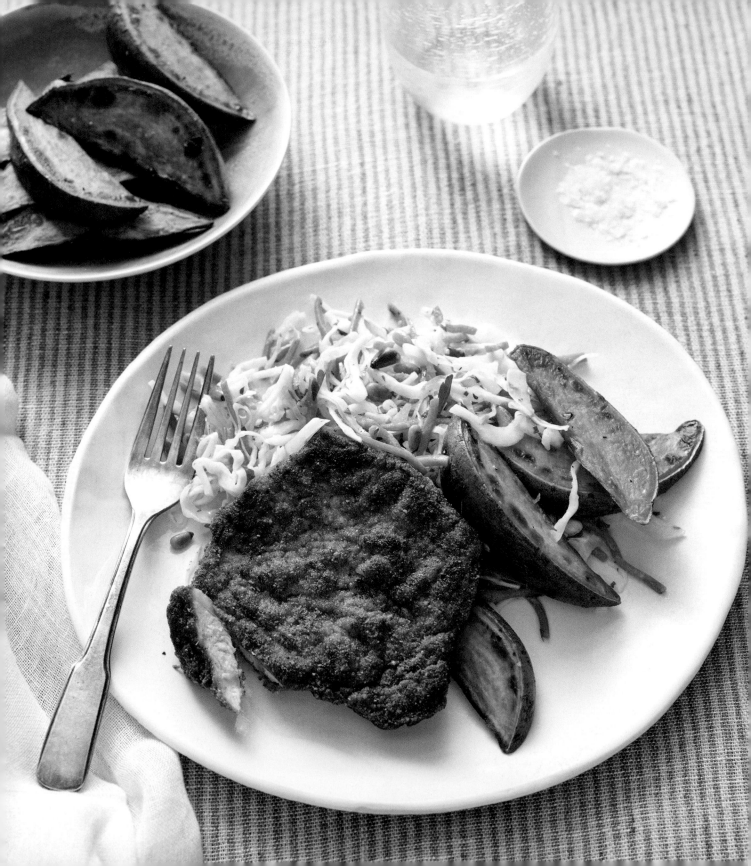

Skillet Pork Chops with Sweet Potatoes

SERVES 4

Pounding the chops to ¼-inch thickness helps them cook super-quick. Dredging them in almond or coconut flour seasoned with sage, paprika, and dry mustard gives them a crisp, delicious crust.

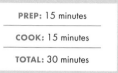

PREP: 15 minutes

COOK: 15 minutes

TOTAL: 30 minutes

FOR THE SIMPLE GREEK SLAW

3 cups shredded cabbage and carrot coleslaw mix

⅓ cup chopped fresh parsley

2 tablespoons pine nuts, toasted (see Tip)

⅓ cup Whole30-compliant lemon-garlic dressing

FOR THE SWEET POTATOES

1 tablespoon coconut oil

1 medium sweet potato, cut into ½-inch-thick wedges

¼ teaspoon salt

⅛ teaspoon black pepper

FOR THE CHOPS

4 (½-inch-thick) boneless pork loin chops (1 pound total) (see Tip)

1 large egg

1 tablespoon extra-virgin olive oil

⅔ cup almond or coconut flour

1 teaspoon ground sage

1 teaspoon paprika

½ teaspoon ground mustard

½ teaspoon salt

¼ teaspoon black pepper

2 tablespoons coconut oil

MAKE THE SLAW: In a medium bowl, toss together the coleslaw mix, parsley, and pine nuts. Drizzle the dressing over the slaw; toss to coat.

MAKE THE POTATOES: Preheat the oven to 200°F.

HEAT the coconut oil in an extra-large skillet over medium heat. Add the sweet potato wedges, salt, and pepper. Cook, covered, turning once halfway through, until the sweet potatoes are tender, 6 to 8 minutes. If necessary, reduce the heat to medium-low to prevent overbrowning. Transfer the potatoes to a serving plate and keep warm in the oven.

COOK THE CHOPS: Meanwhile, place each chop between two pieces of plastic wrap. Use the flat side of a meat mallet to flatten the chops to ¼-inch thickness. In a shallow dish, whisk together the egg and olive oil. In another shallow dish, stir together the flour, sage, paprika, mustard, salt, and black pepper. Dip each chop in the egg, turning to coat. Allow the excess to drip off. Dip in the flour mixture, turning to coat.

IN the same skillet, heat the coconut oil over medium heat. Add the chops to the skillet. Cook until the coating is lightly browned and the interior is slightly pink, 4 to 6 minutes.

SERVE the pork chops and sweet potatoes with the slaw.

TIPS *To toast pine nuts, heat in a dry skillet, stirring, until fragrant and lightly browned, about 2 minutes.*

To save time in the kitchen, ask your butcher to pound the pork chops thin before wrapping them up for you.

Pork Chops with Sweet Potato Colcannon

SERVES 4

FROM *Scott Gooding of The Scott Gooding Project*

Growing up, nothing tasted better than mashed potato, ghee, and salt. Not much has changed except superior salt and swapping white potato for sweet. Colcannon is a traditional Irish recipe, which I've tweaked slightly.

PREP: 15 minutes

COOK: 25 minutes

TOTAL: 40 minutes

1 large (1 pound) sweet potato, peeled and roughly chopped

2 tablespoons Clarified Butter (page 283) or ghee

1 bunch Swiss chard, stalks removed, roughly chopped

1 leek, finely sliced

½ teaspoon salt

½ teaspoon black pepper

4 (1-inch-thick) boneless pork loin chops

FILL a large saucepan with salted water and bring to a boil. Add the sweet potato, reduce the heat to a simmer, and cook until softened, 6 to 8 minutes. Drain the water and heat the potato in the saucepan for 1 minute to remove excess moisture. Transfer to a bowl and cover to keep warm.

IN the same saucepan, heat 1 tablespoons of the butter over low heat. Add the chard, leek, ¼ teaspoon of the salt, and ¼ teaspoon of the black pepper. Cook, stirring, until the leek and chard are softened, 6 to 8 minutes. Remove from the heat and keep warm.

MEANWHILE, in a large skillet, heat the remaining 1 tablespoon butter over high heat. Lightly season the pork chops with the remaining ¼ teaspoon salt and ¼ teaspoon black pepper. Add the chops to the skillet and cook until the internal temperature is 145°F, 3 to 4 minutes on each side.

COMBINE the leeks, Swiss chard, and sweet potato. Serve with the pork chops.

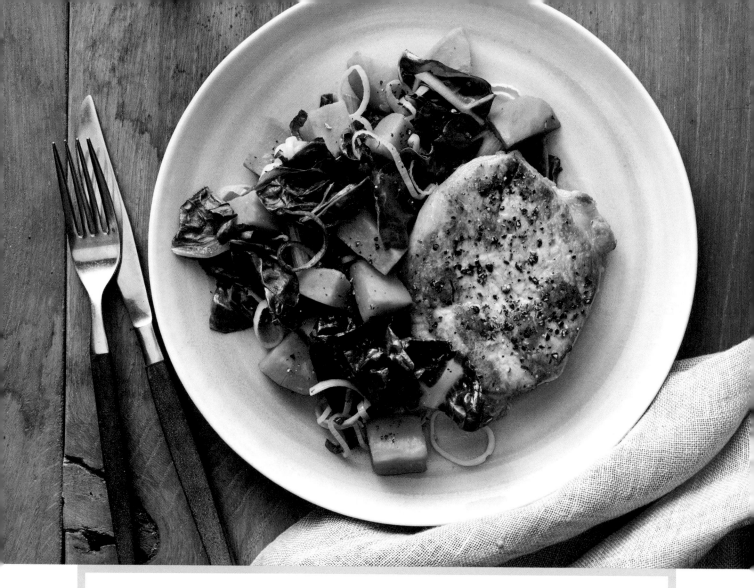

Scott Gooding

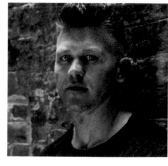

Scott Gooding is an Australian chef and the thought leader behind The Scott Gooding Project, which encourages and inspires people to cook real food at home for themselves and their loved ones. Scott breaks down the barriers to cooking healthy food with his simple, affordable, nourishing recipes. He's a big proponent of a higher-fat, lower-carbohydrate protocol and hopes to contribute to changing the current food landscape, in the name of optimal health for his followers and his son.

Mongolian Beef

SERVES 4

FROM *ChihYu Smith of I Heart Umami*

"Mongolian beef" is the Western name for *Cōng bào niúròu* in Mandarin. The Mandarin name literally means "beef with scallion and ginger stir-fry." This dish is packed with tons of flavor, color, and texture. Most of the Mongolian beef recipes found online are covered with glossy sauces with tons of starch, but with this recipe there's no need to use added sugar, honey, or starch. It will be just as delicious, if not better, for you and your family!

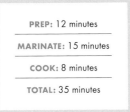

PREP:	12 minutes
MARINATE:	15 minutes
COOK:	8 minutes
TOTAL:	35 minutes

2 tablespoons coconut aminos

1 tablespoon Red Boat fish sauce

2 teaspoons toasted sesame oil

1 pound beef sirloin tips, skirt steak, or boneless short ribs, thinly sliced

1 piece (3 inches) fresh ginger, peeled and cut into matchsticks

2 fresh red chile peppers, seeded and cut into matchsticks or thinly sliced (optional)

3 cloves garlic, minced

3 green onions, cut into 3-inch lengths, white and green parts separated

4 tablespoons Clarified Butter (page 283), ghee, or coconut oil

1 container (5 ounces) mixed greens

COMBINE the coconut aminos, fish sauce, and sesame oil in a large bowl. Add the beef and turn to coat. Cover the bowl and marinate in the refrigerator for 15 to 20 minutes.

MEANWHILE, in a small bowl, combine the ginger, chile peppers, garlic, and white parts of the green onions.

IN a large skillet, melt 1 tablespoon of the butter over medium heat. Add the beef and marinade to the skillet and cook, tossing with tongs occasionally, until no longer pink, 4 to 5 minutes. Transfer the meat and sauce to a bowl.

IN the same skillet, heat the remaining 3 tablespoons butter. Add the ginger mixture and cook over medium heat, stirring, until fragrant, 1 to 2 minutes. Add the meat and green parts of green onions to the skillet; toss to combine.

SERVE the beef and sauce over the mixed greens.

ChihYu Smith

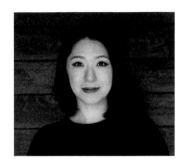

ChihYu Smith is the founder of Cook Once Eat All Week, a paleo meal planning program that helps busy professionals save time and add deliciousness to their paleo and Whole30 cooking. She specializes in Asian-inspired paleo cuisine with no added sugar. Her work has been published throughout the U.S., Europe, and Australia.

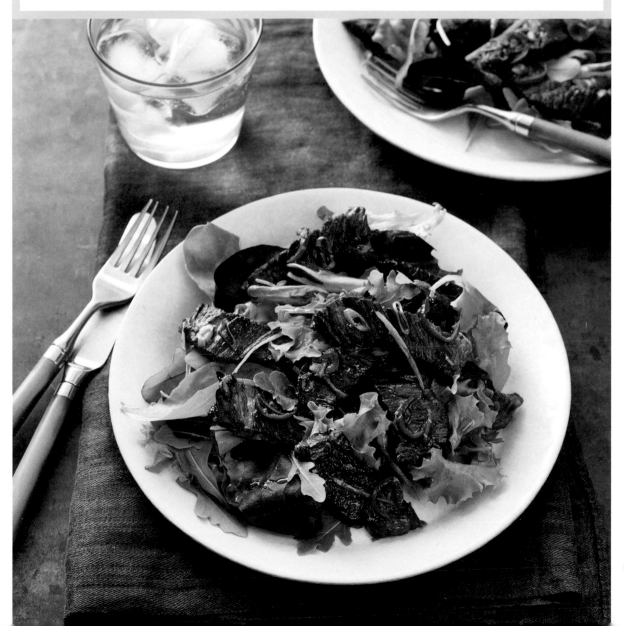

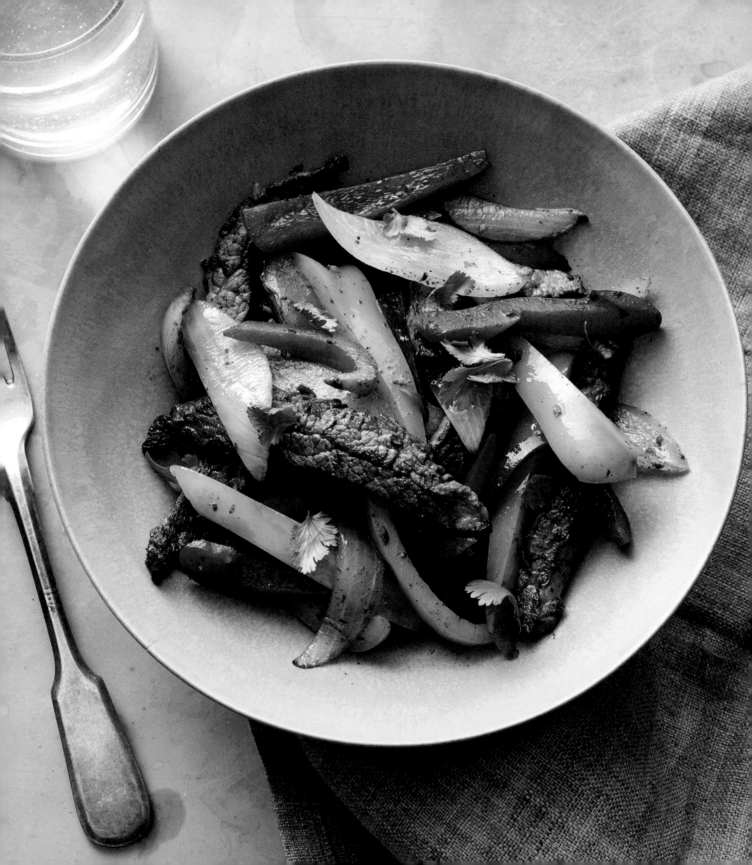

Indian Beef and Bell Pepper Stir-Fry

SERVES 4

If you like your stir-fry strips of beef fairly thin, stick the steak in the freezer for 30 minutes to partially freeze it before slicing. It will make it easier to make even, thin slices.

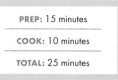

PREP: 15 minutes

COOK: 10 minutes

TOTAL: 25 minutes

1 tablespoon Whole30-compliant garam masala

½ teaspoon garlic salt

2 tablespoons coconut oil

1 medium onion, cut into thin wedges

2 large yellow and/or red bell peppers, cut into strips

1½ pounds strip steak, flank steak, or skirt steak, cut into strips

2 teaspoons minced fresh ginger

Fresh cilantro

IN a small bowl, stir together 3 tablespoons water, the garam masala, and garlic salt; set aside.

HEAT 1 tablespoon of the oil in a large skillet over medium-high heat. Add the onion and cook, stirring, for 1 minute. Add the bell pepper and cook, stirring, until beginning to soften but still crisp, about 3 minutes. Transfer the onion and pepper to a plate and cover to keep warm.

IN the same skillet, heat the remaining 1 tablespoon oil over medium-high heat. Add the meat and ginger and cook, stirring, until meat is desired doneness, 1 to 2 minutes. Stir in the onion and pepper mixture and the garam masala mixture and heat through, about 1 minute. Garnish with the cilantro and serve.

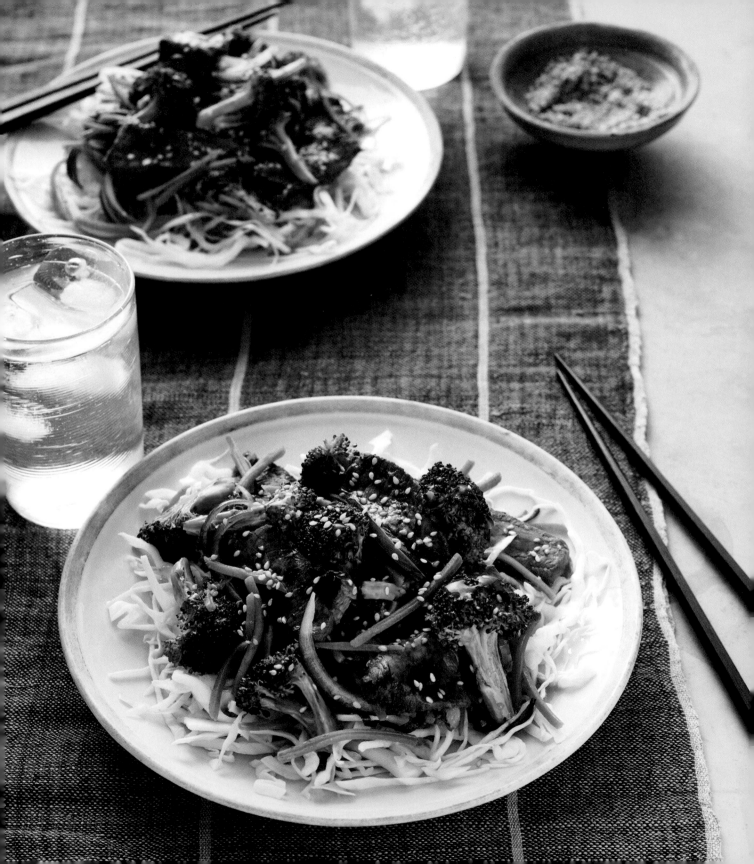

Beef and Broccoli Stir-Fry

SERVES 4

This fresh take on the Chinese restaurant favorite gives you a double dose of tasty veggies—the broccoli, of course, and a bed of quick-sautéed shredded green cabbage in place of the usual rice.

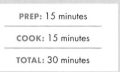

PREP: 15 minutes

COOK: 15 minutes

TOTAL: 30 minutes

2 tablespoons coconut aminos

1 tablespoon minced fresh ginger

4 cloves garlic, minced

¼ teaspoon salt

1 pound boneless top sirloin steak, trimmed and cut against the grain into ⅛-inch slices

4 tablespoons toasted sesame oil

3 cups small broccoli florets

1 medium red onion, quartered and thinly sliced

1 cup packaged shredded carrots, or 2 medium carrots, shredded

1 cup low-sodium Whole30-compliant beef broth or Beef Bone Broth (page 280)

2 teaspoons arrowroot

¼ to ½ teaspoon red pepper flakes

6 cups packaged shredded green cabbage

1 tablespoon sesame seeds, toasted (see Tip)

IN a medium bowl, combine the coconut aminos, ginger, garlic, and salt. Add the beef and mix well. Let the beef stand at room temperature while cooking the vegetables.

IN a large skillet, heat 1 tablespoon of the sesame oil over medium-high heat. Add the broccoli, onion, and carrots. Cook, stirring, until the vegetables are crisp-tender, about 3 minutes. Transfer the vegetables to a bowl and set aside.

ADD 1 tablespoon sesame oil to the skillet. Add half the beef and cook, stirring, until slightly pink in the center, 2 to 3 minutes. Add to the bowl with the vegetables. Add 1 tablespoon sesame oil to the skillet and cook the remaining beef, stirring, until slightly pink in center, 2 to 3 minutes. Return the vegetables and cooked beef to the skillet.

IN a small bowl, whisk together the broth, arrowroot, and pepper flakes until smooth. Push the meat and vegetables to the edges of the skillet. Pour the broth mixture into the center. Cook over medium-high heat, stirring, until thickened, 1 to 2 minutes. Stir the meat and vegetables into the sauce. Transfer the stir-fry to a large serving bowl and cover to keep warm. Carefully wipe out the skillet with paper towels.

ADD the remaining 1 tablespoon sesame oil to the skillet and heat over medium-high heat. Add the cabbage and cook, stirring, until bright green and wilted, 1 to 2 minutes. Spoon the stir-fry over the cabbage, sprinkle with the sesame seeds, and serve.

TIP *To toast sesame seeds, heat in a dry skillet over medium heat, stirring, until fragrant and lightly browned, about 2 minutes.*

Chicken Sauté with Ginger and Basil

SERVES 2

Slicing the sugar snap peas helps them incorporate a little better with the other veggies—shredded carrots and slivered red onion—in this Asian-inspired sauté.

PREP: 15 minutes	
COOK: 15 minutes	
TOTAL: 30 minutes	

2 boneless, skinless chicken breast halves (6 ounces each)

Coarse salt and black pepper

2 tablespoons coconut oil

1 tablespoon fresh lime juice

1 tablespoon minced fresh ginger

½ cup Whole30-compliant chicken broth or Chicken Bone Broth (page 280)

1 cup packaged shredded carrots, or 2 medium carrots, shredded

1 medium red onion, slivered

1 cup sliced sugar snap peas

¼ teaspoon crushed red pepper

2 tablespoons snipped fresh basil

PLACE the chicken breasts between two pieces of plastic wrap and use the flat side of a meat mallet to flatten them to a ¼-inch thickness. Lightly season both sides with salt and pepper.

HEAT 1 tablespoon of the coconut oil in a large skillet over medium heat. Add the chicken and cook until golden, 3 to 4 minutes per side, adding more oil if needed. Remove the chicken from the skillet and cover to keep warm.

ADD the lime juice, ginger, and broth to the skillet, scraping up any browned bits on the bottom of the skillet. Bring to a boil, reduce the heat, and simmer until the pan sauce is reduced to about ¼ cup, 1 to 2 minutes. Remove the skillet from the heat.

MEANWHILE, heat the remaining 1 tablespoon coconut oil in a medium skillet over medium-high heat. Add the carrots, onion, snap peas, and crushed red pepper and cook, stirring, until crisp-tender, about 4 minutes.

ARRANGE the chicken and vegetables on serving plates and drizzle the pan juices over all. Sprinkle with the fresh basil and serve.

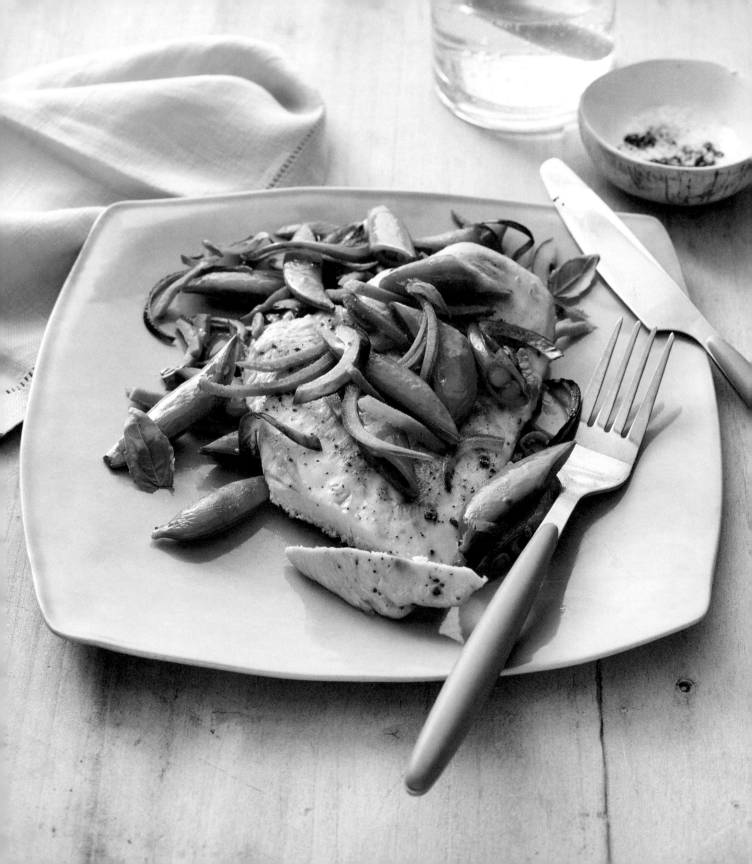

Pork and Pepper Stir-Fry

SERVES 2

A splash of apple cider—a natural pairing with pork—adds a hint of sweetness to the sauce for this dish.

PREP: 15 minutes

COOK: 10 minutes

TOTAL: 25 minutes

2 tablespoons coconut aminos

2 tablespoons apple cider

1 tablespoon rice vinegar

2 cloves garlic, minced

2 teaspoons minced fresh ginger

$\frac{1}{8}$ teaspoon red pepper flakes

2 tablespoons coconut oil

12 ounces pork tenderloin, cut into thin, bite-size strips

1 small red bell pepper, cut into bite-size strips

1 bag (8 ounces) fresh sugar snap peas

2 green onions, sliced on the bias, white and green parts separated

2 teaspoons sesame seeds, toasted (see Tip)

IN a small bowl, mix the coconut aminos, cider, vinegar, garlic, ginger, and pepper flakes; set aside.

HEAT 1 tablespoon of the coconut oil in a large skillet or wok over medium-high heat. Add the pork and cook, stirring, until no longer pink, 2 to 3 minutes. Remove the pork from the skillet.

IN the same skillet, heat the remaining 1 tablespoon coconut oil over medium-high heat. Add the bell pepper, snap peas, and white parts of the green onions. Cook, stirring, until the vegetables are crisp-tender, 3 to 5 minutes. Stir in the coconut aminos mixture. Cook, stirring, for 1 minute more. Return the pork to the skillet and heat through.

SERVE the stir-fry topped with the remaining green onions and the sesame seeds.

TIP *To toast sesame seeds, heat in a skillet over medium heat, stirring, until fragrant and lightly browned, about 2 minutes.*

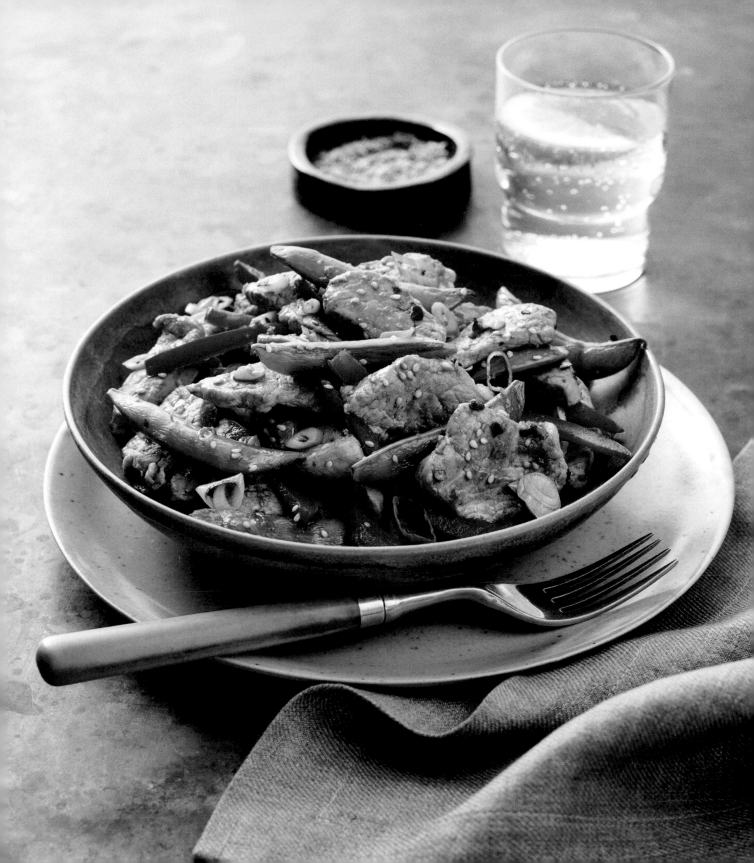

Shrimp Stir-Fry over Cauliflower Grits

SERVES 4

Here's a totally new way to do shrimp and grits. The shrimp is cooked in bacon drippings and flavored with garlic, green onions, lemon juice, and parsley instead of Cajun seasoning—and they're served on incredibly creamy and decadent-tasting cauliflower grits. You will not believe what you're tasting!

PREP: 20 minutes
COOK: 15 minutes
TOTAL: 35 minutes

2 slices Whole30-compliant bacon, chopped

FOR THE CAULIFLOWER GRITS

2 bags (12 ounces each) frozen riced cauliflower, or 6 cups raw cauliflower rice (see opposite)

¼ cup Clarified Butter (page 283) or ghee

2 teaspoons minced garlic

½ teaspoon salt

½ teaspoon black pepper

½ cup Whole30-compliant unsweetened almond milk

FOR THE SHRIMP

1 tablespoon Clarified Butter (page 283) or ghee

1½ pounds peeled and deveined medium shrimp (see Tip)

2 teaspoons minced garlic

½ cup sliced green onions

2 tablespoons fresh lemon juice

2 tablespoons chopped fresh parsley

IN a large skillet, cook the bacon over medium heat until crisp. Transfer to paper towels and set aside. Reserve 1 tablespoon of the drippings in the skillet.

MAKE THE CAULIFLOWER GRITS: While the bacon is cooking, place the riced cauliflower in a large microwave-safe bowl. Cover and cook on high for 5 to 6 minutes or until hot. Let stand 1 minute. Add the butter, garlic, salt, black pepper, and almond milk. Using an immersion blender, blend until fairly smooth. Cover and keep warm while cooking the shrimp.

MAKE THE SHIRMP: Add the butter to the skillet with the bacon drippings. Add the shrimp and cook over medium-high heat, stirring, for 1 minute. Add the garlic and green onions. Cook, stirring, until the shrimp are opaque, about 3 minutes more. Stir in the lemon juice.

SERVE the shrimp on the grits, sprinkled with the bacon and parsley.

TIP *You can also use cooked shrimp in place of the raw shrimp. Add them after the garlic and green onions have softened and cook, stirring, until heated through, 1 to 2 minutes. Stir in the lemon juice.*

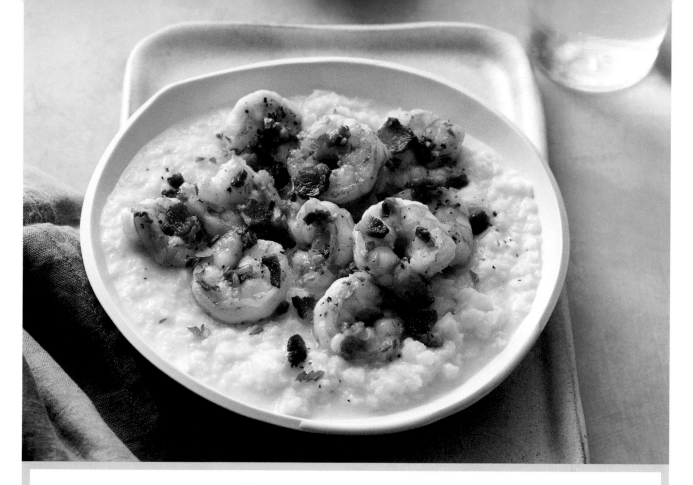

Cauliflower Rice and Crumbles

Nutritious cauliflower rice or "crumbles" can be used to replace couscous, grains, or rice, and serves as a blank canvas for seasonings. You can buy bags of frozen riced cauliflower or refrigerated cauliflower crumbles in the refrigerated aisle of your supermarket, but it takes just 5 minutes to make your own.

HOMEMADE CAULIFLOWER CRUMBLES: Cut 1 large head cauliflower into large florets. In batches, place the florets in a food processor (don't fill more than three-fourths full). Pulse the florets until processed into crumbles. Remove any unprocessed large pieces from the food processor. Transfer the crumbles or rice to bowl, then reprocess the large pieces. Makes about 7 cups.

HOMEMADE CAULIFLOWER RICE: Process as directed above, but pulse a bit longer, until the cauliflower is in rice-size pieces.

TO COOK CRUMBLES OR RICE: Place cauliflower crumbles or rice in a microwave-safe bowl; drizzle with 1 tablespoon extra-virgin olive oil and stir to coat. Tightly cover the bowl with plastic wrap and cook until just tender, about 3 minutes. Or, heat 1 tablespoon extra-virgin olive oil in a large skillet over medium-high heat. Add the cauliflower and cook until just tender, 3 to 5 minutes.

Place any leftover cauliflower crumbles or rice in airtight container and freeze for up to 3 months. Thaw at room temperature for 10 minutes just before using.

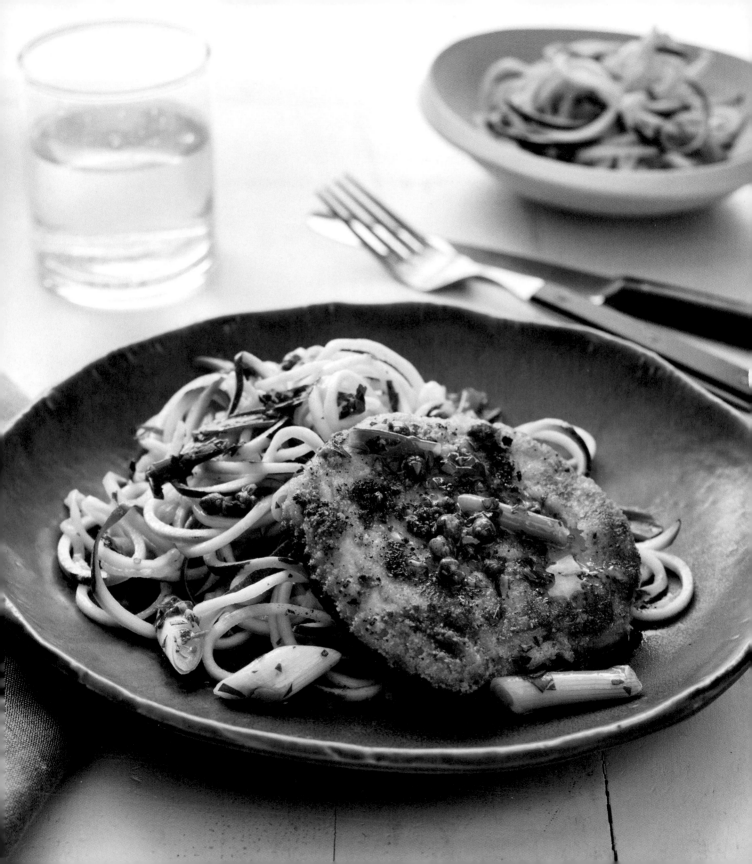

Almond-Crusted Pork Piccata with Zucchini Noodles

SERVES 4

The Italian word *piccata* refers to a thin scallop of meat—usually veal—but here it's pork. The classic ingredients in piccata—lemon, capers, and parsley—give this dish a bright and briny flavor.

PREP: 15 minutes
COOK: 15 minutes
TOTAL: 30 minutes

4 (¾-inch-thick) boneless pork loin chops (see Tip)

1 large egg

1 cup almond flour

½ teaspoon salt

½ teaspoon black pepper

3 tablespoons Clarified Butter (page 283) or ghee

2 packages (10.7 ounces each) zucchini noodles; or 3 medium zucchini, spiralized, long noodles snipped if desired

¾ cup Whole30-compliant chicken broth or Chicken Bone Broth (page 280)

6 green onions, cut into 1-inch pieces

¼ cup chopped fresh parsley

Grated zest and juice of 1 lemon

1 tablespoon capers

PREHEAT the oven to 200°F.

PLACE each chop between two pieces of plastic wrap. Use the flat side of a meat mallet to flatten the chops to ¼-inch thickness. Combine the flour, salt, and pepper in another shallow dish. Dip each chop into the egg, turning to coat. Allow the excess to drip off, then dip into the flour mixture, turning to coat.

MELT 2 tablespoons of the butter in an extra-large skillet over medium-high heat. Add the pork and cook until browned and cooked through, 3 to 4 minutes per side. Transfer the pork to a platter and keep warm in the oven.

MELT the remaining 1 tablespoon of butter in the skillet. Add the spiralized zucchini and cook, stirring, until crisp-tender, about 3 minutes. Transfer the noodles to the platter and cover to keep warm.

ADD the broth to the skillet and bring to a boil. Add the green onions and cook, stirring, until the broth is reduced slightly, about 2 minutes. Stir in the parsley, lemon zest and juice, and capers. Drizzle the sauce over the pork and noodles.

TIP *To save time in the kitchen, ask your butcher to pound the pork chops before wrapping them up for you.*

Pork Scaloppini with Mushroom-Tarragon Cream Sauce

SERVES 2

FROM *Ronny Joseph of Primal Gourmet*

I served this recipe to my family twice. Both times they couldn't tell that it was dairy-free! The secret is to reduce the coconut milk until it is at least three-quarters its original volume. Also, don't be afraid to season with a healthy pinch of salt and pepper. The dish is quite hearty and can be served on its own. Or, to cut through the cream sauce, serve with some fresh, peppery arugula dressed in a bit of lemon juice.

PREP: 10 minutes

COOK: 15 minutes

TOTAL: 25 minutes

2 thick, boneless center-cut pork chops (4 to 6 ounces each)

Salt

Black pepper

2 tablespoons Clarified Butter (page 283) or ghee

1 tablespoon extra-virgin olive oil

8 ounces cremini mushrooms, sliced

1 clove garlic, minced

⅔ cup Whole30-compliant coconut milk (see Tip)

1 tablespoon chopped fresh tarragon

CUT each pork chop in half horizontally to make a total of four thin pieces. Place each between two sheets of plastic wrap and use the flat side of a meat mallet to flatten to an ⅛-inch thickness. (Your butcher can do this for you.) Season both sides of the chops with ¼ teaspoon salt and ¼ teaspoon pepper.

HEAT the butter in a heavy large skillet over medium-high heat. As soon as the butter begins to smoke, carefully add the chops to the pan. Cook, turning once, until browned, 2 to 4 minutes. Transfer the chops to a serving platter and cover with foil to keep warm.

ADD the olive oil to the same skillet and reduce the heat to medium. Add the mushrooms, ⅛ teaspoon salt, and ⅛ teaspoon pepper and cook, stirring frequently, until the mushrooms are tender and browned, 4 to 5 minutes longer. Add the garlic and cook for 1 minute. Add the coconut milk and scrape up any browned bits on the bottom of the skillet. Bring to a boil, reduce the heat, and simmer, 3 minutes longer. Stir in the tarragon. Spoon the sauce over the chops and serve.

TIP *Canned coconut milk separates in the can with the cream rising to the top. Make sure to whisk the coconut milk well before measuring.*

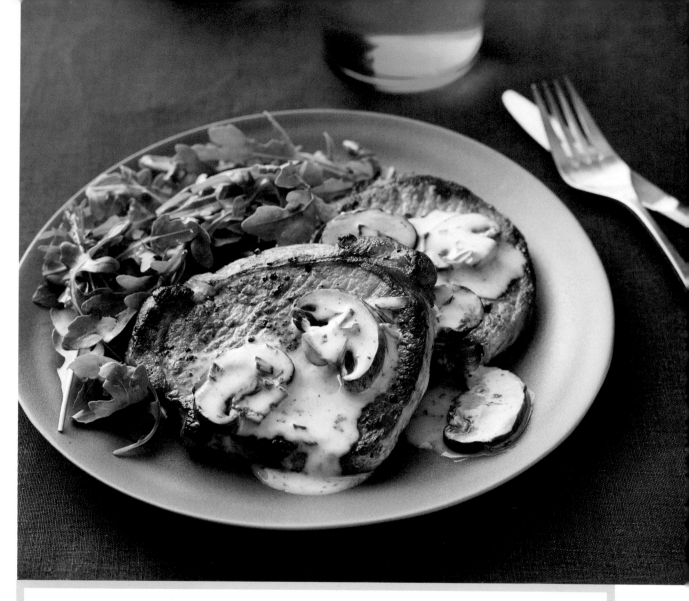

Ronny Joseph

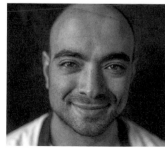

Ronny Joseph is a self-taught cook, food photographer, and coffee enthusiast. In 2013, after a lifetime of struggling with obesity, body image, and failed diets, he began a paleo journey that helped him lose more than 40 pounds and inspired him to launch his blog, Primal Gourmet. His goal is to share real-food recipes that are easy and healthy but don't sacrifice flavor.

Zucchini-Basil Chicken Hash

SERVES 2

FROM *Sarah Steffens of Savor and Fancy*

While it's pretty romantic to dream up multiple-course meals to prepare for lavish evenings spent with loved ones, most nights dinner is all about getting protein, veggies, and fat onto a plate and taking a moment to enjoy its immediate and nourishing impact on the body, mind, and soul. This one-skillet meal was whipped up on one of those evenings when dinner was simply a matter of what was in the refrigerator, but I've since made it again and again. Feel free to use chicken breast in lieu of thighs, but the higher fat content in the thighs is a part of what makes this hash that much more delicious—and likely what will cause you to also make this dish again and again.

PREP: 20 minutes

COOK: 10 minutes

TOTAL: 30 minutes

2 tablespoons coconut oil

¼ cup finely chopped red onion

2 green onions, thinly sliced

2 cloves garlic, minced

2 medium zucchini, trimmed and diced

1¼ pounds boneless, skinless chicken thighs, diced

1 teaspoon dried oregano, crushed

1 teaspoon salt

2 tablespoons balsamic vinegar

¼ cup thinly sliced fresh basil

MELT the coconut oil in a large skillet over medium heat. Add the red onion, green onions, and garlic and cook, stirring, until tender and starting to brown, about 1 minute. Add the zucchini and cook, stirring occasionally, until softened and starting to brown, 4 to 5 minutes.

ADD the chicken, oregano, and salt and cook, stirring occasionally, until the chicken is cooked through and starting to brown, 5 to 6 minutes. Gently stir in the vinegar and basil and serve.

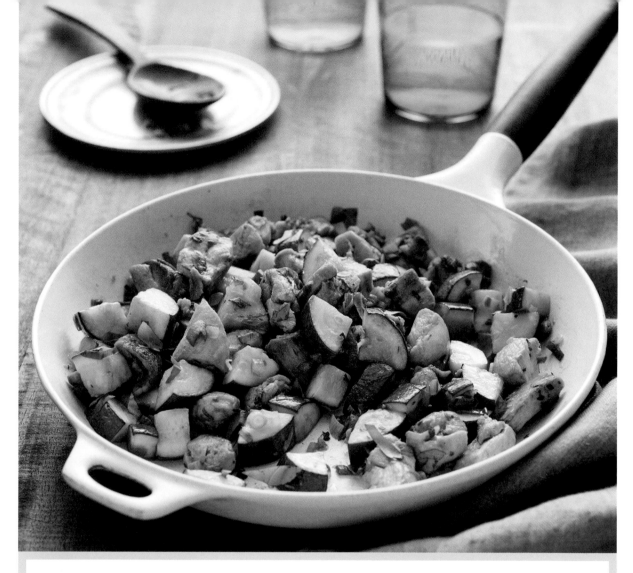

Sarah Steffens

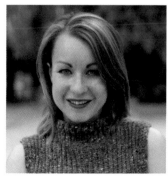

After years of experimenting with nutrition and recipes in her own kitchen, Sarah began working as a personal chef in Los Angeles, cooking meals that support her clients' intention to physically and mentally thrive. She has catered several independent film sets, optimizing the energy and well-being of each creative crew. When Sarah is not cooking Whole30 and Autoimmune Protocol (AIP) meals, she is sharing recipes on her blog, Savor and Fancy, exploring mid-century sites in L.A., taking photographs, listening to an audiobook, or hiking at Griffith Park.

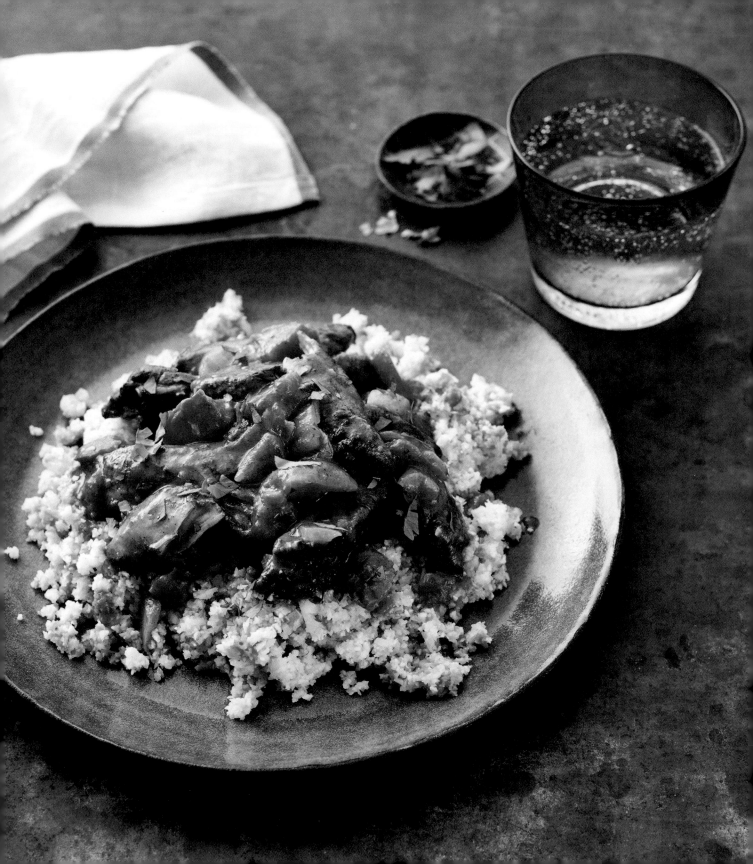

Skillet Butter Chicken

SERVES 4

Also called Chicken Makhani, this Indian-style Butter Chicken inspires silence as you're eating—it's *that* good. While the traditional version is made with cream and yogurt, we think the coconut milk in this Whole30 version makes it even yummier! If you like things spicy, increase the cayenne a bit.

PREP: 15 minutes

COOK: 20 minutes

TOTAL: 35 minutes

1 ¼ pounds boneless, skinless chicken thighs, cut into 1-inch pieces

1 tablespoon garam masala

½ teaspoon salt

⅛ teaspoon cayenne pepper

2 tablespoons Clarified Butter (page 283) or ghee

1 medium onion, chopped

3 cloves garlic, minced

1 tablespoon minced fresh ginger

1 can (14.5 ounces) Whole30-compliant diced tomatoes, undrained

1 cup Whole30-compliant coconut milk (see Tip)

1 package (12 ounces) frozen riced cauliflower and sweet potato

2 tablespoons chopped fresh cilantro

IN a medium bowl, toss the chicken with the garam masala, salt, and cayenne. In an extra-large skillet, heat the butter over medium-high heat. Add the chicken and cook, stirring occasionally, until browned, 4 to 6 minutes. Stir in the onion and cook, stirring occasionally, until the onion is softened, 2 to 3 minutes. Add the garlic and ginger and cook, stirring, for 1 minute.

STIR in the diced tomatoes and juice and bring to a boil. Reduce the heat and simmer until the chicken is cooked through, 10 to 12 minutes longer. Stir in the coconut milk and heat through, about 1 minute.

MEANWHILE, prepare the riced cauliflower and sweet potato according to package directions.

SPOON the butter chicken over the cooked cauliflower and sweet potato, top with the cilantro, and serve.

TIP *Canned coconut milk separates in the can with the cream rising to the top. Make sure to whisk the coconut milk well before measuring.*

Bacon and Eggs with Sweet Potato Noodles

SERVES 2 GENEROUSLY

The salty-smokiness from the bacon and the sweetness from the sweet potatoes is a fabulous flavor combo. This dish makes a smashing supper and—if you use packaged sweet potato noodles—is easy enough to whip up for breakfast any day of the week.

PREP: 10 minutes

COOK: 20 minutes

TOTAL: 30 minutes

4 slices Whole30-compliant bacon

1 small red onion, chopped

2 tablespoons Clarified Butter (page 283), ghee, or extra-virgin olive oil

2 packages (10.7 ounces each) sweet potato noodles, or 2 medium sweet potatoes, peeled and spiralized

2 teaspoons chopped fresh thyme

½ teaspoon salt

½ teaspoon black pepper

4 large eggs

IN a large skillet, cook the bacon over medium heat until crisp, about 10 minutes. Transfer with a slotted spoon to paper towels to drain. Reserve 2 tablespoons of the drippings in the skillet.

ADD the onion to the skillet and cook, stirring, until softened, about 3 minutes. Add the butter and melt. Add the sweet potato noodles and season with the thyme, salt, and pepper. Gently toss to combine, then cook over medium-high heat, stirring occasionally, 5 minutes. Crumble the bacon and sprinkle over the noodles.

MAKE four indentations in the noodles that are about 2 inches apart. Carefully crack one egg into each indentation. Cover and cook until the whites are set and the yolks start to thicken, or to desired doneness, 2 to 3 minutes.

Mussels in Spicy Tomato Sauce with Squash Ribbons

SERVES 4

Mussels may not be something you think about making for dinner on a busy weeknight, but these shellfish cooked in a spicy tomato sauce and intertwined with crisp-tender ribbons of summer squash takes just 20 minutes to prep and 10 minutes to cook.

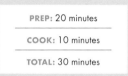

PREP: 20 minutes

COOK: 10 minutes

TOTAL: 30 minutes

2 tablespoons extra-virgin olive oil

4 medium shallots, finely chopped

4 cloves garlic, minced

1 can (28 ounces) Whole30-compliant diced tomatoes

½ to 1 teaspoon red pepper flakes

½ teaspoon salt

½ teaspoon black pepper

2 pounds mussels, scrubbed and debearded

2 medium yellow summer squash, trimmed and shaved into ribbons (see Tip)

2 tablespoons fresh lemon juice

½ cup chopped fresh basil

HEAT 1 tablespoon of the olive oil in an extra-large skillet over medium heat. Add the shallots and garlic and cook, stirring, just until softened, about 2 minutes. Add the tomatoes, pepper flakes, salt, and pepper and bring to a boil. Add the mussels. Cover and cook until the mussels are just starting to open, 3 to 4 minutes.

STIR in the squash ribbons. Continue to cook, stirring occasionally, until the mussels have opened and the squash is crisp-tender, 1 to 2 minutes. Discard any mussels that do not open. Drizzle the lemon juice and remaining 1 tablespoon olive oil over the mussels and squash, top with the basil, and serve.

TIP *To make squash ribbons, use a vegetable peeler to shave 3 ribbons from 1 side of the squash. Turn the squash 90 degrees and shave 3 ribbons from that side. Repeat turning the squash and shaving ribbons until you reach the seeds. Discard the core.*

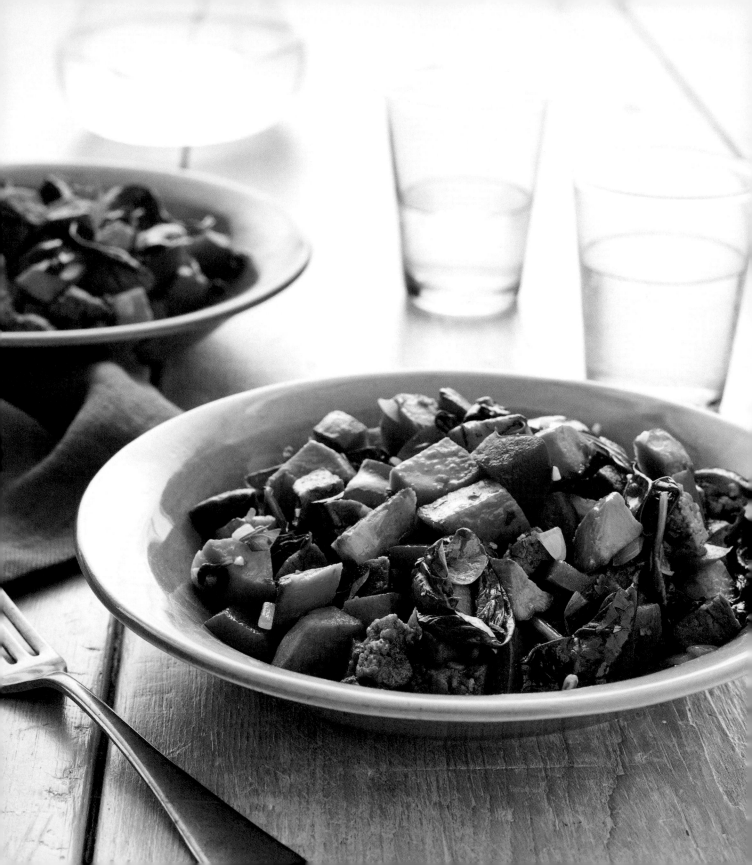

Chorizo and Sweet Potato Skillet

SERVES 2 GENEROUSLY

FROM *Brian Kavanaugh of The Sophisticated Caveman*

Skillets make for easy one-pot meals any time of day, but they're especially handy at breakfast. This skillet combines chorizo and sweet potato for a sweet and spicy, no-hassle dish that comes together in no time. If you've been eating eggs on eggs on eggs, this dish will be a welcome early-morning change, but you can always add an over-medium egg on top to make it extra healthy.

PREP: 15 minutes

COOK: 20 minutes

TOTAL: 35 minutes

2 tablespoons coconut oil

3 medium sweet potatoes, peeled and cut into ½-inch cubes

1 medium yellow onion, diced

1 large red bell pepper, diced

1 clove garlic, minced

½ pound Whole30-compliant cooked chorizo links, halved lengthwise and diced

4 cups loosely packed baby spinach

¼ cup loosely packed chopped fresh cilantro

HEAT the coconut oil in a large skillet over medium heat. Add the sweet potatoes and cook, covered, for 5 minutes. Uncover and cook, stirring frequently, until the potatoes are just tender, 5 to 8 minutes.

ADD the onion and pepper and cook, stirring frequently, for 5 minutes. Add the garlic, chorizo, and spinach and cook, stirring occasionally, until the spinach is wilted and the chorizo is heated through, about 4 minutes. Stir in the cilantro and serve.

Seared Salmon Fillets with Ginger-Caramelized Pineapple

SERVES 4

Coconut oil in a very hot skillet gives the tops of these salmon fillets a beautiful crisp, golden crust.

PREP: 5 minutes

COOK: 15 minutes

TOTAL: 20 minutes

2 tablespoons Clarified Butter (page 283) or ghee

4 pineapple rings, halved

1 teaspoon minced fresh ginger

½ teaspoon black or white sesame seeds

4 skin-on salmon fillets (5 to 6 ounces each) (see Tip)

½ teaspoon salt

¼ teaspoon black pepper

1 tablespoon coconut oil

Chopped green onion (optional)

IN a large nonstick skillet, heat the butter over medium-high heat. Add the pineapple, ginger, and sesame seeds and cook, turning once, until the pineapple is golden, 6 to 8 minutes. Transfer to a plate and cover to keep warm. Carefully wipe out the skillet.

SPRINKLE the salmon with the salt and pepper. Heat the same pan over medium heat until very hot. Add the coconut oil and heat until you see ripples across the surface. Place the salmon in the skillet, skin side down. Cook, without touching, until the salmon has cooked about three-fourths of the way up the fillets, 4 to 5 minutes (see Tip). Using a spatula, carefully turn the salmon over. Cook until the salmon just barely starts to flake when pulled apart with two forks, 2 to 3 minutes longer.

SERVE the salmon with the caramelized pineapple and drizzle any pan juices over the top. If desired, top with green onion.

TIPS *For best results, remove the salmon fillets from the refrigerator about 15 minutes before cooking so they can come to room temperature.*

Most of the cooking of the salmon will take place while the salmon is skin-side down in the pan. The color of the fillet will begin to lighten as it cooks, starting at the bottom and moving upward.

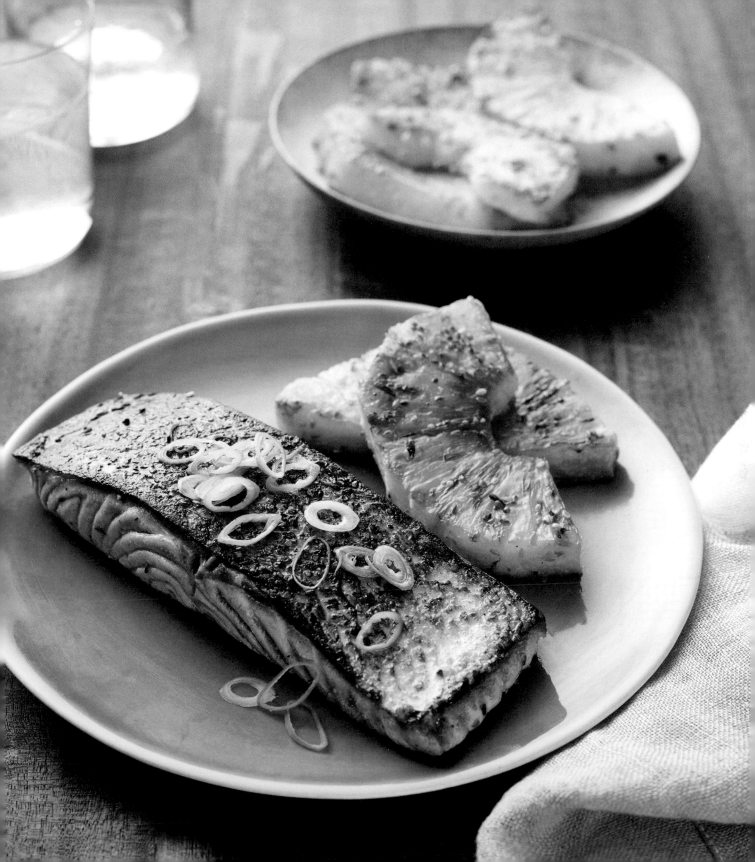

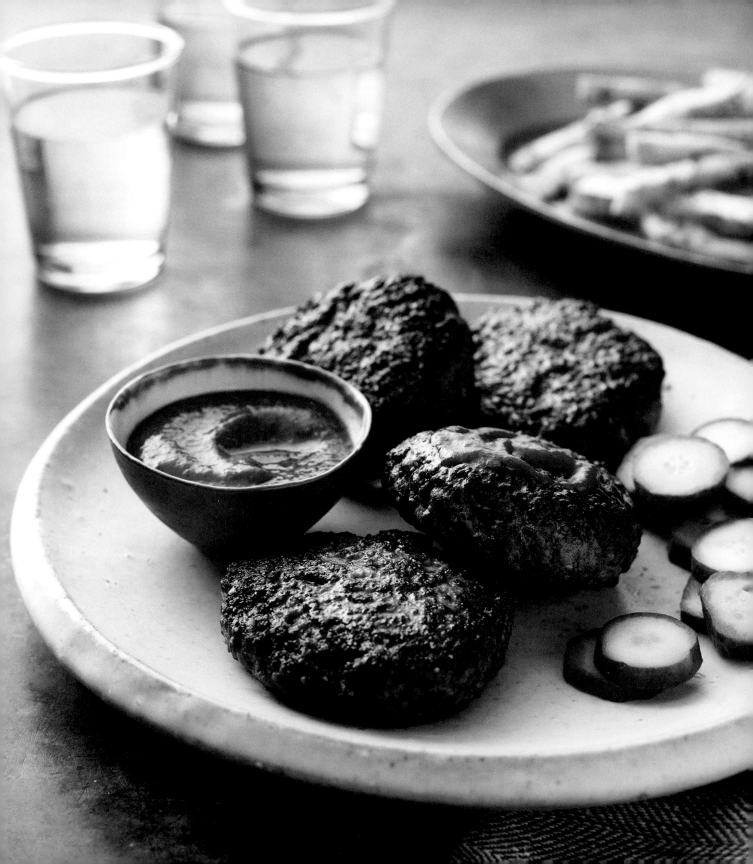

Skillet Grass-Fed Burgers with Roasted-Red-Pepper Ketchup

SERVES 4

Grass-fed beef is leaner and more flavorful—and it actually has more heart-healthy omega-3 acids—than beef that comes from animals raised on a diet of grains. If you can find it, use it in these satisfying burgers topped with spicy homemade ketchup.

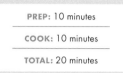

PREP: 10 minutes

COOK: 10 minutes

TOTAL: 20 minutes

FOR THE ROASTED-RED-PEPPER KETCHUP

1 tablespoon unsulfured golden raisins

½ (7-ounce) jar roasted red peppers, drained

3 tablespoons extra-virgin olive oil

2 tablespoons cider vinegar

2 tablespoons Whole30-compliant tomato paste

¼ teaspoon salt

¼ teaspoon ground chipotle pepper or smoked paprika

FOR THE BURGERS

1 tablespoon extra-virgin olive oil

1 pound ground beef

½ teaspoon coarse salt

½ teaspoon black pepper

Whole30-compliant dill pickles (optional)

MAKE THE KETCHUP: Place the raisins and 2 tablespoons hot water in a blender container; let stand for 5 minutes. Add the roasted peppers, oil, vinegar, tomato paste, salt, and ground chipotle. Cover and blend until smooth. Use immediately, or place in an airtight container and refrigerate for up to 3 days.

MAKE THE BURGERS: Heat the olive oil in heavy large skillet or cast-iron griddle over medium-high heat. Shape the meat into four ¾-inch-thick patties. Sprinkle each patty with the salt and pepper. Cook the patties, turning once, until the internal temperature is 160°F, about 8 minutes.

SERVE the patties with some of the red-pepper ketchup and, if desired, pickles.

Red Curry Shrimp Skillet

SERVES 4

Red curry paste is a magical (and thankfully, generally compliant!) ingredient. Just a spoonful or two infuses a dish with amazing layers of flavor. The most familiar brand is made with just red chili, garlic, lemongrass, galangal (Thai ginger), salt, onion, makrut lime, coriander, and pepper.

PREP: 20 minutes

COOK: 15 minutes

TOTAL: 35 minutes

1 tablespoon coconut oil

1 small onion, chopped

2 cloves garlic, minced

2 teaspoons minced fresh ginger

1 can (14 ounces) Whole30-compliant coconut milk

2 tablespoons Whole30-compliant Thai red curry paste

1 tablespoon coconut aminos

1 pound peeled and deveined large shrimp (see Tip)

4 cups fresh baby spinach

1 tablespoon fresh lime juice, plus lime wedges for serving

1 package (16 ounces) cauliflower crumbles, or 4 cups raw cauliflower rice (see page 75)

Torn fresh basil

Lime wedges

IN a large skillet, heat the oil over medium heat. Add the onion and cook, stirring occasionally, until tender, 3 to 4 minutes. Add the garlic and ginger and cook, stirring, until fragrant, about 1 minute. Stir in the coconut milk, curry paste, and coconut aminos. Bring to a boil, then reduce the heat and simmer for 5 minutes. Add the shrimp and cook, stirring occasionally, until opaque, about 5 minutes. Remove from the heat and stir in the spinach and lime juice.

MEANWHILE, prepare the cauliflower crumbles according to the package directions. Serve the shrimp curry over the cauliflower rice. Top with the fresh basil and serve with lime wedges.

TIP *To make this recipe even faster, use cooked shrimp in place of the raw shrimp, and cook just 1 to 2 minutes or until heated through.*

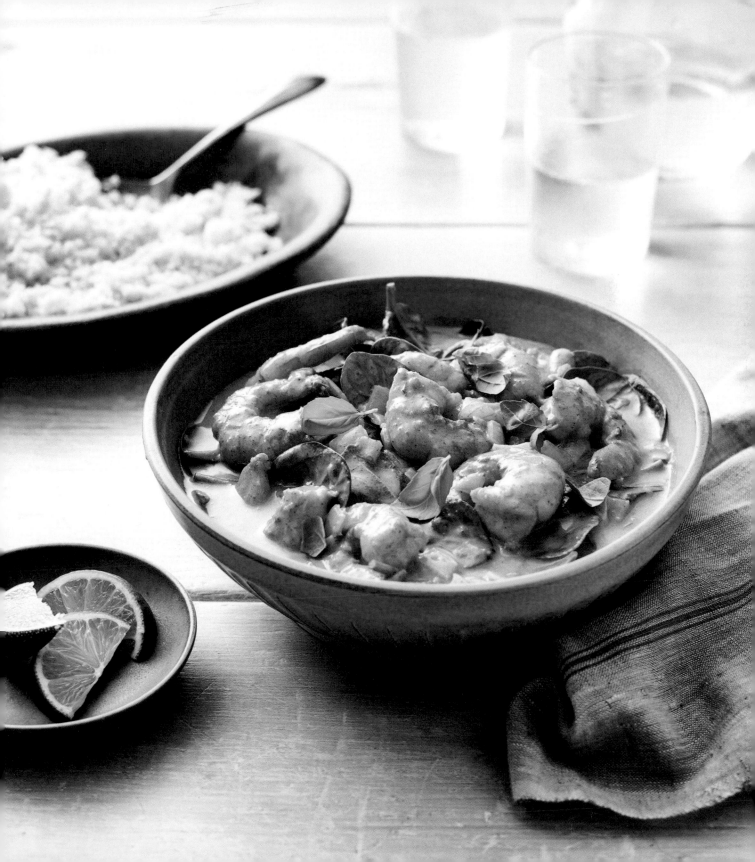

Skillet Turkey and Squash Chili

SERVES 4

This recipe is proof that with just a few clean prepared products, you can make a really tasty dish in nearly no time. This chili benefits from the smoky flavor of fire-roasted tomatoes, a blend of fresh or frozen carrots, celery, and onion—and the crowning touch: a spoonful of prepared guacamole.

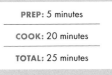

PREP: 5 minutes

COOK: 20 minutes

TOTAL: 25 minutes

1 tablespoon extra-virgin olive oil

1 pound ground turkey

2 cloves garlic, minced

1 package (14 ounces) fresh or frozen diced carrots, celery, and onion blend

2 tablespoons chili powder

2 teaspoons ground cumin

½ teaspoon salt

1 package (12 ounces) chopped butternut squash

1 can (28 ounces) Whole30-compliant fire-roasted diced tomatoes, undrained

Toppings such as Whole30-compliant guacamole, chopped fresh cilantro, sliced green onions, finely chopped jalapeño, and/or lime wedges (optional)

HEAT the olive oil in a large skillet over medium-high heat. Add the turkey and garlic and cook, breaking up the meat with a wooden spoon, until the turkey is browned, about 5 minutes. Add the carrot mixture, chili powder, cumin, and salt and cook, stirring occasionally, until the vegetables are tender, 5 minutes.

ADD the squash and tomatoes and bring to a boil. Reduce the heat and simmer, stirring occasionally, until the squash is tender, 10 to 12 minutes. Serve with the toppings, if desired.

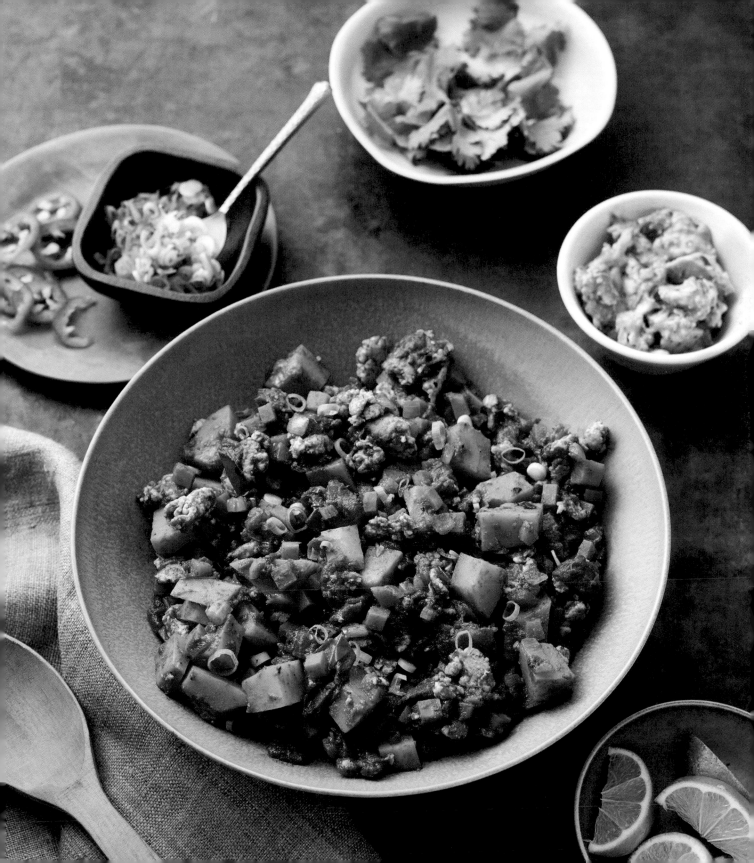

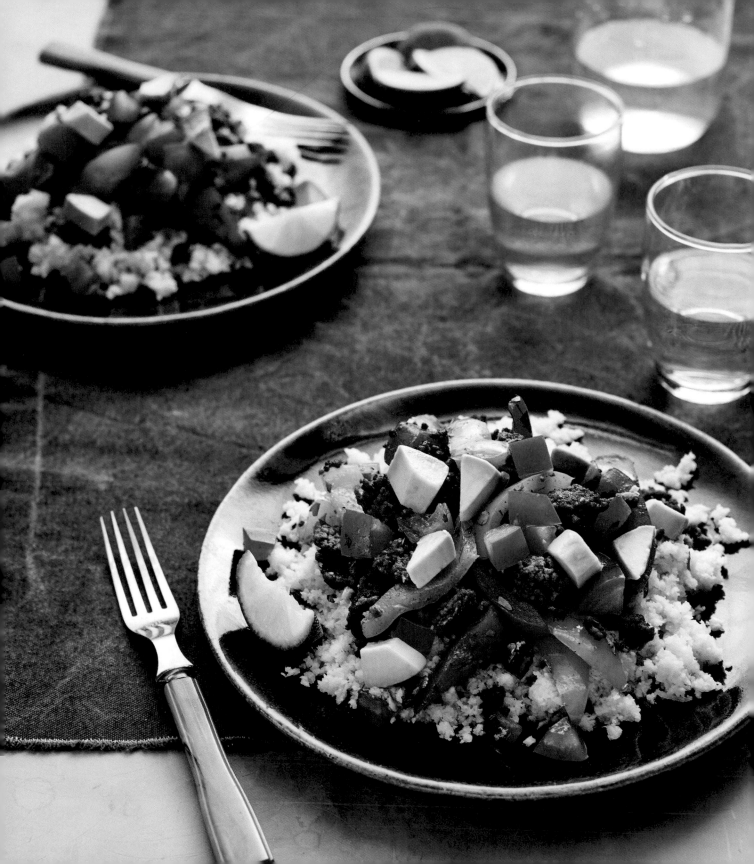

Fajita Beef Skillet

SERVES 4

All the flavors of traditional beef fajitas—sweet peppers, onion, garlic, chili powder, cumin, and cilantro come together in this dish that ingeniously swaps ground beef for the skirt or flank steak. Meat that doesn't need slicing means dinner's on the table that much faster!

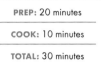

PREP: 20 minutes

COOK: 10 minutes

TOTAL: 30 minutes

1 pound ground beef

1 tablespoon extra-virgin olive oil

1 small red onion, coarsely chopped

1 small red bell pepper, coarsely chopped

1 small yellow bell pepper, coarsely chopped

2 cloves garlic, minced

½ teaspoon salt

2 teaspoons chili powder

¼ teaspoon ground cumin

⅛ teaspoon cayenne pepper

1 tablespoon fresh lime juice

2 tablespoons chopped fresh cilantro

1 package (16 ounces) cauliflower crumbles, or 4 cups raw cauliflower rice (see page 75)

Diced avocado and/or diced fresh tomato (optional)

Lime wedges

IN a large skillet, cook the beef over medium-high heat, breaking it up with a wooden spoon, until browned, about 5 minutes. Drain off any fat and transfer the beef to a bowl.

HEAT the olive oil in the same skillet over medium heat. Add the onion, bell peppers, garlic, and salt and cook, stirring occasionally, until the vegetables are crisp-tender, 4 to 6 minutes. Stir in the beef, chili powder, cumin, and cayenne and heat through for about 1 minute. Stir in the lime juice. Remove the skillet from the heat and stir in the cilantro.

MEANWHILE, prepare the cauliflower crumbles according to the package directions.

SPOON the beef and vegetables over the cauliflower and top with avocado and/or tomato if desired; serve with lime wedges.

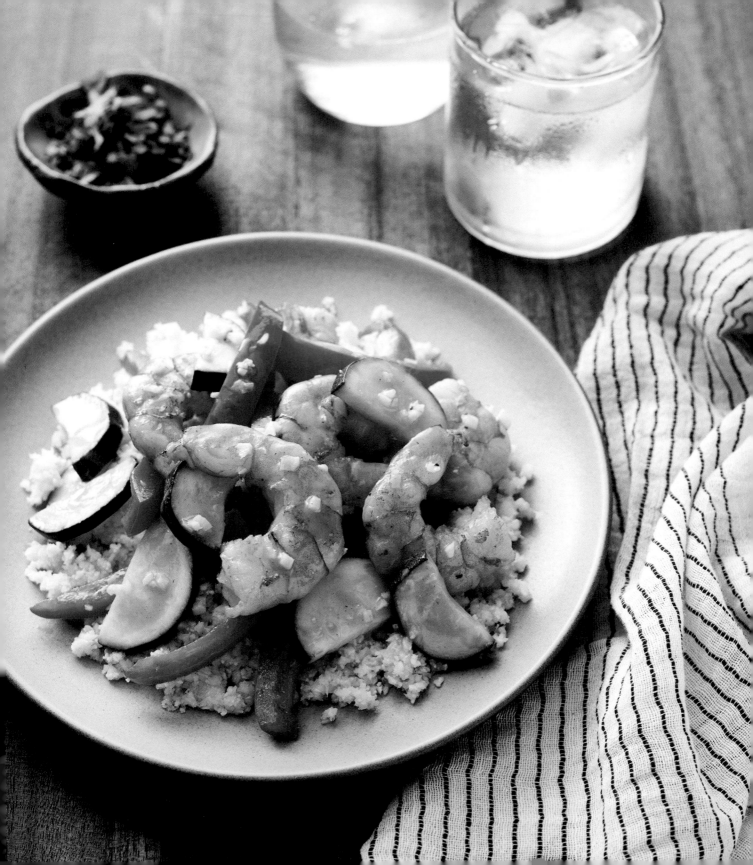

Lemon-Garlic Shrimp and Veggies

SERVES 4

A flash-in-the-pan sauce made with clarified butter and lemon juice gives this fresh dish light, bright flavor.

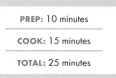

PREP: 10 minutes

COOK: 15 minutes

TOTAL: 25 minutes

1 tablespoon olive oil

1 medium zucchini, trimmed, halved lengthwise, and cut into half-moons

1 medium red bell pepper, cut into thin strips

1 pound peeled and deveined extra-large shrimp (see Tip)

3 cloves garlic, minced

¼ cup Clarified Butter (page 283) or ghee

¼ cup fresh lemon juice

½ teaspoon salt

¼ teaspoon black pepper

1 package (16 ounces) cauliflower crumbles, or 4 cups raw cauliflower rice (see page 75)

¼ cup chopped fresh parsley (optional)

HEAT the olive oil in a large skillet over medium-high heat. Add the zucchini and pepper strips and cook, stirring occasionally, for 3 minutes. Add the shrimp and garlic and cook, turning the shrimp and stirring vegetables once, until the shrimp are opaque, 5 to 6 minutes. Transfer the shrimp mixture to a bowl and cover to keep warm.

TO make the lemon pan sauce, reduce the heat to medium and melt the butter in the skillet. Add the lemon juice, salt, and black pepper, bring to a boil, and whisk until smooth.

MEANWHILE, cook the cauliflower crumbles according to the package directions.

SPOON the shrimp and vegetables over the cauliflower. Drizzle with the lemon sauce, sprinkle with parsley if desired, and serve.

TIP *To make this recipe even faster, use cooked shrimp instead of raw, and cook with the vegetables just 1 to 2 minutes, or until heated through.*

North African Chicken Skillet with Sweet Potato Noodles

SERVES 4

What makes this North African? The combination of warm spices—smoked paprika and cinnamon—with the sweetness of dates and orange juice. Toasted almonds provide a nutty crunch.

PREP: 15 minutes	
COOK: 10 minutes	
TOTAL: 25 minutes	

1¼ to 1½ pounds boneless, skinless chicken breasts

1½ teaspoons smoked paprika

1 teaspoon salt

¾ teaspoon ground cinnamon

2 tablespoons extra-virgin olive oil

3 medium shallots, sliced

1 package (10 ounces) sweet potato noodles, or 1 large sweet potato, peeled and spiralized

1 can (14.5 ounces) Whole30-compliant diced tomatoes, undrained

½ cup chopped pitted unsweetened dates

¼ cup fresh orange juice

Sliced almonds, toasted (see Tip), optional

Finely chopped fresh parsley, optional

PLACE each chicken breast between two pieces of plastic wrap and use the flat side of a meat mallet to flatten to an even ½-inch thickness. Sprinkle both sides of the chicken with the paprika, salt, and cinnamon.

HEAT the olive oil in an extra-large heavy skillet over medium-high heat. Add the chicken and shallots. Cook, turning once, until the chicken is lightly browned but not cooked through, 2 to 4 minutes. Transfer the chicken to a plate and cover with foil to keep warm.

ADD the sweet potato noodles, tomatoes, dates, and orange juice to the skillet with the shallots; stir to combine. Return the chicken to the skillet. Bring to a boil over medium heat, cover, and reduce the heat to low. Cook until the chicken is no longer pink and the sweet potato noodles are just tender, 6 to 8 minutes. Serve with sliced almonds and parsley, if desired.

TIP *To toast almonds, heat in a skillet over medium heat, stirring, until fragrant and lightly browned, about 2 minutes.*

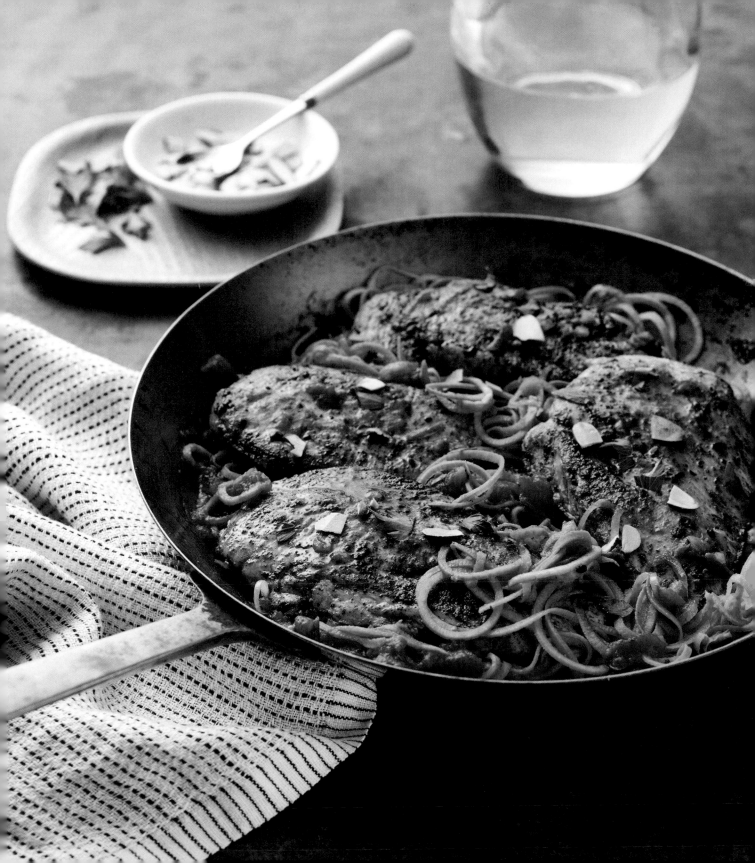

Orange Chicken with Cauliflower Rice

SERVES 4

This version of the Chinese-restaurant favorite will not make you feel bloated and sluggish—there's no breaded, deep-fried chicken swimming in a sugary-sweet sauce served on a carb bomb of white rice. It's just chicken breast and lots of veggies in a light, fresh sauce made with fresh orange juice and zest, coconut aminos, rice vinegar, garlic, and ginger thickened with a little tapioca flour.

PREP: 20 minutes
COOK: 10 minutes
TOTAL: 30 minutes

1 teaspoon grated orange zest

¾ cup fresh orange juice

1 tablespoon coconut aminos

1 teaspoon rice vinegar

2 cloves garlic, minced

1 teaspoon minced fresh ginger

¼ teaspoon salt

1 teaspoon tapioca flour, or 2½ teaspoons arrowroot powder

1 tablespoon Clarified Butter (page 283) or ghee

1½ pounds boneless, skinless chicken breasts, cut into 1-inch pieces

1 bag (12 ounces) fresh broccoli, carrots, and snow peas stir-fry vegetables

1 package (16 ounces) cauliflower crumbles, or 4 cups raw cauliflower rice (see page 75)

2 green onions, sliced

IN a small bowl, mix together the orange zest and juice, coconut aminos, rice vinegar, garlic, ginger, and salt. In another small bowl, whisk together 2 teaspoons cold water and the tapioca flour until smooth.

HEAT the butter in a large skillet over medium-high heat. Add the chicken and cook, stirring, until fully cooked, 5 to 6 minutes. Transfer the chicken to a plate and cover to keep warm.

STIR the orange juice mixture into the same skillet and bring to a boil, stirring, over medium-high heat. Whisk in the tapioca flour mixture until smooth. Add the stir-fry vegetables and cook, stirring frequently, until the vegetables are crisp-tender and the sauce has thickened slightly, 4 to 6 minutes. Stir in the chicken and heat through, about 1 minute.

MEANWHILE, prepare the cauliflower crumbles according to the package directions.

SPOON the chicken and vegetables over the cauliflower, sprinkle with green onions, and serve.

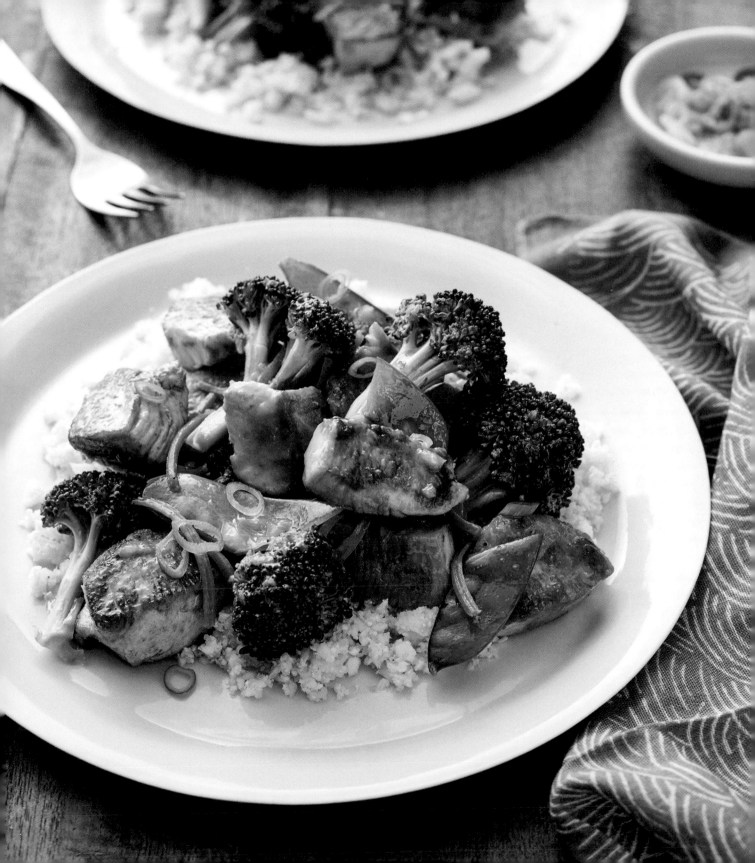

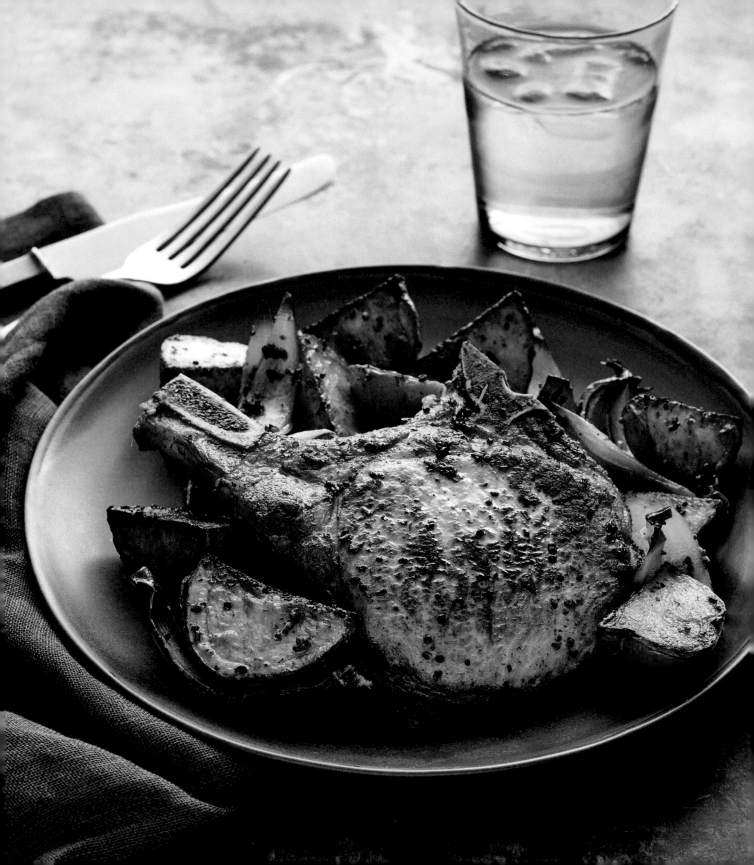

Skillet Rosemary Pork Chops with Potatoes and Onions

SERVES 2

When you're craving some serious comfort food, look no further. It's amazing how much flavor the whole-grain mustard, rosemary, and garlic give to this dish.

> **PREP:** 10 minutes
>
> **COOK:** 20 minutes
>
> **TOTAL:** 30 minutes

3 tablespoons extra-virgin olive oil

1 tablespoon Whole30-compliant whole-grain mustard

2 cloves garlic, minced

1 teaspoon chopped fresh rosemary

¼ teaspoon salt

¼ teaspoon black pepper

8 small red potatoes, quartered

1 small red onion, cut into 8 wedges

2 bone-in pork chops, cut ½ to ¾ inch thick

PREHEAT the oven to 425°F.

IN a small bowl, stir together 1 tablespoon of the olive oil, the mustard, garlic, rosemary, salt, and pepper. In a medium bowl, toss the potatoes and onion with half of the mustard mixture. Brush the remaining mustard mixture on both sides of the chops.

HEAT 1 tablespoon of the olive oil in a large cast-iron or heavy ovenproof skillet over medium-high heat. Add the chops to the skillet and cook, turning once, until browned, about 2 minutes. Transfer the chops to a plate and cover to keep warm.

HEAT the remaining 1 tablespoon olive oil in the same skillet over medium heat. Add the potatoes and onion and cook, stirring occasionally, until browned, about 5 minutes.

ARRANGE the chops in with the potatoes and onions. Transfer the skillet to the oven and bake until the internal temperature of the chops is 145°F and the potatoes are tender, 10 to 15 minutes.

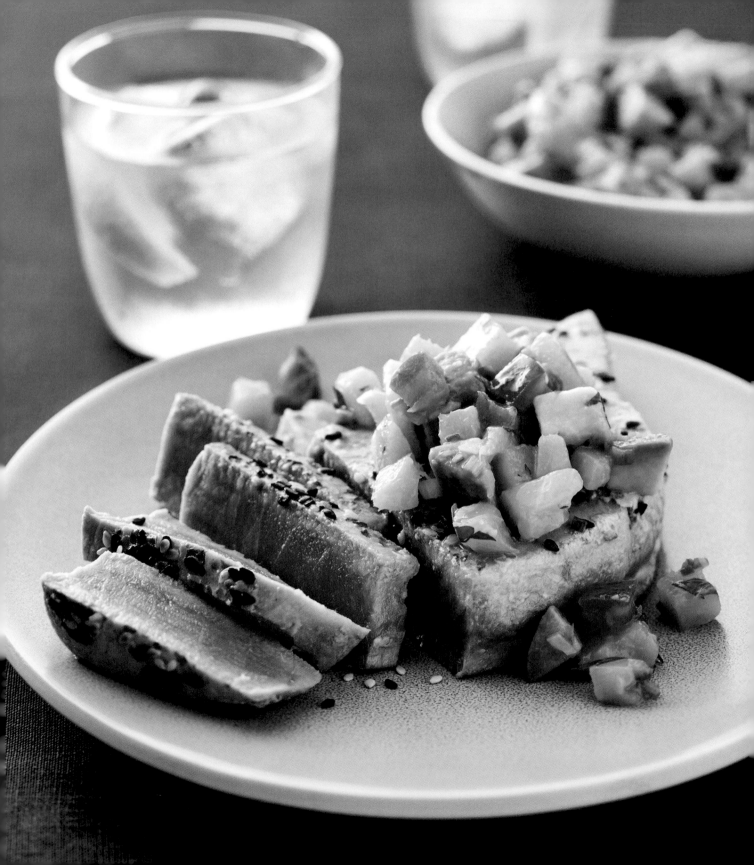

Seared Ahi Tuna with Mango Avocado Salsa

SERVES 2

FROM *Ronny Joseph of Primal Gourmet*

This mango and avocado salsa is bursting with sweet, spicy, and citrusy flavors and is hearty enough to be eaten as a salad. When paired with a delicious source of lean protein, like seared ahi tuna, it makes for the perfect warm-weather lunch. The best part is you can have everything ready in 20 minutes or less.

> **PREP:** 15 minutes
>
> **COOK:** 5 minutes
>
> **TOTAL:** 20 minutes

FOR THE SALSA

1 mango, pitted, peeled, and diced

1 medium tomato, seeded and diced

2 green onions, minced

1 avocado, halved, pitted, peeled, and diced

¼ cup roughly chopped fresh cilantro

½ jalapeño, seeded and minced

Juice of 1 lime

⅛ teaspoon salt

⅛ teaspoon black pepper

FOR THE TUNA

2 ahi tuna steaks (4 to 6 ounces each), about 1 inch thick (see Tip)

Avocado oil

1 teaspoon black sesame seeds

1 teaspoon white sesame seeds

¼ teaspoon salt

¼ teaspoon black pepper

MAKE THE SALSA: In a medium bowl, combine all the salsa ingredients and toss to mix.

MAKE THE TUNA: Brush both sides of the tuna with a small amount of avocado oil. Season both sides with the sesame seeds, salt, and black pepper.

HEAT a large ceramic nonstick skillet or cast-iron skillet over medium-high heat. Add the tuna and sear for 2 minutes on one side. Turn the tuna over and sear the other side for 2 minutes, until browned and crusty on the outside and rare inside. Serve the salsa with the tuna steaks.

TIP *The ahi tuna steaks in this recipe are seared, meaning scorched with intense heat, creating a delicious crust with rare cooked interior. Because it is served rare, be sure to use sushi-grade or other high-quality tuna.*

Shrimp and Asparagus Dinner Omelets

SERVES 2

Why add water to the eggs when making omelets? As the eggs cook, the water creates steam—which translates into fluffier omelets!

PREP: 10 minutes

COOK: 15 minutes

TOTAL: 25 minutes

FOR THE FILLING

1 teaspoon Clarified Butter (page 283), ghee, or extra-virgin olive oil

¼ pound asparagus, trimmed and cut into 1-inch pieces (about 1 cup)

6 ounces cooked peeled and deveined medium shrimp, coarsely chopped

½ cup quartered grape tomatoes

FOR THE OMELETS

5 large eggs

Pinch of salt

Pinch of black pepper

2 teaspoons Clarified Butter (page 283), ghee, or extra-virgin olive oil

2 tablespoons Whole30-compliant pesto or Basil Pesto (page 170)

MAKE THE FILLING: Heat the butter in a small nonstick skillet over medium heat. Add the asparagus and cook, stirring, until crisp-tender, about 3 minutes. Stir in the shrimp and tomatoes and heat through for 1 to 2 minutes. Transfer the filling to a bowl and cover with foil to keep warm.

MAKE THE OMELETS: Whisk together the eggs, 2 tablespoons water, the salt, and pepper in a medium bowl. In the same skillet, heat 1 teaspoon of the butter over medium heat. Add half of the egg mixture. Cook, gently stirring and pushing the cooked portion toward the center with a spatula and allowing the uncooked egg to flow underneath, until the eggs are set and have formed an even layer in the skillet, 30 to 60 seconds. Spoon 1 tablespoon of the pesto over the omelet. Spoon half of the filling over one side of the omelet. Fold the opposite side over the filling. Transfer to a plate and keep warm.

REPEAT to make the second omelet. Serve immediately.

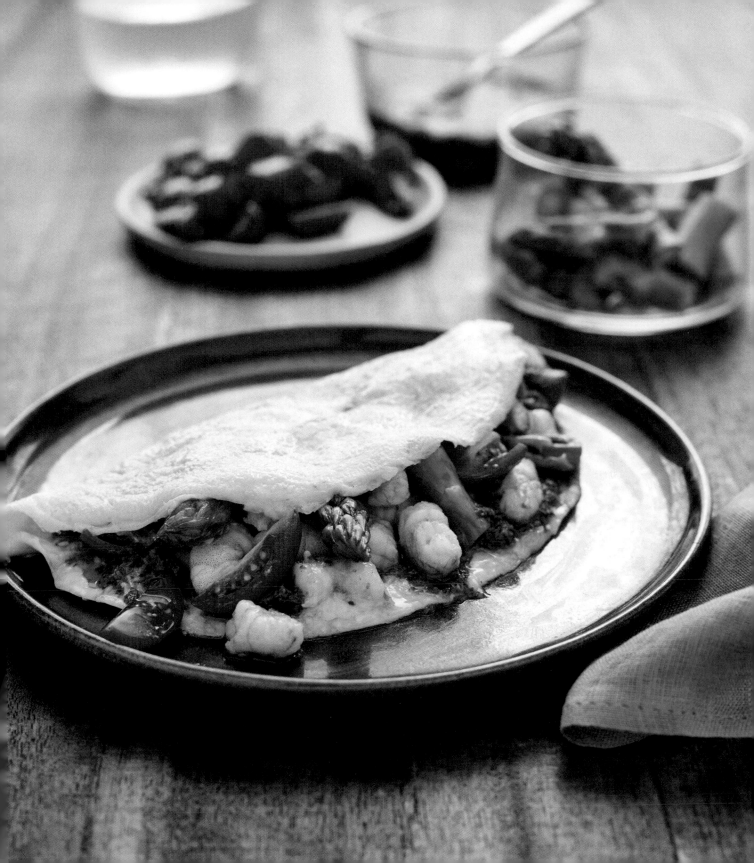

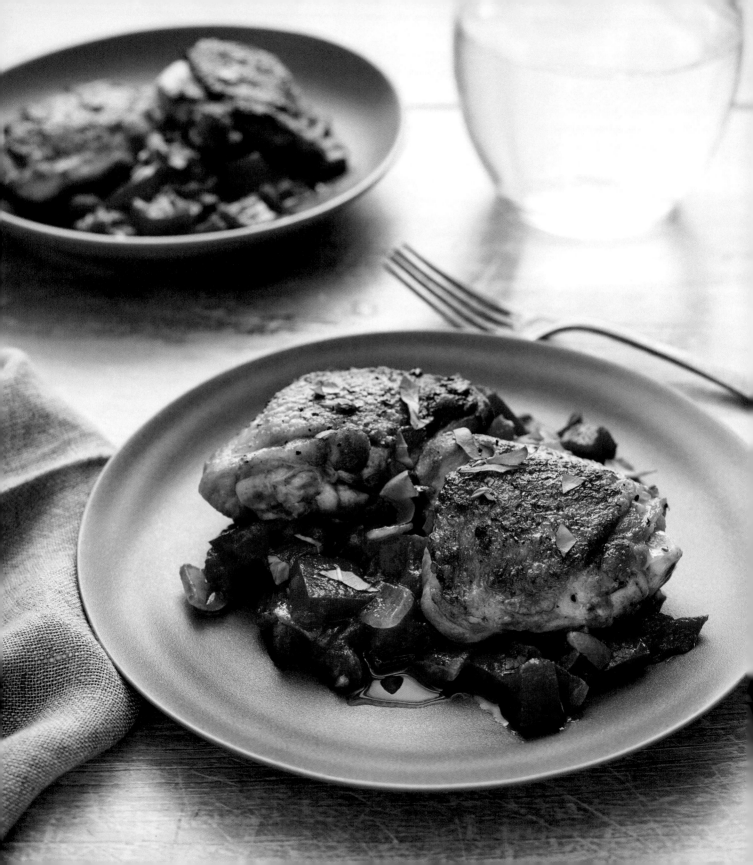

Spicy Red Pepper Chicken Skillet

SERVES 4

Like a little spice? Go with the ¼ teaspoon of red pepper flakes. Like things a little more fiery? Go with the ½ teaspoon. If you have it on hand, the basil will add a touch of slightly sweet, licoricey flavor to the finished dish.

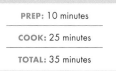

PREP: 10 minutes

COOK: 25 minutes

TOTAL: 35 minutes

2 tablespoons extra-virgin olive oil

1½ pounds bone-in, skin-on chicken thighs

1 teaspoon salt

½ teaspoon black pepper

2 medium red bell peppers, chopped

1 medium onion, chopped

2 cloves garlic, minced

1 can (14.5 ounces) Whole30-compliant diced tomatoes

½ cup Whole30-compliant chicken broth or Chicken Bone Broth (page 280)

¼ to ½ teaspoon red pepper flakes

Sliced fresh basil leaves (optional)

HEAT 1 tablespoon of the olive oil in a large heavy skillet over medium-high heat. Season the chicken with ½ teaspoon of the salt and ¼ teaspoon of the pepper. Add the chicken and cook, turning once, until the skin is browned, about 5 minutes. Transfer to a plate and cover to keep warm.

IN the same skillet, heat the remaining 1 tablespoon olive oil over medium heat. Add the bell peppers, onion, and garlic and cook, stirring frequently, until tender, 3 to 4 minutes. Stir in the tomatoes, broth, pepper flakes, and the remaining ½ teaspoon salt and ¼ teaspoon pepper. Cook until the mixture begins to thicken slightly, 5 to 7 minutes.

RETURN the chicken to the skillet. Cover and reduce the heat to low. Cook until the chicken is no longer pink and the internal temperature is 170°F, 12 to 15 minutes. Serve with basil, if desired.

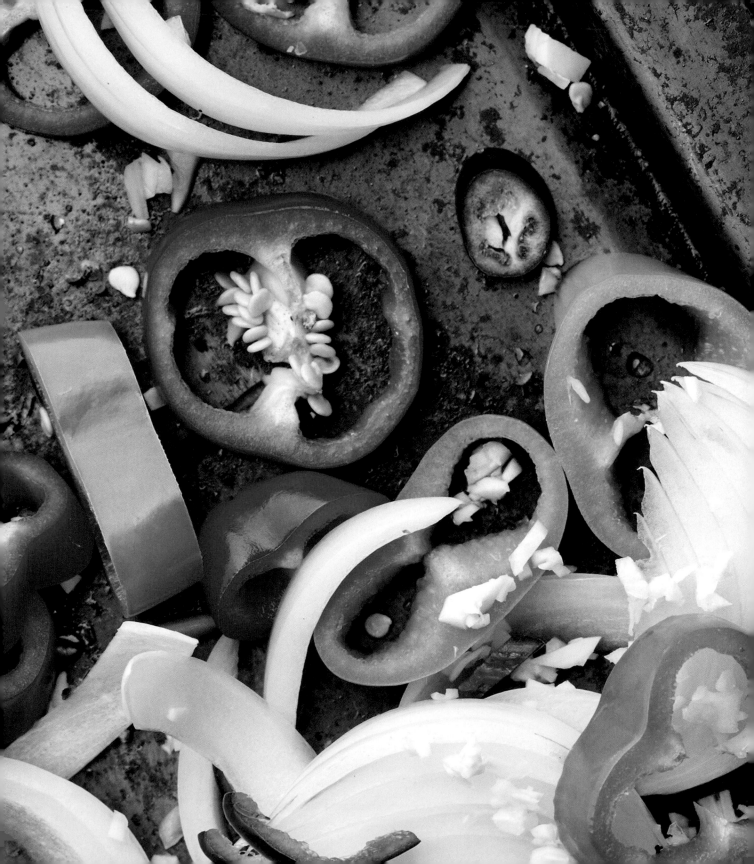

CHAPTER 3

SHEET PAN SUPPERS

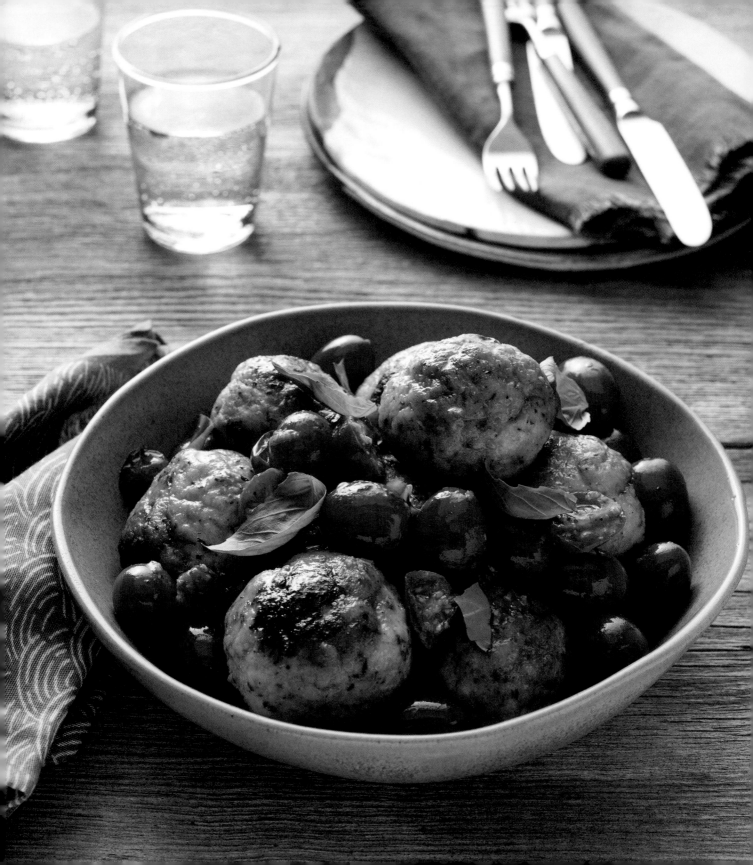

Big Turkey Meatballs with Roasted Cherry Tomatoes

qped

SERVES 3

Not only does forming 8 hefty meatballs rather than 24 or 36 smaller ones save time—it also makes for a fun presentation on a serving platter with the roasted cherry tomatoes and fresh basil.

PREP:	15 minutes
ROAST:	30 minutes
TOTAL:	45 minutes

FOR THE MEATBALLS

1½ pounds ground turkey

1 large egg

½ cup almond flour

2 cloves garlic, minced

2 teaspoons Whole30-compliant Italian seasoning

1 teaspoon fennel seeds, crushed

1 teaspoon black pepper

½ teaspoon salt

1 tablespoon extra-virgin olive oil

FOR THE TOMATOES

2 pints red and/or yellow cherry tomatoes

1 tablespoon extra-virgin olive oil

2 cloves garlic, minced

1 teaspoon Whole30-compliant Italian seasoning

¼ teaspoon salt

¼ teaspoon black pepper

2 tablespoons chopped fresh basil

PREHEAT the oven to 400°F. Line a large rimmed baking pan with parchment paper.

MAKE THE MEATBALLS: In a large bowl, combine the turkey, egg, almond flour, garlic, Italian seasoning, fennel seeds, pepper, salt, and olive oil. Form into 9 meatballs. Arrange the meatballs on the pan, spacing them evenly. Roast for 20 minutes.

MAKE THE TOMATOES: Meanwhile, in a medium bowl, combine the cherry tomatoes, olive oil, garlic, and Italian seasoning. Season with the salt and black pepper.

ADD the cherry tomatoes to the pan around the meatballs. Turn the meatballs and roast for 10 minutes more, or until the tomatoes split and the internal temperature of the meatballs is 165°F.

TOP the meatballs and roasted tomatoes with the fresh basil and serve.

Roasted Salmon with Tomatoes and Fennel

SERVES 4

A combination of garlic, lemon juice, olive oil, capers, dill, and Dijon mustard makes a intensely flavored—and speedy—sauce for both the fish and vegetables.

PREP: 20 minutes	
ROAST: 15 minutes	
TOTAL: 35 minutes	

1½ **pounds skin-on salmon fillet**

3 **cups halved cherry tomatoes**

1 **medium fennel bulb, cored, quartered, and thinly sliced**

½ **teaspoon coarse salt**

½ **teaspoon black pepper**

2 **cloves garlic, minced**

2 **tablespoons fresh lemon juice**

2 **tablespoons extra-virgin olive oil**

2 **tablespoons capers, drained**

2 **teaspoons chopped fresh dill**

2 **teaspoons Whole30-compliant Dijon mustard**

PREHEAT the oven to 400°F. Line a large rimmed baking pan with parchment paper.

RINSE the salmon and pat dry. Place the salmon, tomatoes, and fennel on the pan and sprinkle with the salt and pepper.

IN a small bowl, stir together the garlic, lemon juice, olive oil, capers, dill, and mustard. Drizzle the sauce over the fish, tomatoes, and fennel. Gently stir the tomatoes and fennel to coat.

ROAST until the salmon just barely starts to flake when pulled apart with a fork, 15 to 18 minutes.

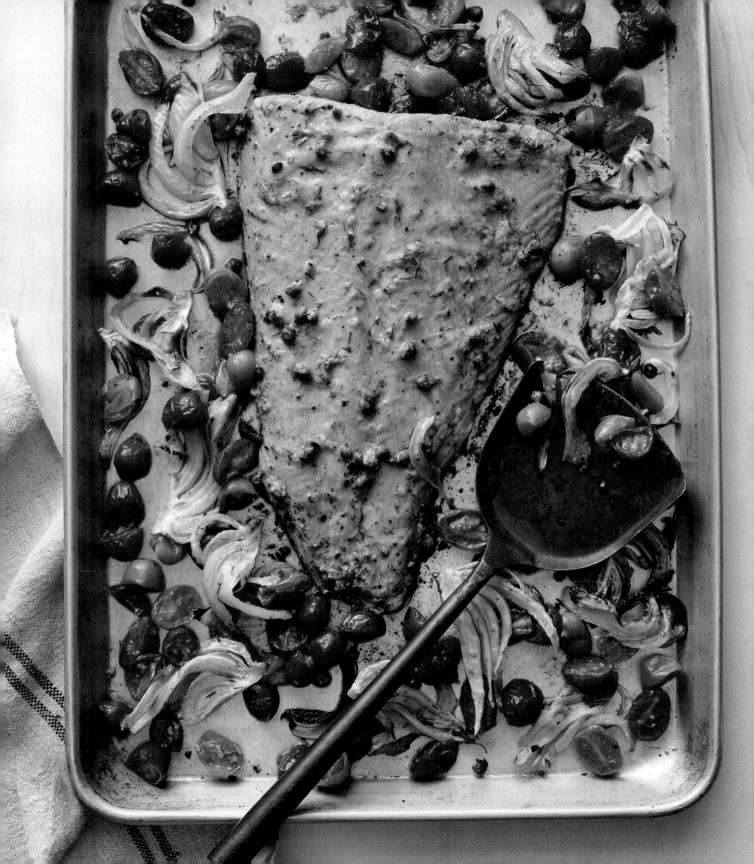

Rosemary-Garlic Chicken with Bacon-Wrapped Cabbage

SERVES 2

If you've never roasted cabbage before, this recipe will inspire you to make it part of your regular repertoire. The wedges turn tender and buttery at high heat—with crisped, lightly browned edges. Wrapping them in bacon before roasting makes them even better!

PREP:	20 minutes
ROAST:	35 minutes
TOTAL:	55 minutes

1 tablespoon extra-virgin olive oil

1 tablespoon finely chopped fresh rosemary

2 teaspoons minced garlic

2 teaspoons finely chopped fresh sage

Grated zest of 1 lemon

1 teaspoon coarse salt

1 teaspoon black pepper

2 bone-in, skin-on chicken breasts (8 to 12 ounces each)

½ small green cabbage, core intact, cut into 4 wedges

4 slices Whole30-compliant bacon

4 teaspoons fresh lemon juice

PREHEAT the oven to 425°F.

COMBINE the olive oil, rosemary, garlic, sage, lemon zest, salt, and ½ teaspoon of the black pepper in a small bowl. Rub the seasoning over the chicken and underneath the skin with your fingers.

PLACE the chicken, skin side up, on one side of a large rimmed baking pan Roast the chicken for 10 minutes.

MEANWHILE, wrap each cabbage wedge with one slice of bacon. Place the cabbage wedges on the other side of the baking pan. Sprinkle with the remaining ½ teaspoon black pepper. Roast until the internal temperature of the chicken is 170°F and the cabbage is tender, about 15 minutes more. Drizzle the chicken and cabbage with the lemon juice and serve.

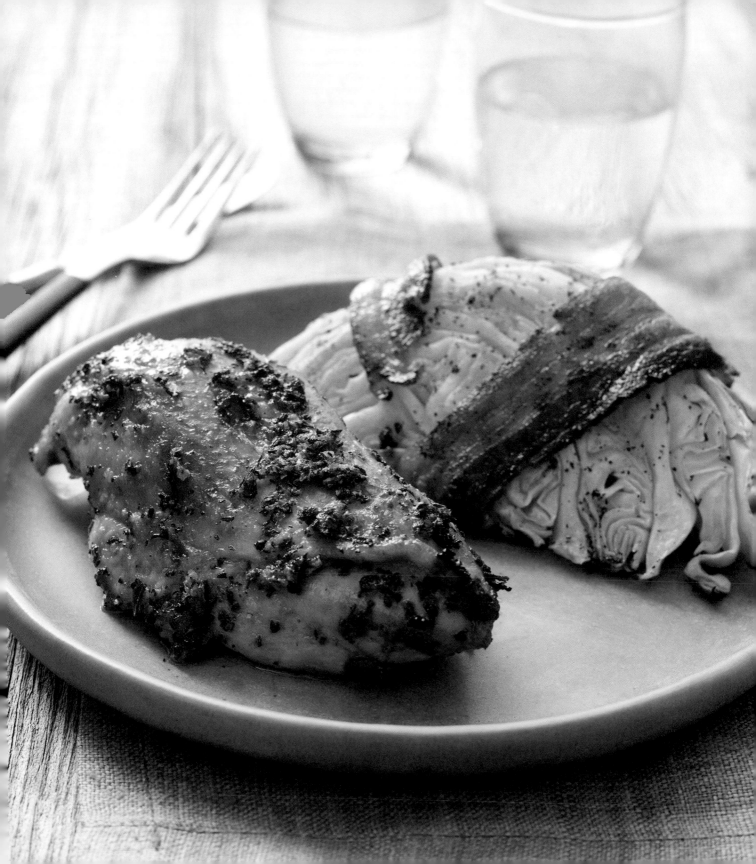

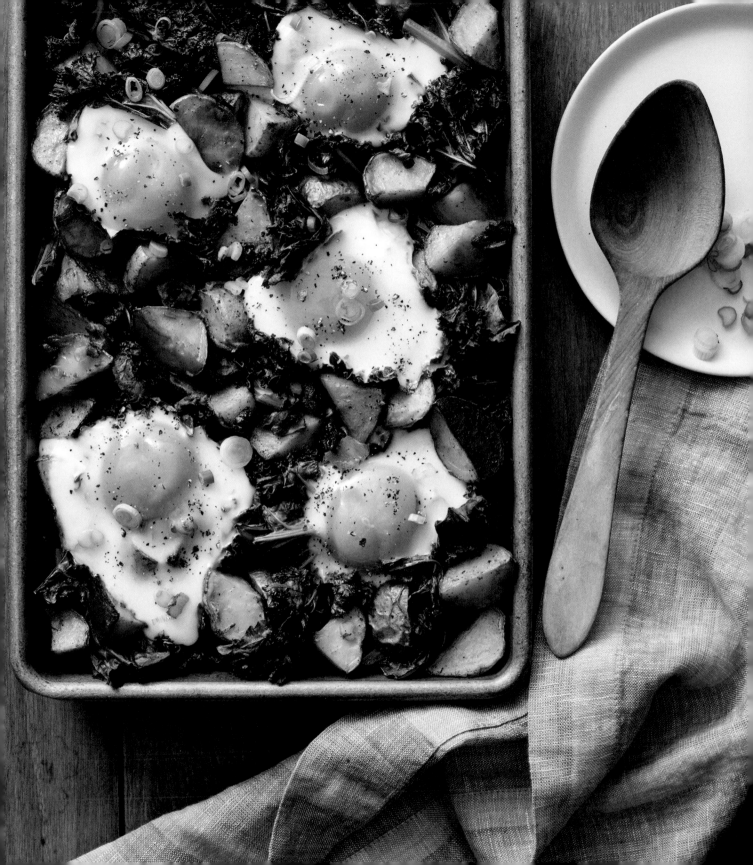

Roasted Potato and Kale Hash with Eggs ✓ good

SERVES 4

The creaminess of the roasted potatoes nicely balances the hearty texture of the kale in this sheet-pan hash. Using pre-chopped kale saves the time of washing, stripping, and chopping the greens.

PREP: 20 minutes	
ROAST: 30 minutes	
TOTAL: 50 minutes	

1 ½ **pounds Yukon Gold potatoes,** cut into ¾-inch pieces

1 **large onion, chopped**

3 **cloves garlic, chopped**

3 **tablespoons extra-virgin olive oil**

1 ½ **teaspoons dried oregano**

1 **teaspoon chili powder**

1 **teaspoon coarse salt**

½ **teaspoon black pepper**

4 **cups chopped kale (see Tip)**

8 **large eggs**

4 **green onions, thinly sliced**

Chopped fresh parsley (optional)

PLACE a rack in the center of the oven. Preheat the oven to 450°F. Line a large rimmed baking pan with parchment paper.

COMBINE the potatoes, onion, garlic, olive oil, oregano, chili powder, salt, and black pepper in a large bowl and toss to coat. Spread on the baking pan. Roast until the potatoes are just tender and starting to brown, about 20 minutes.

REDUCE the oven temperature to 400°F. Add the kale to the pan and stir until the kale wilts, returning the pan to the oven for a few minutes if necessary. Make eight indentations in the hash and carefully break an egg into each indentation. Roast until the egg whites are set, 6-7 ~~8 to 10~~ minutes more. Top with the green onions, sprinkle with chopped parsley if desired, and serve.

TIP *Look for washed and chopped kale near the packaged lettuce in the produce aisle of the supermarket.*

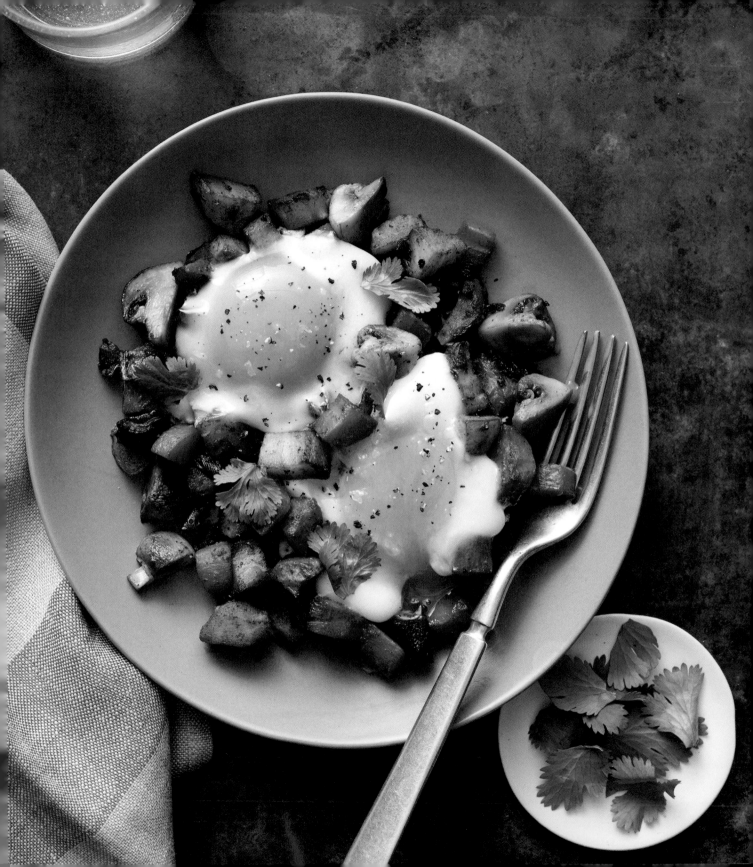

Veggie Hash with Eggs

SERVES 4

A combo of carrots, parsnips, red onion, and mushrooms spiced with cumin, smoked paprika, and chili powder provides a "nest" for eggs roasted just until the whites are set. The yolks are still creamy and provide a rich "sauce" for the veggies.

PREP: 15 minutes

ROAST: 30 minutes

TOTAL: 45 minutes

3 tablespoons extra-virgin olive oil

3 medium carrots, peeled and chopped

3 medium parsnips, peeled and chopped

1 medium red onion, chopped

2 cups quartered button mushrooms

2 cloves garlic, minced

1 teaspoon chili powder

½ teaspoon ground cumin

½ teaspoon smoked paprika

½ teaspoon coarse salt

½ teaspoon black pepper

8 large eggs

2 to 3 tablespoons torn fresh cilantro

PLACE a rack in the center of the oven. Preheat the oven to 425°F. Line a rimmed baking pan with parchment paper.

COMBINE the olive oil, carrots, parsnips, onion, mushrooms, garlic, chili powder, cumin, smoked paprika, salt, and black pepper in a large bowl; toss to coat. Spread the vegetables on the baking pan. Roast for 20 minutes.

MAKE four indentations in the hash and carefully break an egg into each indentation. Roast until the egg whites are set, 8 to 10 minutes more. Top with the cilantro and serve.

Cajun-Style Chicken Legs with Roasted Okra and Peppers

SERVES 2

When it's boiled or steamed, okra can get a little slippery and strange to eat. But as it does for most vegetables, high, dry heat has a magical effect on the crunchy green pods. It stays crisp-tender and browns up beautifully.

PREP: 10 minutes

ROAST: 35 minutes

TOTAL: 45 minutes

1 tablespoon Whole30-compliant salt-free Cajun seasoning

½ teaspoon salt

2 chicken leg quarters (attached drumstick and thigh; 8 to 10 ounces each)

2 tablespoons extra-virgin olive oil

8 ounces fresh okra

1 medium red bell pepper, coarsely chopped

1 medium onion, coarsely chopped

1 stalk celery, sliced

4 cloves garlic, minced

1 teaspoon dried thyme

½ teaspoon black pepper

¼ cup chopped fresh parsley

PREHEAT the oven to 425°F.

COMBINE the Cajun seasoning and salt in a small bowl. Rub the chicken with the seasoning. Place the chicken on half of a large rimmed baking pan. Drizzle with 1 tablespoon of the olive oil. Roast for 15 minutes.

MEANWHILE, combine the okra, bell pepper, onion, celery, garlic, thyme, and black pepper in a large bowl. Drizzle with the remaining 1 tablespoon of the olive oil and toss to coat.

ARRANGE the vegetables on the other half of the baking pan. Roast until the vegetables are tender, and the chicken is no longer pink and the internal temperature is 175°F, about 20 minutes. Sprinkle with the parsley and serve.

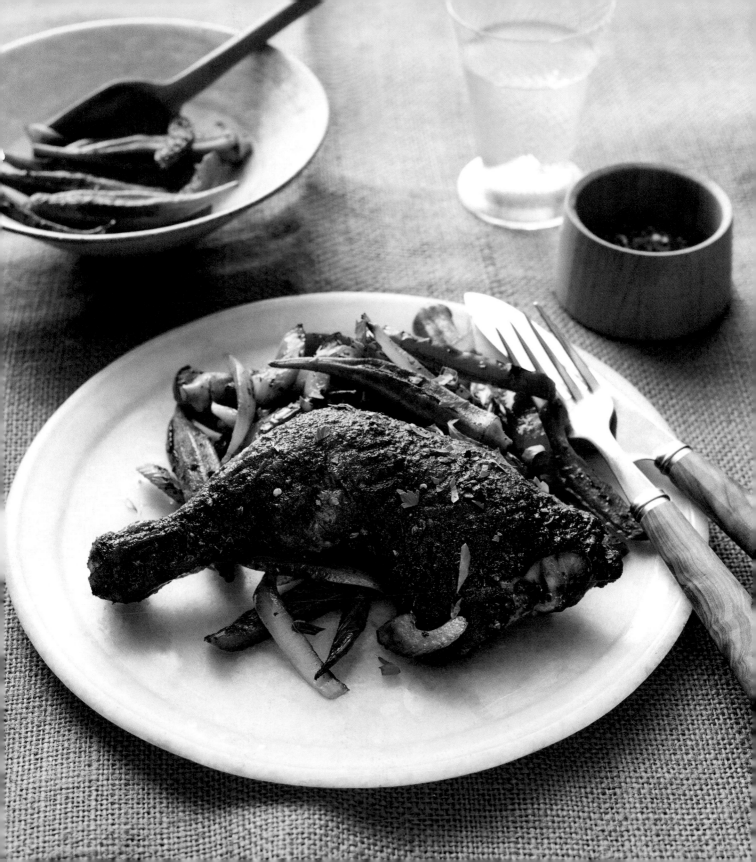

Ancho-Clementine Salmon with Herbed Sweet Potato Fries

SERVES 4

Ancho chile powder is made from dried poblano peppers. It has a rich, fruity, and slightly smoky flavor that is wonderful paired with the citrusy sweetness of the clementines.

PREP: 10 minutes	
BAKE: 25 minutes	
TOTAL: 35 minutes	

FOR THE FRIES

1½ pounds sweet potatoes, cut into ½-inch-thick sticks

3 tablespoons extra-virgin olive oil

1 teaspoon dried oregano

1 teaspoon garlic powder

1 teaspoon rosemary, crushed

1 teaspoon salt

½ teaspoon black pepper

½ teaspoon dried thyme

FOR THE SALMON

Grated zest and juice of 2 clementines or mandarin oranges

2 teaspoons ground ancho chile powder

1 teaspoon dried oregano

½ teaspoon garlic powder

½ teaspoon salt

4 skin-on salmon fillets (4 to 6 ounces each)

PREHEAT the oven to 425°F. Line a large rimmed baking pan with parchment paper.

MAKE THE FRIES: Combine the sweet potatoes, olive oil, oregano, garlic powder, rosemary, salt, pepper, and thyme. Toss to coat, then arrange the fries in a single layer on half of the pan. Roast for 12 minutes.

FOR THE SALMON: Meanwhile, combine the zest, chile powder, oregano, garlic powder, and salt. Rub onto the salmon fillets.

PLACE the fillets on the other half of the pan. Bake until the salmon just starts to flake with a fork and the fries are tender and golden brown, 12 to 15 minutes. Drizzle the clementine juice over the salmon and serve.

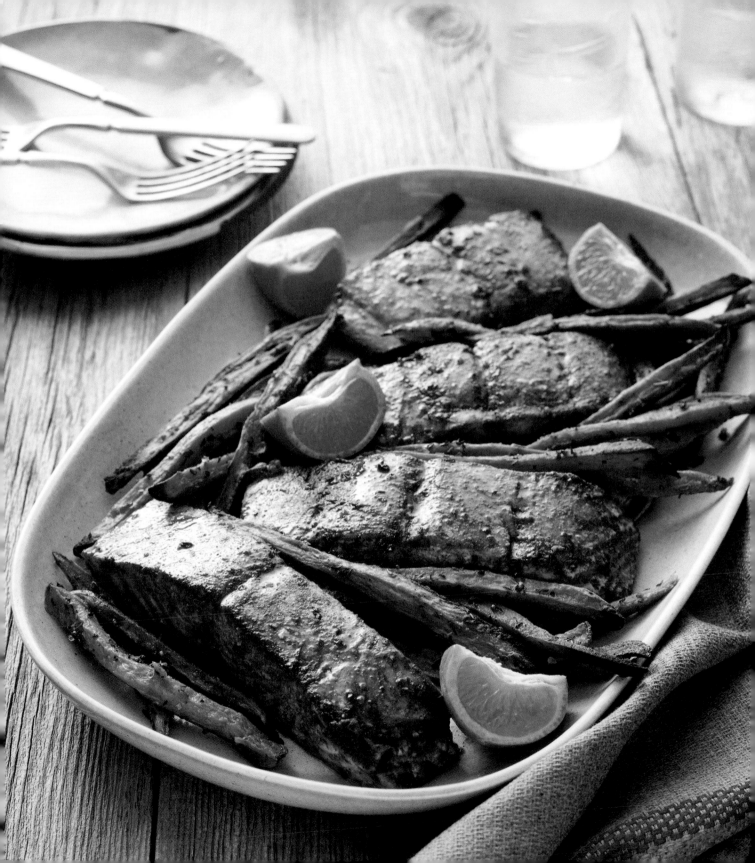

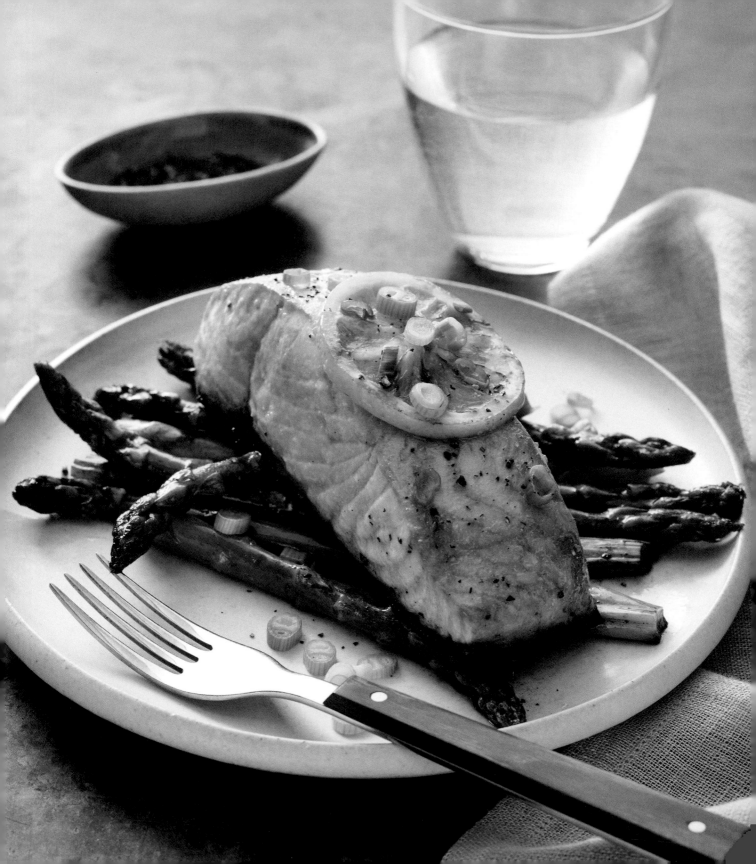

Lemon-Ginger Salmon and Asparagus

SERVES 4

The lemon-ginger lemon dressing that gets tossed with the asparagus and spooned over the salmon before roasting would be delicious on steamed green beans or fresh salad greens as well.

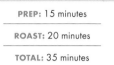

PREP: 15 minutes

ROAST: 20 minutes

TOTAL: 35 minutes

2 tablespoons extra-virgin olive oil

1 tablespoon fresh lemon juice

1 tablespoon coconut aminos

2 teaspoons rice vinegar

2 teaspoons minced fresh ginger

1 clove garlic, minced

¼ teaspoon salt

¼ teaspoon black pepper

1 pound asparagus, trimmed

4 skin-on salmon fillets (6 ounces each)

4 thin slices lemon

Sliced green onions

Lemon wedges (optional)

PREHEAT the oven to 425°F. Line a large rimmed baking pan with parchment paper.

IN a small bowl, stir together the olive oil, lemon juice, coconut aminos, rice vinegar, ginger, garlic, salt, and pepper.

IN a large bowl, toss the asparagus with half of the dressing. Arrange the asparagus in a single layer on the pan and roast for 5 minutes.

PLACE the salmon fillets, skin side down, on top of the asparagus. Top each fillet with a lemon slice. Spoon the remaining dressing over the salmon and lemon.

ROAST the asparagus and salmon for 15 minutes, until the asparagus is just tender browned and the salmon just barely starts to flake when pulled apart with a fork. Serve with green onions and lemon wedges, if desired.

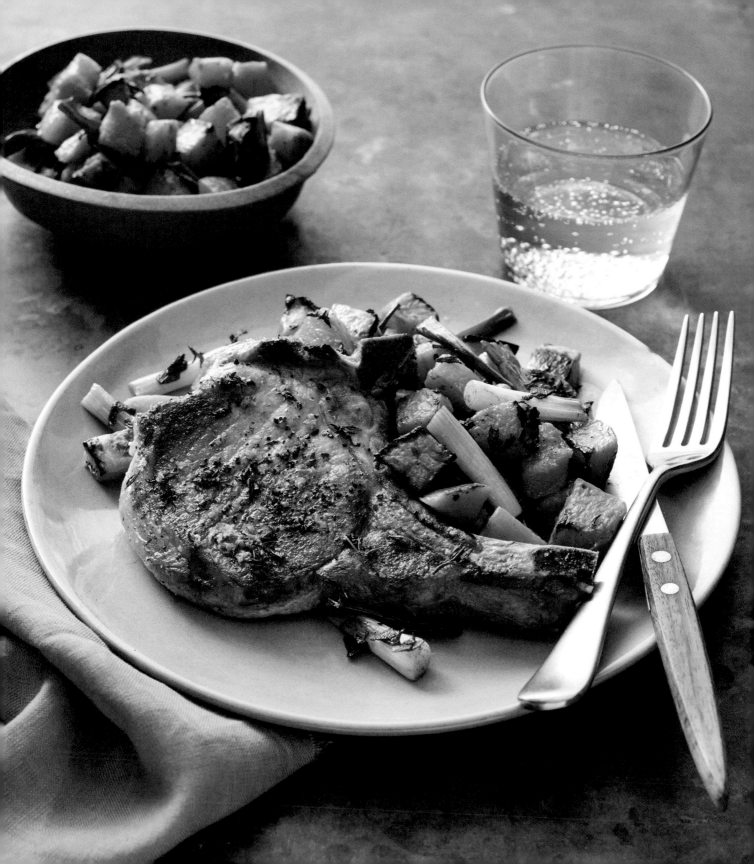

Pork Chops and Squash over Green Onions

SERVES 4

The green onions in this dish get deliciously crispy when roasted—and bathed in the juices of the pork seasoned with lemon and thyme. They are wonderful with the squash, which turns lightly caramelized on the outside and sweet and tender on the inside.

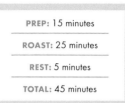

PREP: 15 minutes

ROAST: 25 minutes

REST: 5 minutes

TOTAL: 45 minutes

2 tablespoons extra-virgin olive oil

2 bunches green onions, trimmed and cut into 2-inch pieces

20 fresh sage leaves, coarsely chopped

1 teaspoon coarse salt

¾ teaspoon coarsely ground black pepper

2 teaspoons minced fresh thyme

1 teaspoon grated lemon zest

4 (¾- to 1-inch-thick) bone-in pork chops (about 2 pounds total)

1½ pounds peeled and chopped butternut squash (or other hearty squash such as delicata, which doesn't need to be peeled if using)

PLACE the oven rack in the center of the oven and preheat the oven to 400°F. Brush a large rimmed baking pan with 1 tablespoon of the olive oil. Arrange the green onions on the pan to cover. Sprinkle the sage on top of the green onions.

IN a small bowl, combine ½ teaspoon of the salt, ½ teaspoon of the pepper, the thyme, and lemon zest. Sprinkle the seasoning on the chops; place the chops on one side of the pan.

IN a large bowl, combine the squash with the remaining 1 tablespoon olive oil, the remaining ½ teaspoon salt, and the remaining ¼ teaspoon pepper and toss to coat. Place the squash on the other half of the pan.

ROAST the pork and squash for 20 minutes. Turn on the broiler and broil 4 inches from the heat source for 5 minutes, until the internal temperature of the pork reaches 145°F. Let the pork rest for 5 minutes before serving.

Sheet Pan Shrimp with Sesame Broccoli

SERVES 2

Be sure the shrimp are nice and dry after rinsing so that the mixture of garlic, butter, and coconut aminos clings to them.

PREP: 10 minutes	
ROAST: 35 minutes	
TOTAL: 45 minutes	

4 cups broccoli florets

2 teaspoons toasted sesame oil

⅛ teaspoon salt

⅛ teaspoon red pepper flakes

1 lemon, thinly sliced, seeds removed

12 ounces peeled and deveined extra-large shrimp (see Tip)

2 cloves garlic, minced

2 tablespoons Clarified Butter (page 283) or ghee, melted

1 tablespoon coconut aminos

PREHEAT the oven to 400°F. Line a large rimmed baking pan with parchment paper.

IN a large bowl, toss together the broccoli, sesame oil, salt, and pepper flakes. Spread the broccoli and lemon slices on half of the pan. Roast for 20 to 25 minutes, until the broccoli begins to brown. Stir the broccoli and turn the lemon slices over.

MEANWHILE, in the same large bowl, toss together the shrimp, garlic, butter, and coconut aminos.

ADD the shrimp in single layer to the other half of the pan. Roast the broccoli, lemon slices, and shrimp for 8 to 12 minutes, until the shrimp are opaque.

TIP *For a pretty presentation, purchase peeled and deveined shrimp with the tails on.*

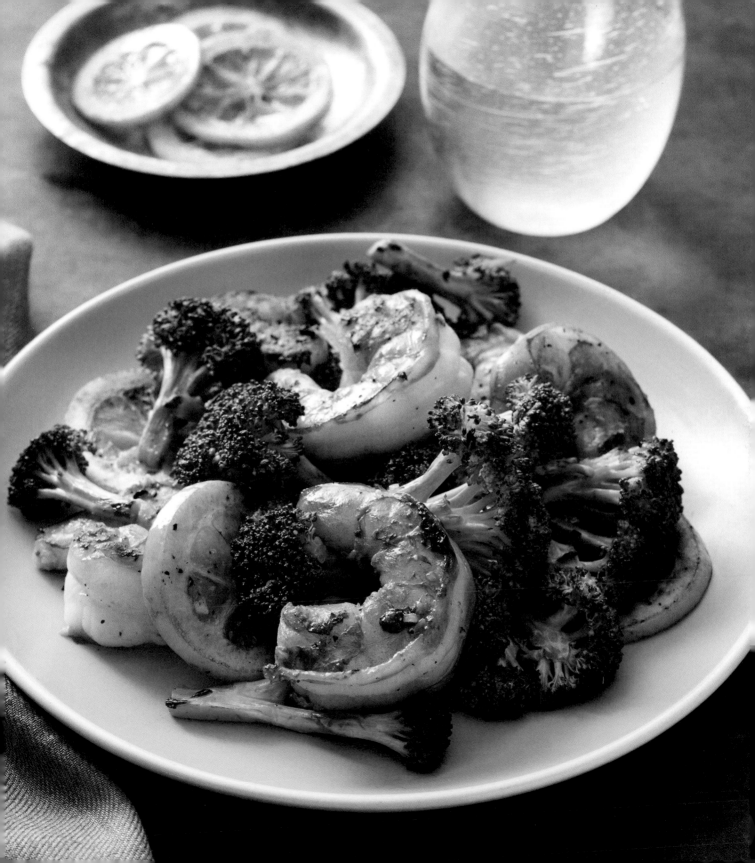

Zucchini-Wrapped Cod with Roasted Brussels Sprouts

SERVES 4

FROM *Laura Miner of the Cook at Home Mom*

When you want your dinner to look and feel fancy, but you're limited on time, this dinner is for you. It's light and bright, totally perfect for warm weather and squash season. If cod isn't available, you can substitute any other white fish.

PREP: 20 minutes

ROAST: 20 minutes

TOTAL: 40 minutes

4 cod fillets (6 ounces each)

¾ teaspoon coarse salt

¾ teaspoon black pepper

2 to 3 small zucchini, ends trimmed

3 tablespoons extra-virgin olive oil or avocado oil

1 lemon, cut into 8 slices

1 teaspoon fresh thyme leaves

4 cups Brussels sprouts, trimmed and halved

PREHEAT the oven to 400°F. Line a rimmed baking pan with parchment paper.

RINSE the cod and pat dry. Sprinkle with ½ teaspoon of the salt and ½ teaspoon of the black pepper.

SLICE the zucchini into $1/16$-inch-thick long ribbons using a vegetable peeler or mandoline, turning the zucchini to avoid the seeds. Wrap the ribbons around the fillets, overlapping slightly, and tuck each end under the fillet. Place on half of the baking pan and drizzle with 1 tablespoon of the olive oil. Place two lemon slices on top of each fillet and sprinkle with the thyme.

IN a medium bowl, drizzle the Brussels sprouts with the remaining 2 tablespoons olive oil and sprinkle with the remaining ¼ teaspoon salt and ¼ teaspoon black pepper. Toss to coat. Place the Brussels sprouts, cut sides down, on the other half of the pan.

ROAST for 15 to 20 minutes, until the fish just barely starts to flake when pulled apart with a fork and the Brussels sprouts are browned.

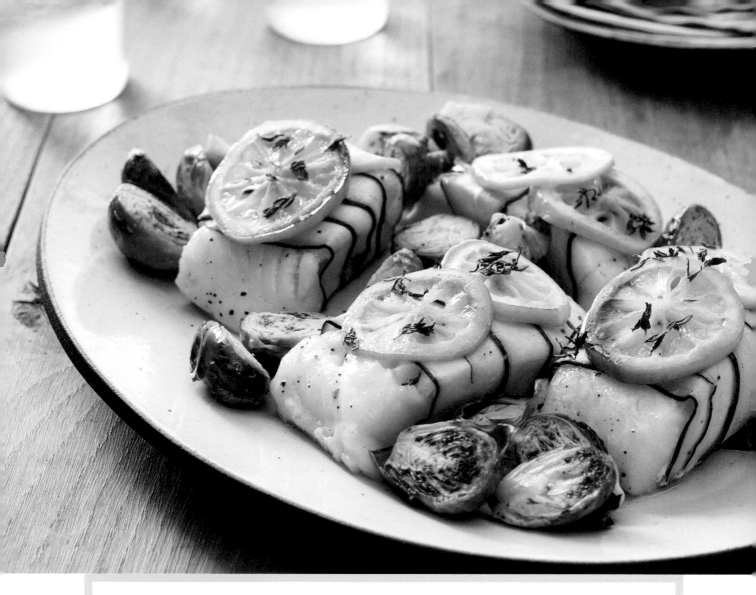

Laura Miner

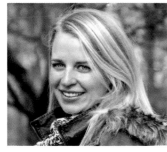

Laura Miner is the Cook at Home Mom, a self-taught chef who loves to help families prepare and enjoy simple, delicious meals together.

Her recipes use lots of fresh and seasonal ingredients, putting a healthy spin on family favorites.

Fajita Chicken and Shrimp with Peppers

SERVES 4

These classically flavored fajitas have all of the attributes of the original—but this chicken-and-shrimp combo is conveniently cooked on a single sheet pan in the oven. You can walk away while everything roasts—and there's no grease splatter to clean up on the stovetop when you're done.

PREP:	15 minutes
ROAST:	15 minutes
TOTAL:	30 minutes

2 tablespoons extra-virgin olive oil

2 teaspoons chili powder

1 teaspoon salt

½ teaspoon ground cumin

⅛ teaspoon ground cayenne

1 pound boneless, skinless chicken breasts, cut into ½-inch slices

2 medium red, orange, and/or yellow bell peppers, cut into ½-inch slices

1 red onion, halved and sliced

1½ pounds peeled and deveined medium shrimp

Lime wedges

Chopped fresh cilantro (optional)

PREHEAT the oven to 425°F.

IN a large bowl, stir together the olive oil, chili powder, salt, cumin, and cayenne. Add the chicken, bell peppers, and onion and toss to coat. Arrange the chicken and vegetables in a single layer on a large rimmed baking pan. Bake for 10 minutes.

STIR the shrimp into the chicken and vegetables. Roast until the chicken is cooked through, the shrimp is opaque, and the vegetables are tender, 5 to 6 minutes. Serve with lime wedges and, if desired, cilantro.

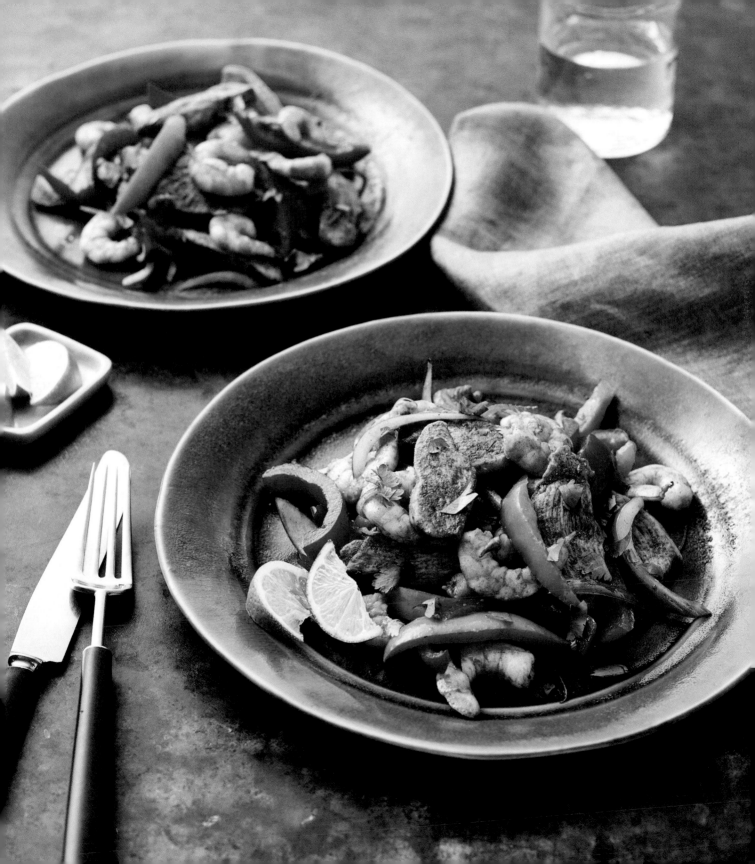

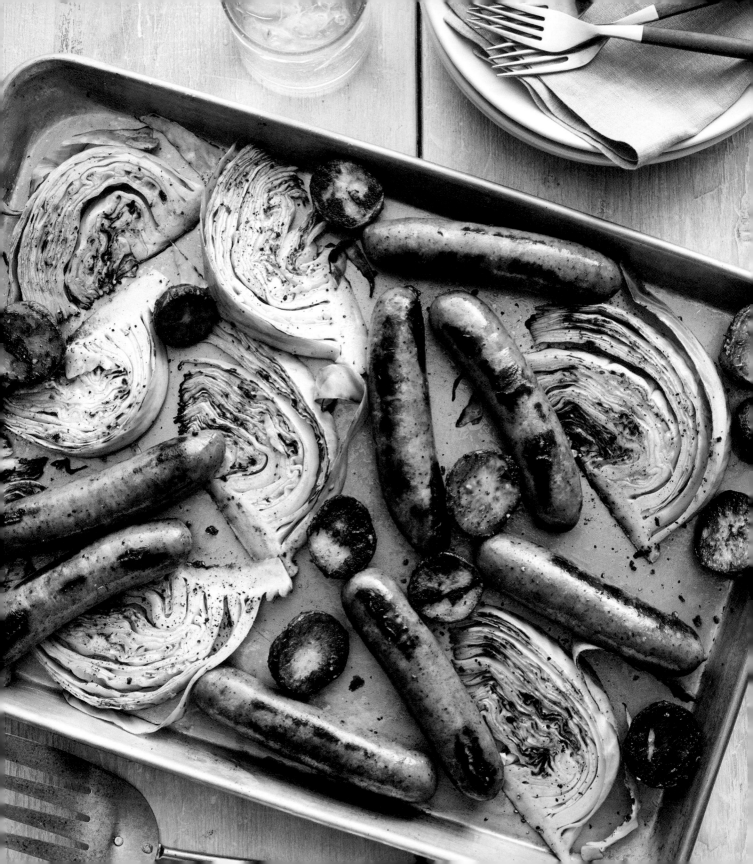

Roasted Sausages with Potatoes and Cabbage

SERVES 4

This hearty German-inspired one-pan dish is perfect for a cool fall night. The vegetables are tossed in a mixture of melted butter, Dijon mustard, and garlic before being roasted—along with chicken and apple sausages—to crispy perfection.

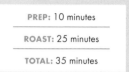

PREP: 10 minutes

ROAST: 25 minutes

TOTAL: 35 minutes

2 tablespoons Clarified Butter (page 283) or ghee

2 teaspoons Whole30-compliant Dijon mustard

2 cloves garlic, minced

½ teaspoon salt

¼ teaspoon black pepper

1 medium head green cabbage, core intact, cut into 8 wedges

8 small red potatoes, halved

2 packages (12 ounces each) Whole30-compliant chicken and apple sausages

PREHEAT the oven to 425°F.

IN a large bowl, stir together the butter, mustard, garlic, salt, and pepper. Add the cabbage and potatoes and gently toss to coat.

ARRANGE the vegetables and sausages on a large rimmed baking pan in a single layer. Roast, stirring once, until the vegetables are tender and browned, 25 to 30 minutes.

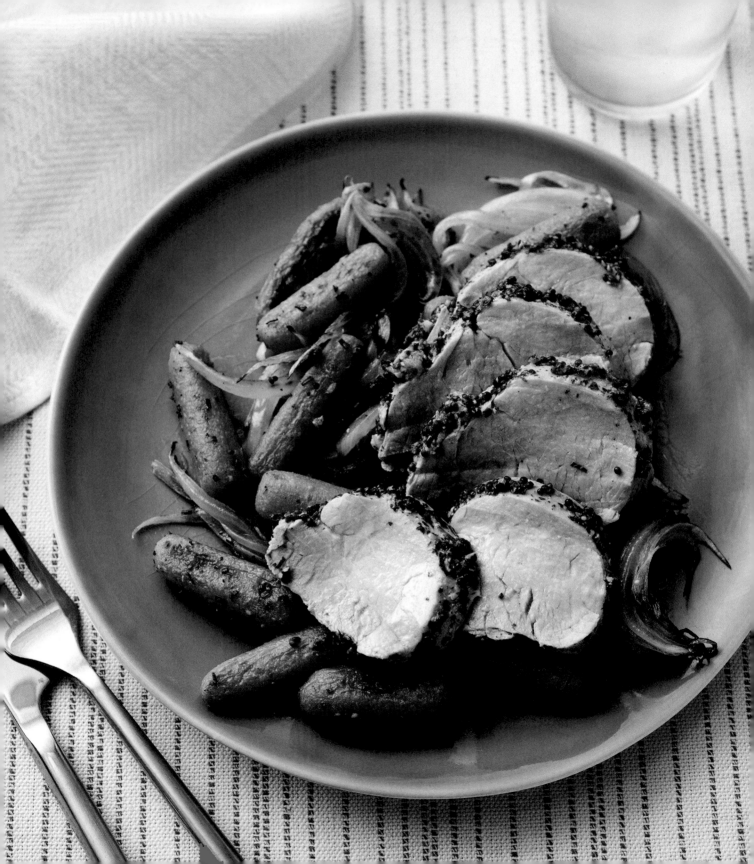

Mustard-Rubbed Pork Tenderloin with Rosemary Baby Carrots

SERVES 4

Baby carrots aren't just for crunching on raw at lunch or snack time. Here, they're roasted, with onion wedges, as a simple-to-prep side to juicy pork tenderloin.

PREP:	10 minutes
ROAST:	40 minutes
TOTAL:	50 minutes

¼ cup Whole30-compliant coarse-grain mustard

1 tablespoon finely chopped fresh parsley

1 teaspoon black pepper

1 teaspoon salt

½ teaspoon grated lemon zest

1 pork tenderloin (about 1¼ pounds)

1 bag (16 ounces) baby-cut carrots

1 medium sweet onion, cut into thin wedges

2 tablespoons avocado oil or extra-virgin olive oil

1 tablespoon finely chopped fresh rosemary

2 cloves garlic, minced

PREHEAT the oven to 425°F. Line a rimmed baking pan with parchment paper.

IN a small bowl, stir together the mustard, parsley, pepper, ½ teaspoon of the salt, and the lemon zest. Spread the mixture all over the tenderloin. Place the tenderloin on the pan.

IN a large bowl, toss the carrots and onion with the oil, rosemary, garlic, and the remaining ½ teaspoon salt. Place the vegetables around the tenderloin.

ROAST the tenderloin until the internal temperature is 145°F, 25 to 30 minutes. Transfer the pork to a cutting board and cover with foil. Continue to roast the vegetables until tender, about 10 minutes longer.

THINLY slice the pork and serve with the vegetables.

Coffee au Poivre Steaks with Spiral Potatoes

SERVES 4

The French term *au poivre* usually refers to a steak that's generously coated in cracked black pepper and then grilled or pan-seared. This recipe takes that concept and applies it to steaks coated in a rub made of finely ground coffee beans, hot chili powder, smoked paprika, sea salt, and mustard powder and broiled. The crispy spiral potatoes served alongside are can't-stop-eating-them good!

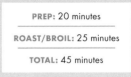

PREP: 20 minutes

ROAST/BROIL: 25 minutes

TOTAL: 45 minutes

FOR THE STEAKS

1½ tablespoons finely ground coffee beans or ground instant coffee

1½ tablespoons hot chili powder

2 teaspoons smoked paprika

1 teaspoon sea salt

½ teaspoon mustard powder

4 (1-inch-thick) rib eye steaks, trimmed of fat (about 8 ounces each)

FOR THE POTATOES

3 medium russet potatoes, peeled and spiralized into noodles

1½ to 2 tablespoons avocado oil or melted coconut oil

1 teaspoon garlic powder

1 teaspoon salt

¼ to ½ teaspoon black pepper

ADJUST the oven racks so one is about 4 inches from the broiler heat and the other is lower in the oven. Preheat the oven to 425°F. Line a rimmed baking pan with foil.

PREPARE THE STEAKS: In a small bowl, combine the ground coffee, chili powder, paprika, salt, and mustard powder. Place the steaks on the un-heated rack of a broiler pan or baking pan. Rub the steaks all over with the coffee mixture.

MAKE THE POTATOES: Place the potato noodles on the lined baking pan and pat dry with a paper towel. In a small bowl, combine the oil, garlic powder, salt, and pepper; drizzle over the potatoes and gently toss to coat. Roast the potato noodles on the lower oven rack, tossing once halfway through, for 20 minutes.

TURN the oven to broil, leaving the potatoes on the lower rack. Place the steaks on the upper rack. Broil the steaks, turning once halfway through, for 12 to 14 minutes for medium-rare (internal temperature is 145°F) or to desired doneness. Remove the pan with the steaks from the oven, and let steaks rest for 5 minutes while finishing potatoes.

MOVE the pan with the potatoes to the upper rack position and broil, watching carefully and tossing occasionally, until golden and crisp, about 5 minutes.

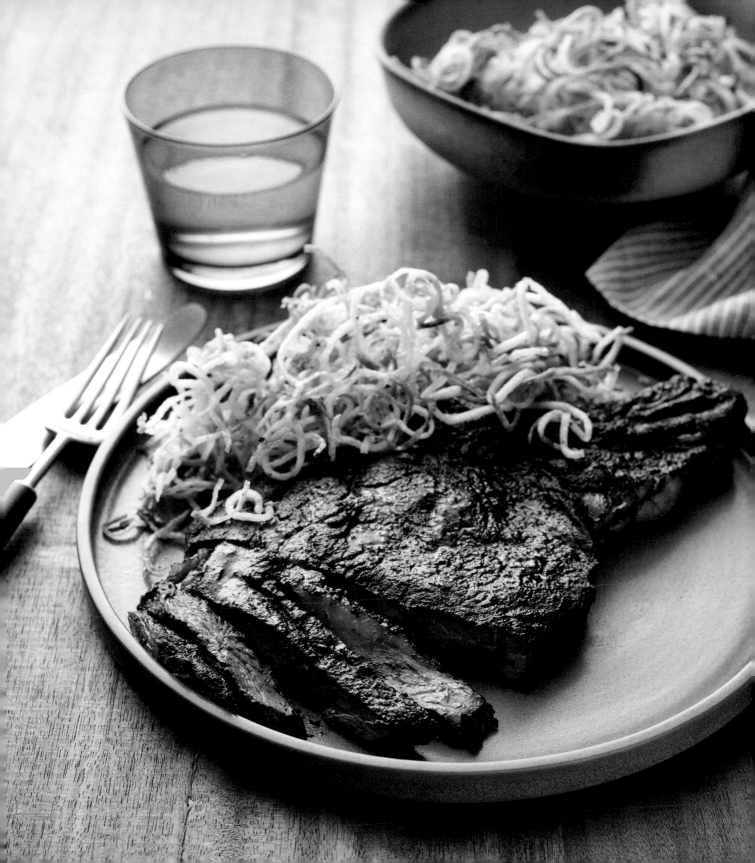

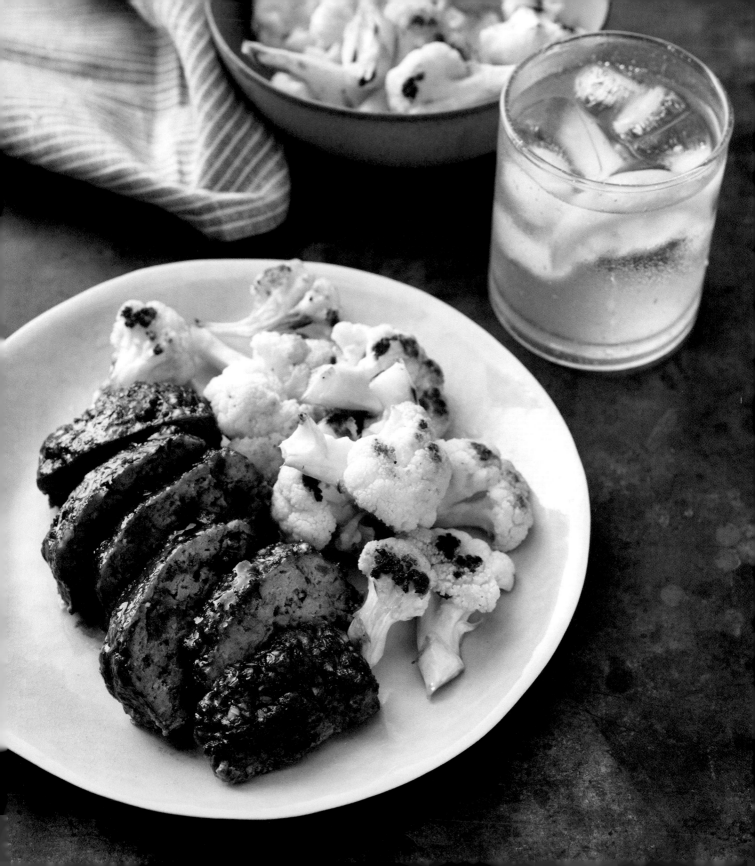

Apricot-Lamb Loaves with Roasted Cauliflower

SERVES 4

These mini meat loaves can be made with lamb—which is wonderful with apricot—but if you're not a fan of lamb, they're delicious made with ground beef too.

PREP: 15 minutes

BAKE: 45 minutes

TOTAL: 1 hour

12 unsulphured dried apricots, finely chopped

6 cups bite-sized cauliflower florets

2 tablespoons olive oil

2 teaspoons salt

1 large egg, lightly beaten

⅓ cup chopped green onion

2 tablespoons chopped fresh cilantro

2 ¼ teaspoons chili powder

1 ½ pounds lean ground lamb or lean ground beef

1 tablespoon balsamic vinegar

PREHEAT the oven to 375°F. Line a rimmed baking pan with parchment paper.

PLACE the apricots in a small saucepan and add enough water to cover. Bring to a boil. Remove from the heat and let stand while preparing the cauliflower.

IN a large bowl, toss together the cauliflower, olive oil, and ½ teaspoon of the salt. Arrange on one end of the pan and bake for 10 minutes. Remove from the oven and stir.

MEANWHILE, using the same bowl, stir together the egg, green onion, cilantro, chili powder, and remaining 1½ teaspoons salt. Drain the apricots well. Add the drained apricots and lamb to the egg mixture and gently mix well. Divide the lamb mixture into four equal portions. Shape each portion into a 4 x 2-inch loaf. Place the loaves on the other end of the pan. Bake, stirring the cauliflower once, until the cauliflower is tender and the internal temperature of the meat loaves is 160°F, 30 to 35 minutes.

DRIZZLE the lamb loaves with the balsamic vinegar and serve with the cauliflower.

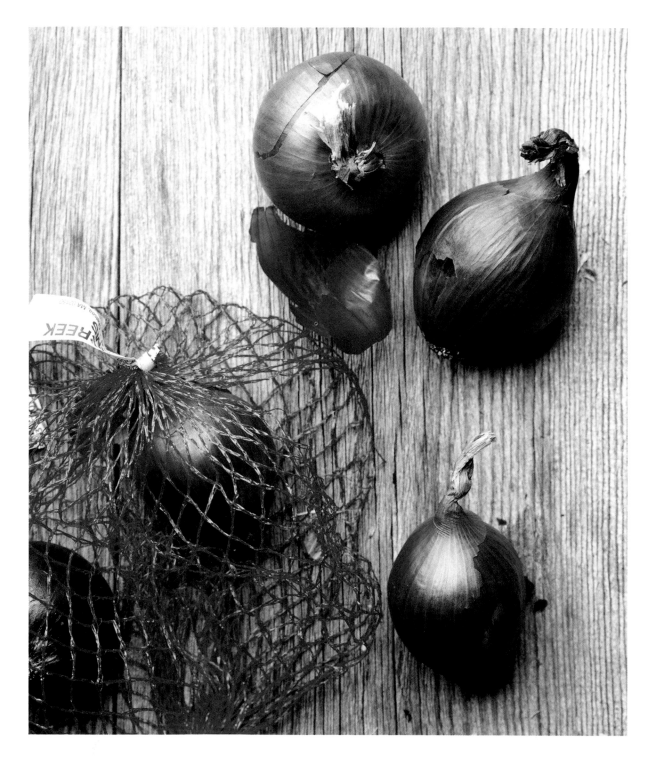

One-Pan Meatballs with Potatoes and Broccoli

SERVES 2

This recipe is an example of how an efficient use of time helps you turn out a terrific dinner with very little effort or stress. While the potatoes and broccoli roast, stir and shape the meatballs. Add them to the sheet pan with the veggies, then clean up in the 15 minutes it takes for the meatballs to cook. And then there's only one pan to deal with when dinner is done!

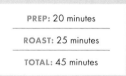

PREP:	20 minutes
ROAST:	25 minutes
TOTAL:	45 minutes

FOR THE POTATOES AND BROCCOLI

2 medium Yukon Gold potatoes (about 8 ounces total), scrubbed and cut into ½-inch-thick wedges

2 cups broccoli florets

1 clove garlic, thinly sliced

¼ teaspoon salt

2 tablespoons extra-virgin olive oil

FOR THE MEATBALLS

1 large egg

2 tablespoons almond flour

1 teaspoon dried Italian seasoning

¼ teaspoon salt

⅛ teaspoon red pepper flakes

8 ounces ground beef

1 ounce thinly sliced pancetta, chopped

¼ cup finely chopped onion

¾ cup Whole30-compliant tomato-basil pasta sauce, warmed

Lemon wedges

PREHEAT the oven to 425°F. Line a large rimmed baking pan with foil.

PREPARE THE POTATOES AND BROCCOLI: Place the potatoes and broccoli on the pan, sprinkle with the garlic and salt, and drizzle with the olive oil. Toss to coat and spread in an even layer on half of the pan. Roast for 10 minutes.

PREPARE THE MEATBALLS: Meanwhile, in a medium bowl, whisk together the egg, almond flour, Italian seasoning, salt, and pepper flakes. Add the ground beef, pancetta, and onion. Mix with your hands just until combined, then shape into 6 meatballs.

ARRANGE the meatballs on the other side of the pan. Roast until the vegetables are tender and the meatballs' internal temperature is 160°F, about 15 minutes longer.

TOSS the meatballs with the warmed pasta sauce. Serve with the vegetables and lemon wedges.

Sheet Pan Barbecue Pork Chops with Potatoes

SERVES 2

Add a quick slaw to this meat-and-potatoes dish and you've got a complete meal. Try a packaged shredded broccoli or cabbage slaw tossed with a purchased compliant dressing or one of the following homemade dressings: Asian Citrus Dressing (page 277), Everyday Whole30 Salad Dressing (page 278), Apple-Mustard Vinaigrette (page 277), or Blender Green Goddess Dressing (page 275).

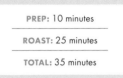

PREP: 10 minutes

ROAST: 25 minutes

TOTAL: 35 minutes

½ **pound small new potatoes, quartered**

1 **tablespoon extra-virgin olive oil**

¼ **teaspoon dried thyme**

½ **teaspoon salt**

¼ **teaspoon black pepper**

2 **bone-in pork loin chops (¾ inch thick)**

1 **tablespoon Clarified Butter (page 283) or ghee, melted**

¼ **cup Whole30-compliant barbecue sauce, plus more for serving if desired**

PREHEAT the oven to 425°F. Line a large rimmed baking pan with parchment paper.

IN a large bowl, combine the potatoes, olive oil, thyme, ¼ teaspoon of the salt, and ⅛ teaspoon of the pepper. Spread the potatoes on half of the pan and roast for 10 minutes; stir.

BRUSH the pork chops with the melted butter and sprinkle with the remaining ¼ teaspoon salt and ⅛ teaspoon pepper. Add the chops to the pan and roast for 10 minutes. Brush both sides of the chops with the barbecue sauce. Roast until the chops' internal temperature is 145°F and the potatoes are tender and golden brown, about 5 minutes longer. Let the chops rest for 5 minutes.

SERVE the chops and potatoes with additional barbecue sauce, if desired, and season to taste with salt and pepper.

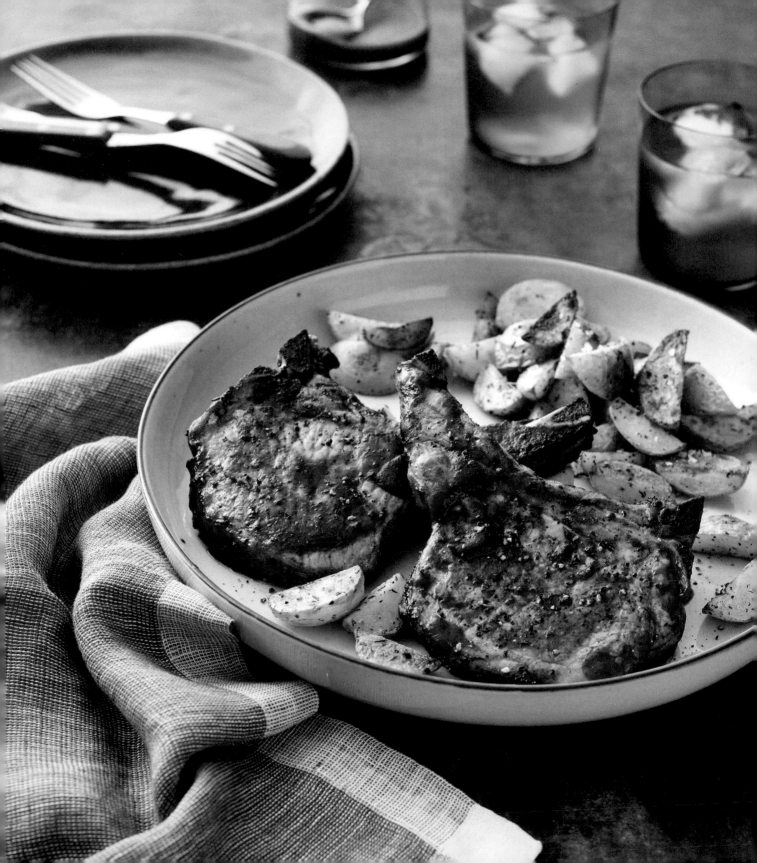

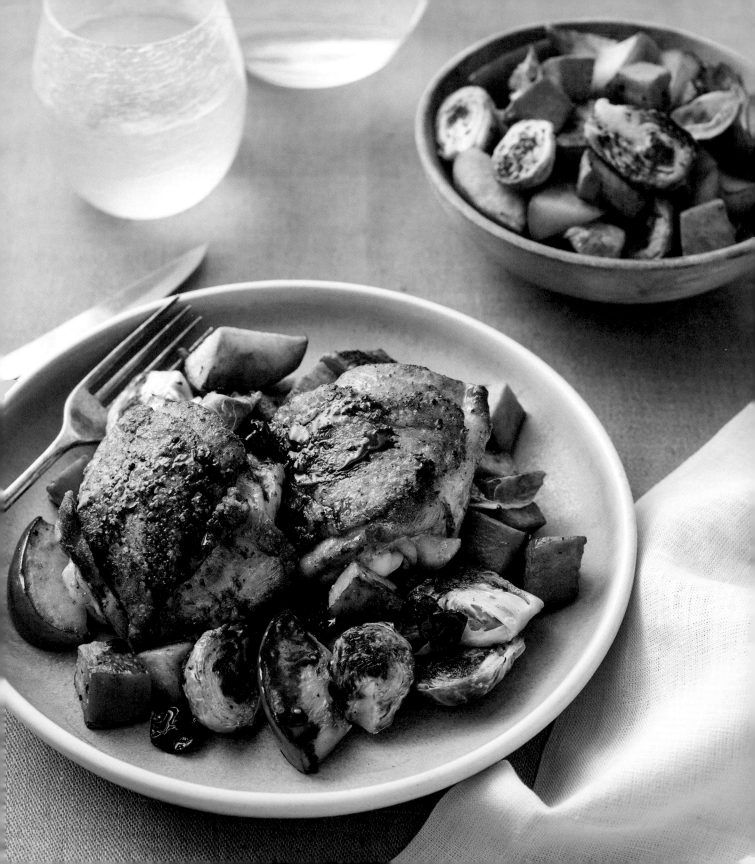

Roasted Chicken Thighs with Harvest Vegetables and Apples

SERVES 4

You can use any cooking apple in this recipe, but our favorite is Granny Smith. They hold their shape well when exposed to heat and we like how their tartness balances out the sweetness of the dried cherries and sweet potatoes.

PREP: 15 minutes

BROIL/ROAST: 30 minutes

TOTAL: 45 minutes

1 ¼ to 1 ½ pounds bone-in chicken thighs

¾ teaspoon coarse salt

½ teaspoon black pepper

1 medium sweet potato, peeled and cut into 1-inch pieces

2 cups trimmed and halved Brussels sprouts

3 small sprigs fresh rosemary

2 tablespoons extra-virgin olive oil

1 cup balsamic vinegar

¼ cup no-sugar-added dried cherries

2 medium cooking apples, quartered, cored, and chopped

PREHEAT the broiler.

PLACE the chicken thighs, skin side up, on one half of a large rimmed baking pan. Sprinkle with ¼ teaspoon of the salt and ¼ teaspoon of the pepper. Broil 5 to 6 inches from the heat until the skin is lightly browned, 4 to 5 minutes. Remove the pan and place on a wire rack. Set the oven temperature to 425°F.

ADD the sweet potato, Brussels sprouts, and 2 sprigs of the rosemary to the other half of the baking pan in an even layer. Drizzle with the olive oil and sprinkle with the remaining ½ teaspoon salt and ¼ teaspoon pepper. Toss to coat. Return to the oven and roast, uncovered, for 20 minutes.

MEANWHILE, in a small saucepan, bring the vinegar just to boiling. Boil gently, uncovered, until the vinegar is reduced to ½ cup, 6 to 8 minutes. Add the dried cherries and the remaining sprig of rosemary and cook for 1 minute longer. Remove from the heat; let cool until ready to serve.

ADD the apples to the vegetables. Roast until the internal temperature of a chicken thigh registers 175°F and the vegetables are tender and lightly browned, 5 to 8 minutes.

TO serve, remove the rosemary sprig from the balsamic sauce and spoon over the chicken.

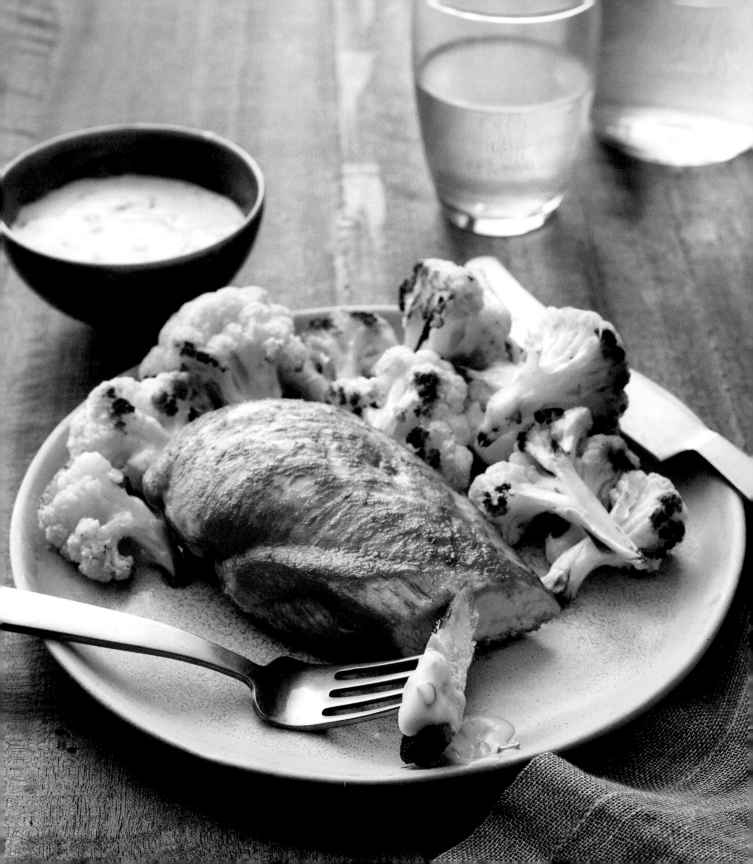

Sheet Pan Buffalo Chicken with Cauliflower

SERVES 2

You don't have to give up your favorite bar snack just because you can't go to the bar—and this is actually a very tasty entree! Crisp-roasted cauliflower is swapped in for the raw celery and carrots in the traditional version. Serve those too, if you like. You can't get too many veggies on the Whole30!

PREP:	10 minutes
ROAST/COOK:	35 minutes
TOTAL:	45 minutes

4 cups cauliflower florets

1 tablespoon extra-virgin olive oil

¼ teaspoon salt

⅛ teaspoon black pepper

2 tablespoons Clarified Butter (page 283) or ghee, melted

2 boneless, skinless chicken breasts

2 tablespoons Whole30-compliant Buffalo sauce, plus more for serving if desired

¼ cup Whole30-compliant creamy ranch dressing or Whole30 Ranch Dressing (page 282)

PREHEAT the oven to 425°F. Line a large rimmed baking pan with parchment paper.

IN a large bowl, combine the cauliflower, olive oil, salt, and pepper; mix well. Spread the cauliflower on three-fourths of the pan and roast for 15 minutes.

MEANWHILE, heat 1 tablespoon of the butter in a medium skillet over medium-high heat. Add the chicken and cook, turning once, until golden brown, 5 to 6 minutes.

IN the same bowl, stir together the remaining 1 tablespoon butter and the Buffalo sauce. Add the browned chicken and coat with the sauce. Add the chicken to the pan. Continue roasting until the internal temperature of the chicken is 170°F and the cauliflower is tender and lightly browned, 20 to 25 minutes longer.

SERVE the chicken and cauliflower with the ranch dressing for dipping. If desired, drizzle the chicken with additional Buffalo sauce.

Chicken Thighs with Stuffed Mushrooms

SERVES 4

A delicious concoction of dried tomatoes, fresh thyme, and garlic gets tucked under the skin of these chicken thighs before they're roasted to crispy perfection. They're served with a side of mushrooms stuffed with smoky sausage, kale, and more dried tomatoes and garlic.

PREP: 15 minutes	
COOK: 30 minutes	
TOTAL: 45 minutes	

FOR THE CHICKEN

2 tablespoons finely diced drained oil-packed dried tomatoes

1 teaspoon extra-virgin olive oil

1 clove garlic, minced

1 teaspoon fresh thyme leaves

½ teaspoon coarse salt

¼ teaspoon black pepper

1¼ to 1½ pounds bone-in chicken thighs

FOR THE MUSHROOMS

4 medium portobello mushrooms (about 1 pound total) (see Tip)

4 ounces Whole30-compliant smoked kielbasa, diced

1 cup chopped fresh kale

2 tablespoons finely diced drained oil-packed dried tomatoes

1 tablespoon oil from oil-packed dried tomatoes

2 cloves garlic, minced

PREHEAT the oven to 425°F. Line a large rimmed baking pan with parchment paper.

MAKE THE CHICKEN: In a small bowl, combine the dried tomatoes, olive oil, garlic, thyme, salt, and black pepper. For each thigh, run a finger under the skin to lift it off the meat, but leaving it attached along the sides. Spoon some of the thyme mixture under the skin. Place the thighs on one side of the pan. Roast for 5 minutes.

MAKE THE MUSHROOMS: Meanwhile, remove the stems and gills from the mushrooms. Use a damp paper towel to wipe the mushrooms clean. Add the mushrooms, gill sides down, to the pan. Roast until the mushrooms are just tender, 15 to 18 minutes.

MEANWHILE, in a medium bowl, combine the kielbasa, kale, tomatoes, tomato oil, and garlic. Turn the mushrooms over. Spoon the kielbasa filling into the mushrooms. Roast until the chicken is no longer pink and a thermometer inserted in the thigh registers 175°F and the mushrooms are just tender, 10 to 15 minutes longer.

 TIP *Use a spoon to scrape the gills from the mushrooms.*

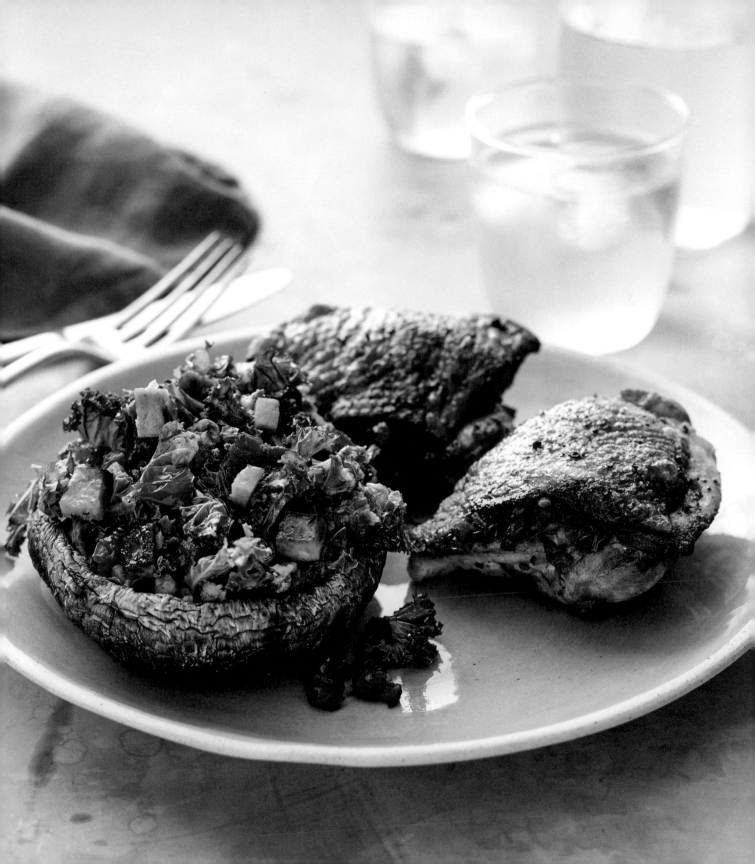

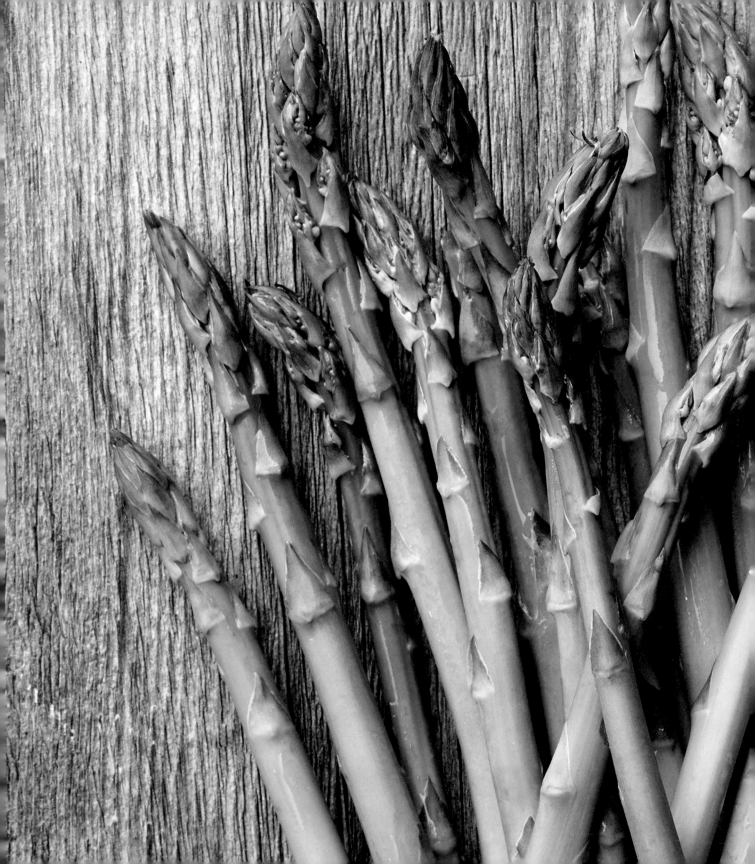

CHAPTER 4

SOUPS, STEWS, AND NOODLE BOWLS

Mexican Shrimp and Zoodle Soup

SERVES 4

Chili powder has a slightly higher proportion of ground chiles to other ingredients—usually cumin, oregano, and garlic powder—than Mexican seasoning does, but otherwise, they are very much the same. Both work equally well in this zippy soup.

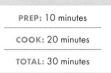

PREP: 10 minutes

COOK: 20 minutes

TOTAL: 30 minutes

1 tablespoon extra-virgin olive oil

1 large onion, chopped

2 large jalapeños, seeded and finely chopped

¼ teaspoon kosher salt

¼ cup Whole30-compliant tomato paste

1 tablespoon Whole30-compliant Mexican seasoning or chili powder

5 cups Whole30-compliant chicken broth or Chicken Bone Broth (page 280)

1 pound peeled and deveined small shrimp (see Tip)

1 package (10.7 ounces) zucchini noodles; or 2 small zucchini, spiralized, long noodles snipped if desired

1 cup chopped fresh cilantro

Chopped avocado

Lime wedges

HEAT the olive oil in a 4-quart Dutch oven or stockpot over medium heat. Add the onion, jalapeños, and salt and cook, stirring occasionally, until softened, 6 to 8 minutes. Stir in the tomato paste and Mexican seasoning. Cook, stirring, for 1 minute. Add the broth and bring to a boil.

STIR in the shrimp and zucchini noodles. Cook until the shrimp are opaque and the zucchini is crisp-tender, about 5 minutes. Stir in the chopped cilantro. Serve the soup with chopped avocado and lime wedges.

TIP *For an even easier dinner, buy cooked small shrimp: Add them after cooking the noodles for 3 minutes, and then cook for just a minute or two longer, until the shrimp are heated through.*

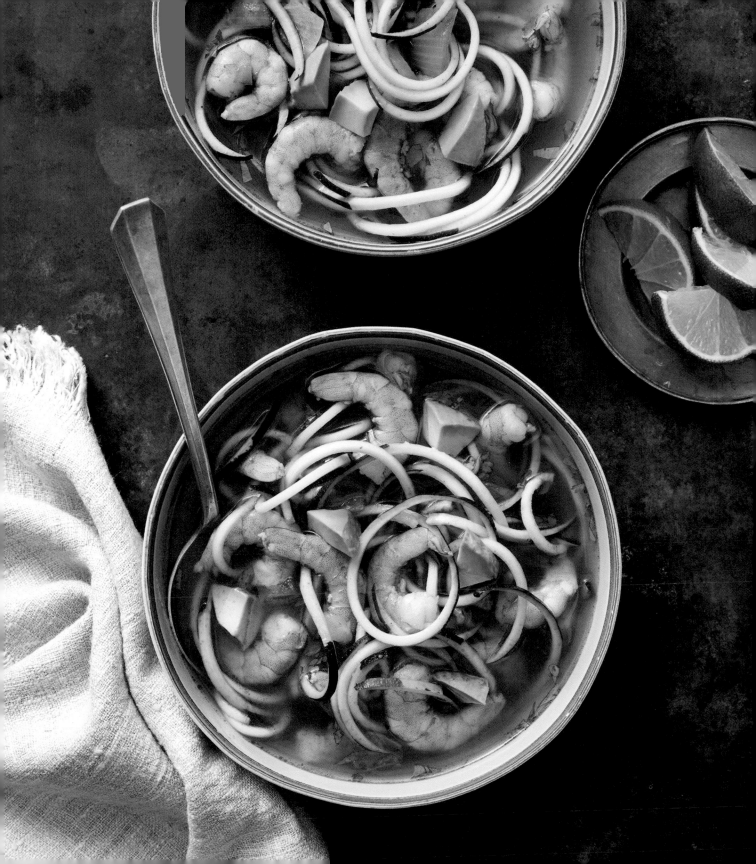

Thai Chicken Sweet-Potato-Noodle Bowls

SERVES 4

This colorful dish has very clean, fresh flavors—just sweet pepper, sweet potato noodles, and chicken in chicken broth with a generous helping of herbs. For the most interesting taste, use a blend of basil and mint.

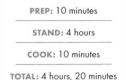

PREP: 10 minutes

STAND: 4 hours

COOK: 10 minutes

TOTAL: 4 hours, 20 minutes

FOR THE CASHEW-COCONUT CREAM

1 cup raw unsalted cashews

¾ cup Whole30-compliant coconut milk (see Tip)

⅛ teaspoon salt

FOR THE SWEET POTATO NOODLES AND CHICKEN

6 cups Whole30-compliant chicken or vegetable broth or Chicken Bone Broth (page 280)

¼ teaspoon salt

1 (10-ounce) package sweet potato spirals or 1 medium sweet potato, spiralized

1 medium red bell pepper, seeded and cut into bite-size pieces

½ jalapeño, seeded and finely chopped

3 cups shredded cooked chicken breast (see Tip)

1 cup coarsely chopped fresh basil and/or mint

MAKE THE CASHEW-COCONUT CREAM: Rinse the cashews and drain. Place in a bowl and add enough water to cover by 1 inch. Cover the bowl and let stand for 4 hours or up to overnight. Drain the cashews and rinse under cold water. Place the cashews, coconut milk, and salt in a high-speed blender. Cover and blend until smooth. Add cold water, 1 tablespoon at a time, to reach drizzling consistency.

MAKE THE SWEET POTATO NOODLES AND CHICKEN: In a large saucepan, bring the broth and salt to a boil. Add the sweet potato, bell pepper, and jalapeño and simmer for 3 minutes. Remove from the heat and stir in the chicken. Let stand until heated through, 2 minutes.

DIVIDE the herbs among four bowls. Ladle the soup over the herbs. Drizzle each with about 1 tablespoon of the Cashew-Coconut Cream.

TIPS *Canned coconut milk separates in the can with the cream rising to the top. Be sure to whisk the coconut milk well before measuring.*

This is a great way to use up leftover roasted, grilled, or steamed skinless, boneless chicken breast.

The Cashew-Coconut Cream can be made up to 1 week ahead. Cover and store in an airtight container in the refrigerator. Cashew cream makes a delicious vegan substitute for cream and sour cream. Makes about 2 cups.

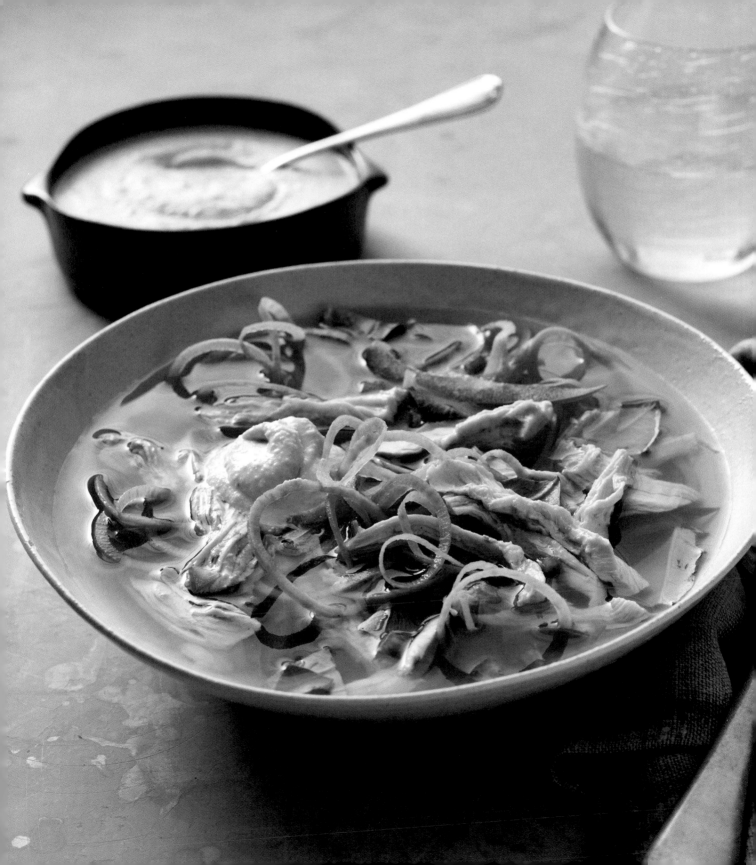

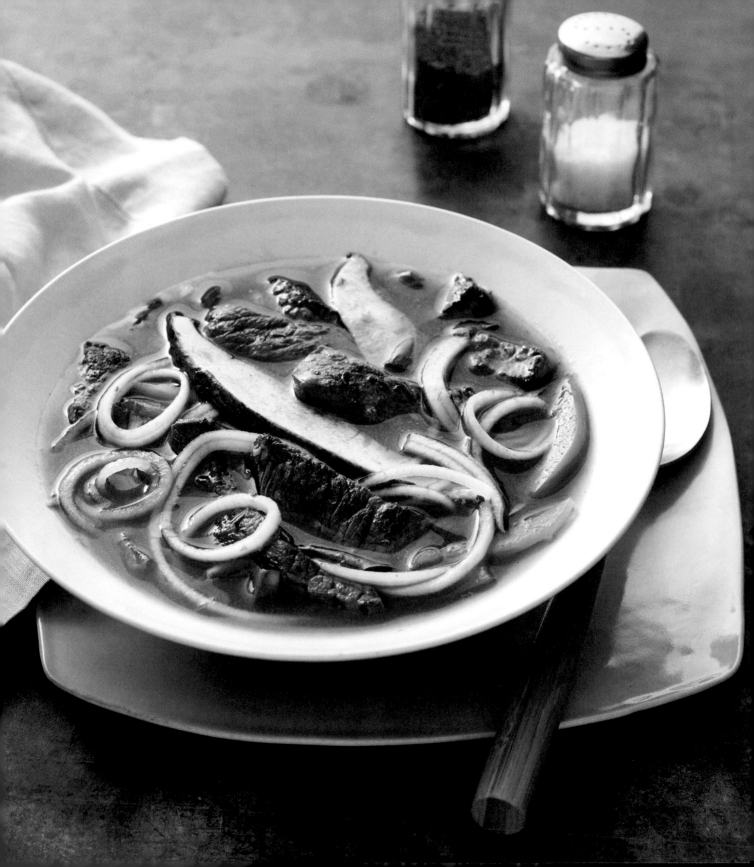

Steak and Portobello Rutabaga-Noodle Bowls

SERVES 6

Although they're edible, the gills on portobello mushrooms can turn an entire dish black and muddy-looking. It's almost always best to remove them before cooking.

PREP: 15 minutes

COOK: 20 minutes

TOTAL: 35 minutes

1 ½ pounds beef stir-fry strips

2 teaspoons Whole30-compliant Italian seasoning

½ teaspoon salt

½ teaspoon black pepper

2 tablespoons olive oil

1 bag (14 ounces) frozen bell pepper and onion blend

4 cups Whole30-compliant beef broth or Beef Bone Broth (page 280)

1 can (14.5 ounces) Whole30-compliant diced tomatoes with garlic and onion

2 portobello mushrooms, gills removed (see Tip), halved and sliced

1 medium rutabaga, spiralized or diced

1 cup fresh basil leaves

SEASON the meat with the Italian seasoning, salt, and pepper. Heat 1 tablespoon of the olive oil over medium-high heat in a large pot. Add half of the meat and cook, stirring occasionally, until browned but still pink in the center, 2 to 3 minutes. Transfer the meat to a bowl. Add the remaining 1 tablespoon olive oil to the pot and cook the remaining meat. Transfer the meat to the bowl.

ADD the frozen bell pepper and onion blend to the pot. Cook over medium heat, stirring occasionally, until tender, 3 to 4 minutes. Add the broth and tomatoes and bring to a boil.

ADD the mushrooms and rutabaga noodles and bring to a low boil. Cook until the mushrooms and rutabaga are just tender, 6 to 7 minutes. Return the meat to the pot, stir in the basil, and serve.

TIP *Use a spoon to scrape the gills from the mushrooms.*

Smoky Scallop Noodle Bowls

SERVES 2

The smokiness in this dish comes from smoked paprika, which is made from a type of mild pepper that's dried over wood-burning fires. We love it—you get so much flavor from a single ingredient!

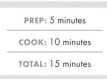

PREP: 5 minutes

COOK: 10 minutes

TOTAL: 15 minutes

1 pound small sea scallops

1 tablespoon smoked paprika

½ teaspoon salt

2 tablespoons Clarified Butter (page 283), ghee, or extra-virgin olive oil

2 cloves garlic, sliced

2 cups cherry tomatoes

1 cup Whole30-compliant chicken broth or Chicken Bone Broth (page 280)

1 tablespoon fresh lemon juice

2 packages (10.7 ounces each) zucchini noodles; or 2 medium zucchini, spiralized, long noodles snipped if desired

1 tablespoon chopped fresh parsley

RINSE the scallops and pat dry with a paper towel. Sprinkle the paprika and salt on the scallops. In a large heavy skillet, heat 1 tablespoon of the butter over medium-high heat. Add the scallops and sear on each side for 1 minute. (The scallops will not be cooked through at this point.) Remove the scallops from the skillet and cover to keep warm.

ADD the garlic and tomatoes to the skillet and cook over medium-high heat, stirring, until the tomatoes are lightly charred and start to burst, about 3 minutes. Add the broth, lemon juice, and scallops and cook until the scallops are just cooked, about 2 minutes.

MEANWHILE, in a large skillet, cook the zucchini noodles in the remaining 1 tablespoon butter until just tender, 1 to 2 minutes. Serve the scallops, tomatoes, and broth over the noodles in bowls. Top with the fresh parsley and serve.

Hearty Chinese Egg Drop Soup

SERVES 2

FROM *ChihYu Smith of I Heart Umami*

Egg drop soup is a super-common dish in many Asian households. Each region (and even household) has a slightly different take on the traditional soup. Some like to use chicken broth, while others use vegetable broth. I decided to make a heartier soup by adding ground chicken so that if you're hungry after work, the soup is very quick to put together and will fill you up in a hurry.

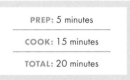

PREP: 5 minutes

COOK: 15 minutes

TOTAL: 20 minutes

2 teaspoons Clarified Butter (page 283) or ghee

2 green onions, chopped, white and green parts separated

2 teaspoons minced fresh ginger

½ pound ground chicken or turkey

1 cup sliced stemmed fresh shiitake mushrooms

½ teaspoon salt

3 cups Whole30-compliant chicken broth or Chicken Bone Broth (page 280)

2 tablespoons coconut aminos

½ teaspoon ground cumin

3 large eggs

Toasted sesame oil

HEAT the butter in a medium saucepan over medium-high heat. Add the white parts of the green onions and the ginger and cook, stirring, until fragrant, about 2 minutes. Add the ground chicken, mushrooms, and salt and cook until the chicken is no longer pink and the mushrooms are tender, 8 to 10 minutes. Add the broth, coconut aminos, and cumin, bring to a boil, then reduce the heat to a simmer.

IN a small bowl, whisk the eggs for 30 seconds. Holding a fork over the saucepan, slowly pour the eggs through the tines of the fork and whisk the broth gently as you pour. Let the soup stand for a few seconds to finish cooking the eggs.

TOP with the green parts of the green onions, drizzle with sesame oil, and serve.

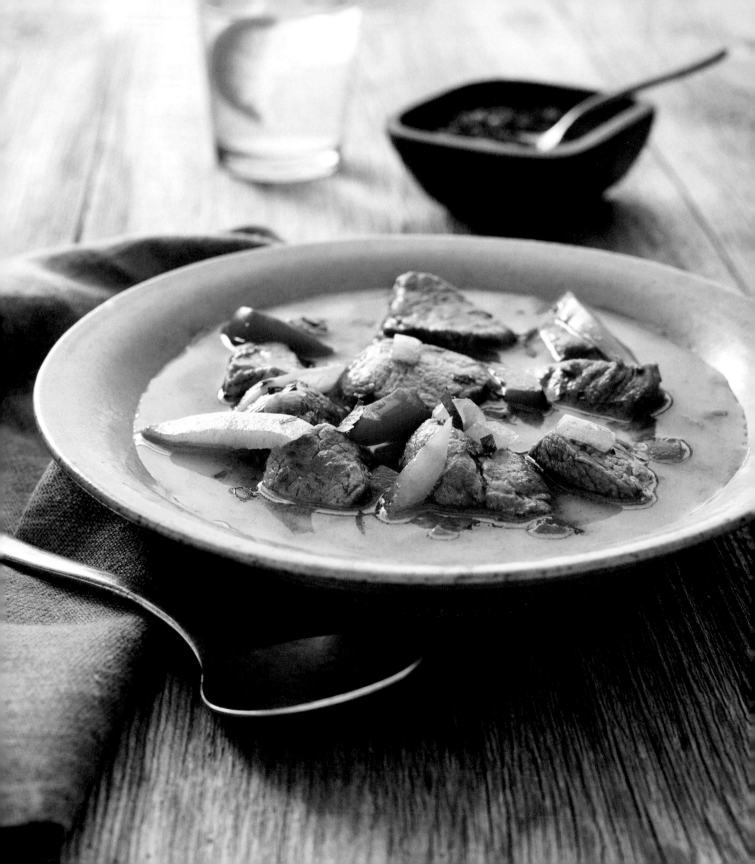

Quick Pork and Pepper Paprikash

SERVES 4

A quick cashew cream stands in for sour cream in this Hungarian-style dish. Be sure to use raw, unsalted cashews to make the cream.

PREP:	15 minutes
COOK:	25 minutes
TOTAL:	40 minutes

¾ cup chopped unsalted raw cashews

1¼ pounds pork tenderloin, cut into 1-inch pieces

½ teaspoon salt

½ teaspoon black pepper

2 tablespoons extra-virgin olive oil

1 package (14.4 ounces) frozen pepper stir-fry blend

2 tablespoons sweet paprika

1 teaspoon dried marjoram

3 tablespoons Whole30-compliant tomato paste

4 cups Whole30-compliant chicken broth or Chicken Bone Broth (page 280)

Chopped fresh parsley

FOR cashew cream, place the cashews in a small bowl and add boiling water to cover. Cover and let stand for 15 minutes. Drain and rinse the cashews. Combine the cashews and ½ cup fresh water in a blender. Puree until smooth, 3 to 4 minutes.

MEANWHILE, season the pork with the salt and black pepper. In a Dutch oven or large pot, heat the olive oil over medium-high heat. Add the pork and cook, stirring occasionally, until the pork begins to brown, about 5 minutes. Add the pepper stir-fry, paprika, and marjoram. Continue to cook, stirring occasionally, until the peppers are softened, about 5 minutes. Stir in the tomato paste and cook, stirring, 1 minute. Stir in the broth and bring to a boil. Reduce the heat to medium-low and simmer for 10 minutes. Remove from the heat. Stir in the cashew cream. Top each serving with parsley.

Apple-Butternut Squash Soup

SERVES 4

It doesn't get much more autumnal than this creamy, sweet, and golden-hued side-dish soup. Fresh ginger and cardamom provide a hit of warm spice.

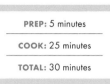

PREP: 5 minutes

COOK: 25 minutes

TOTAL: 30 minutes

2 tablespoons Clarified Butter (see page 283), ghee, or coconut oil

2 medium yellow onions, coarsely chopped

2 bags (10 ounces each) frozen diced butternut squash

2 medium apples (such as Braeburn or Fuji), halved, cored, and roughly chopped

2 tablespoons minced fresh ginger

1 teaspoon ground cardamom

1 teaspoon salt

½ teaspoon black pepper

4 cups chicken broth or Chicken Bone Broth (page 280)

⅔ cup Whole30-compliant coconut milk (see Tip)

2 tablespoons snipped fresh chives

IN a large saucepan, heat the butter over medium heat. Add the onion and cook, stirring often, until caramelized, 10 to 12 minutes. Add the squash and apples and cook, stirring, until browned and tender, 8 to 10 minutes. Stir in the ginger, cardamom, salt, and pepper. Add the broth, raise the heat, and bring to a boil. Reduce the heat and stir in the coconut milk.

CAREFULLY transfer the soup to a blender, in batches if necessary, and let cool briefly; pulse a few times, then blend until smooth. (Or use an immersion blender to blend the soup in the pot.) Top each serving with snipped chives.

TIP *Canned coconut milk separates in the can with the cream rising to the top. Be sure to whisk the coconut milk well before measuring.*

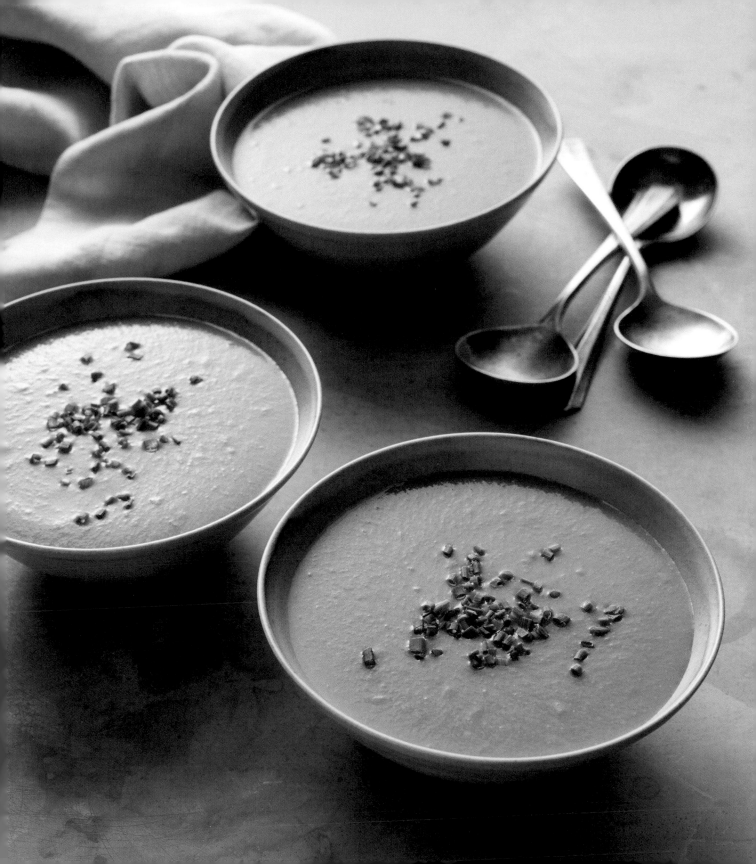

Veggie Noodle Soup with Basil Pesto

SERVES 4

When you're craving veggies, this light and summery soup packed with tomatoes, green beans, carrots, and zucchini noodles is immensely satisfying. The nutritional yeast in the pesto provides a cheesy flavor without cheese—genius!

PREP: 30 minutes
COOK: 15 minutes
TOTAL: 45 minutes

FOR THE PESTO

1 cup lightly packed fresh basil leaves

¼ cup roasted almonds or toasted pine nuts

1 tablespoon nutritional yeast (optional)

¼ teaspoon salt

¼ teaspoon black pepper

1 clove garlic, chopped

⅓ cup extra-virgin olive oil

FOR THE SOUP

1 tablespoon extra-virgin olive oil

1 medium onion, chopped

1 clove garlic, minced

4 cups Whole30-compliant chicken broth or Chicken Bone Broth (page 280)

1 can (14.5-ounces) Whole30-compliant diced tomatoes, undrained

½ pound fresh green beans, trimmed and cut into 1-inch pieces

½ teaspoon salt

¼ teaspoon black pepper

2 large, thick carrots, spiralized

1 package (16 ounces) very small cooked peeled deveined shrimp

1 package (10.7 ounces) zucchini noodles; or 2 small zucchini, spiralized

MAKE THE PESTO: In a food processor, combine the basil leaves, almonds, nutritional yeast (if using), salt, pepper, and garlic. Cover and pulse until finely chopped. With the food processor running, add the oil and process until well combined and nearly smooth.

MAKE THE SOUP: In a large pot, heat the olive oil over medium-high heat. Add the onion and garlic and cook, stirring frequently, until the onions are softened, about 3 minutes. Stir the broth, tomatoes, green beans, salt, and pepper into the pot and bring to a boil. Reduce the heat, cover, and simmer until the beans are crisp-tender, about 5 minutes. Add the carrot noodles and cook for 3 minutes. Add the shrimp and the zucchini noodles and cook until noodles are just tender, about 2 minutes more. Ladle the soup into bowls and top with some of the pesto.

TIP *Store leftover pesto in an airtight container in the refrigerator for up to 24 hours. Or, spoon 2 teaspoons pesto into each compartment of an ice cube tray. Cover tightly with foil and freeze. After frozen, transfer the pesto cubes to a resealable plastic bag and freeze for up to 1 month. To use, remove one portion of the pesto and bring to room temperature.*

Green Chile Pork Stew

SERVES 6

Don't be put off by the total time on this recipe. Almost all of it is inactive time when the stew is bubbling on the stove and you can be doing other things.

PREP: 10 minutes

COOK: 1 hour

TOTAL: 1 hour, 10 minutes

2 pounds boneless pork shoulder, cut into 1-inch pieces

½ teaspoon coarse salt

½ teaspoon black pepper

3 tablespoons Clarified Butter (page 283), ghee, or coconut oil

1 medium onion, chopped

2 cloves garlic, minced

4 cups Whole30-compliant chicken broth or Chicken Bone Broth (page 280)

2 cans (4.5 ounces each) chopped green chiles, undrained

1 pound small red potatoes, cut into ¾-inch pieces

1 small red bell pepper, cut into matchsticks

Snipped fresh cilantro (optional)

SEASON the pork with the salt and black pepper. Heat 1 tablespoon of the butter in a large pot over medium-high heat. Add half of the pork and cook, stirring occasionally, until browned on all sides, about 5 minutes. Transfer the pork to a plate. Add 1 tablespoon butter to the pot and repeat to cook the remaining pork.

ADD the remaining 1 tablespoon butter to the pot. Add the onion and cook, stirring, until tender, 2 to 3 minutes. Add the garlic and cook, stirring frequently, until fragrant, about 30 seconds. Add the broth, green chiles, and pork, bring to a boil, then reduce the heat to medium-low. Cook, covered, until the pork is tender, about 30 minutes.

ADD the potatoes and bell pepper to the pot and bring the stew to a boil. Cook, uncovered, until the potatoes are tender and the stew is slightly thickened, 8 to 10 minutes. Top servings with cilantro.

Mexican Chicken Soup

SERVES 4

Glossy, dark green poblano peppers have just a touch of heat and a wonderful fruity flavor. They help give this soup—along with fire-roasted tomatoes and chili powder—terrific toasty, smoky flavor. The sliced avocado on top provides creamy richness.

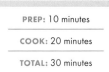

PREP: 10 minutes

COOK: 20 minutes

TOTAL: 30 minutes

1 tablespoon extra-virgin olive oil

½ cup chopped onion

1 medium poblano pepper, seeded and chopped

1 medium yellow or red bell pepper, chopped

2 cloves garlic, minced

½ teaspoon salt

4 cups Whole30-compliant chicken broth or Chicken Bone Broth (page 280)

1 can (14.5 ounces) Whole30-compliant fire-roasted diced tomatoes, undrained

2 teaspoons chili powder

3 cups shredded cooked chicken

Chopped fresh cilantro

1 avocado, halved, pitted, peeled, and sliced

Lime wedges

HEAT the olive oil in a large pot over medium-high heat. Add the onion, poblano, bell pepper, garlic, and salt. Cook, stirring frequently, until the vegetables are crisp-tender, 3 to 5 minutes.

STIR the broth, tomatoes, and chili powder into the pot and bring to a boil. Reduce the heat and simmer for 10 minutes. Add the chicken and heat through, about 1 minute.

SERVE the soup with cilantro, avocado, and lime wedges.

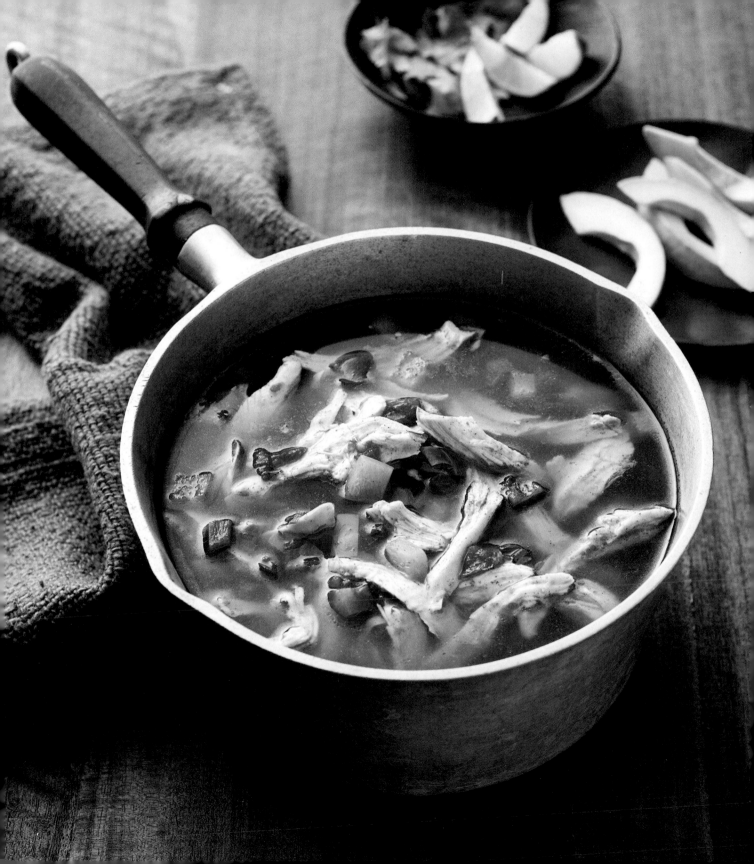

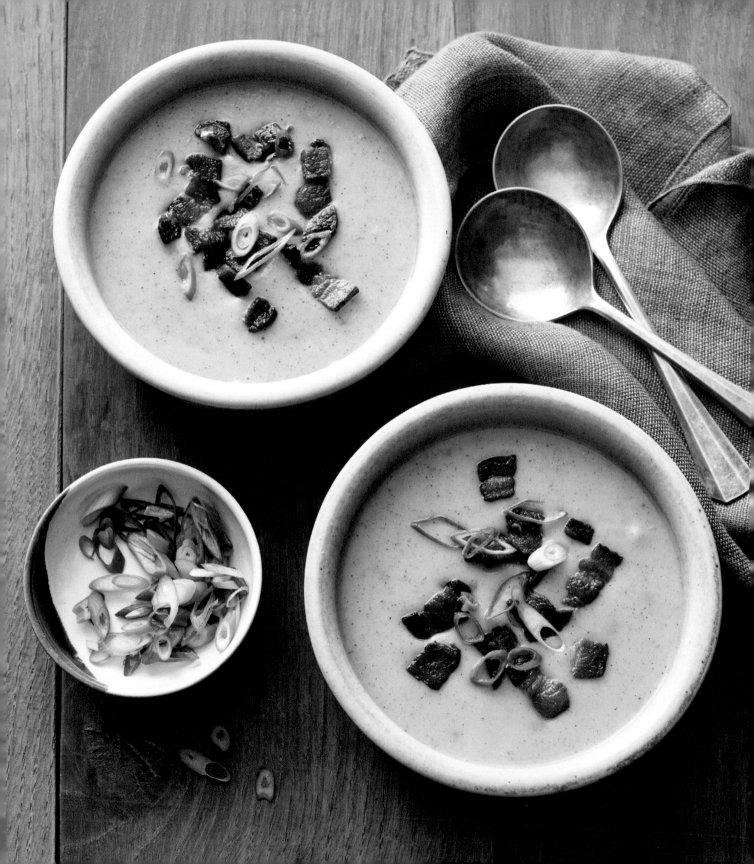

Creamy Turnip and Leek Soup

SERVES 4

FROM *Sarah Steffens of Savor and Fancy*

I never thought I would crave turnips or leeks, but maybe that was because I never prepared them as they are in this soup. Pureed soups have become a staple in my home because they are easy to make and pleasurable to consume. Zucchini blended into this dish gives it a velvety texture and you can never go wrong by garnishing any soup with crispy bacon and freshly minced scallion. Discover turnips and leeks for yourself in a whole new way and never look back!

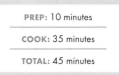

PREP: 10 minutes

COOK: 35 minutes

TOTAL: 45 minutes

4 slices Whole30-compliant bacon, diced

2 leeks, white parts only, cut into 1-inch pieces

2 turnips, peeled and chopped (about 3½ cups)

1 medium zucchini, ends removed and diced

1 can (14.5 ounces) Whole30-compliant coconut milk

1 cup Whole30-compliant chicken broth or Chicken Bone Broth (page 280)

1 teaspoon garlic powder

1 teaspoon onion powder

1 teaspoon dried rosemary

1 teaspoon salt

2 green onions, minced

IN a large pot, cook the bacon over medium-high heat until crisp, about 3 minutes. Use a slotted spoon to remove the bacon and drain on paper towels. Reserve the drippings in the pot.

REDUCE the heat to medium. Add the leeks to the pot and cook, stirring, until softened, about 3 minutes. Add the turnips and zucchini and continue to cook, stirring, until tender, about 5 minutes. Stir in the coconut milk, broth, garlic powder, onion powder, rosemary, and salt. Simmer the soup, covered, for 20 minutes.

CAREFULLY transfer the soup to a blender, in batches if necessary, and let cool briefly; blend until the soup is smooth and creamy. (Or use an immersion blender to blend the soup in the pot.) Top servings with the bacon and green onions.

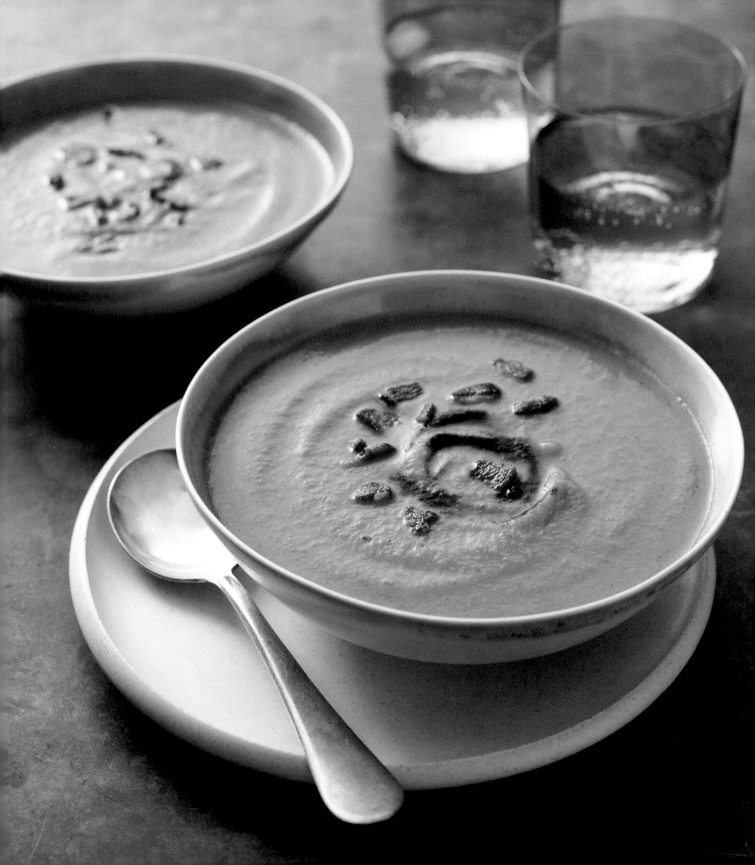

Carrot-Parsnip Soup with Bacon Crumble

SERVES 4 GENEROUSLY

Using a bag of petite baby carrots cuts down on the peeling and chopping needed to be done to make this creamy curried soup.

PREP: 10 minutes	
COOK: 20 minutes	
TOTAL: 30 minutes	

1 package (12 ounces) petite baby carrots

1 small onion, peeled and quartered

1 tablespoon extra-virgin olive oil

4 cups Whole30-compliant chicken broth or Chicken Bone Broth (page 280)

2 large parsnips, peeled and coarsely chopped

2 apples, peeled, cored, and chopped

1 tablespoon curry powder

½ teaspoon salt

1 cup apple cider

Balsamic vinegar

2 slices Whole30-compliant bacon, cooked and finely chopped

USING a food processor, coarsely chop the carrots and onion. Heat the olive oil in a large pot over medium heat. Add the onion and carrots and cook, stirring frequently, until the onion is softened, about 5 minutes. Stir in the broth, parsnips, apples, curry powder, and salt and bring to a boil. Reduce the heat and simmer until the parsnips are tender, about 15 minutes. Stir in the cider.

CAREFULLY transfer the soup to a blender, in batches if necessary, and let cool briefly; blend until the soup is smooth. (Or use an immersion blender to blend the soup in the pot.) Ladle the soup into bowls, drizzle with balsamic vinegar, and sprinkle with the bacon.

Winter Greens and Potato Soup with Poached Eggs

SERVES 4

This soup is inspired by the Brazilian potato and kale soup called *caldo verde* ("green broth"). Some versions add sausage into the mix. This one has poached eggs.

PREP: 10 minutes	
COOK: 30 minutes	
TOTAL: 40 minutes	

2 tablespoons extra-virgin olive oil, plus more for serving

2 small to medium leeks, halved lengthwise and sliced (1½ cups)

½ teaspoon salt

½ teaspoon black pepper

3 cloves garlic, minced

6 cups Whole30-compliant chicken broth or Chicken Bone Broth (page 280)

3 medium russet potatoes, peeled and diced

6 cups chopped greens, such as kale, collard greens, or mustard greens (see Tip)

½ cup packed chopped fresh parsley

Grated zest and juice of 1 lemon

8 large eggs

HEAT the olive oil over medium heat in a large pot. Add the leeks, salt, and pepper and cook, stirring occasionally, until the leeks are softened but not browned, about 4 minutes. Add the garlic and cook, stirring, for 1 minute. Stir in the broth and potatoes and bring to a boil. Reduce the heat, cover, and simmer until the potatoes are tender, about 10 minutes.

ADD the greens and cook over medium-high heat, stirring occasionally, until the greens are wilted, about 2 minutes. Reduce the heat to low and stir in the parsley and lemon zest. Break an egg into a small bowl and slide it into the soup. Repeat with the remaining eggs. Cover and simmer until the eggs are cooked to desired doneness, 4 to 6 minutes.

DRIZZLE each serving with lemon juice and olive oil. Season with salt and pepper to taste.

TIP *Look for washed and chopped greens near the packaged lettuce in the produce aisle of the supermarket.*

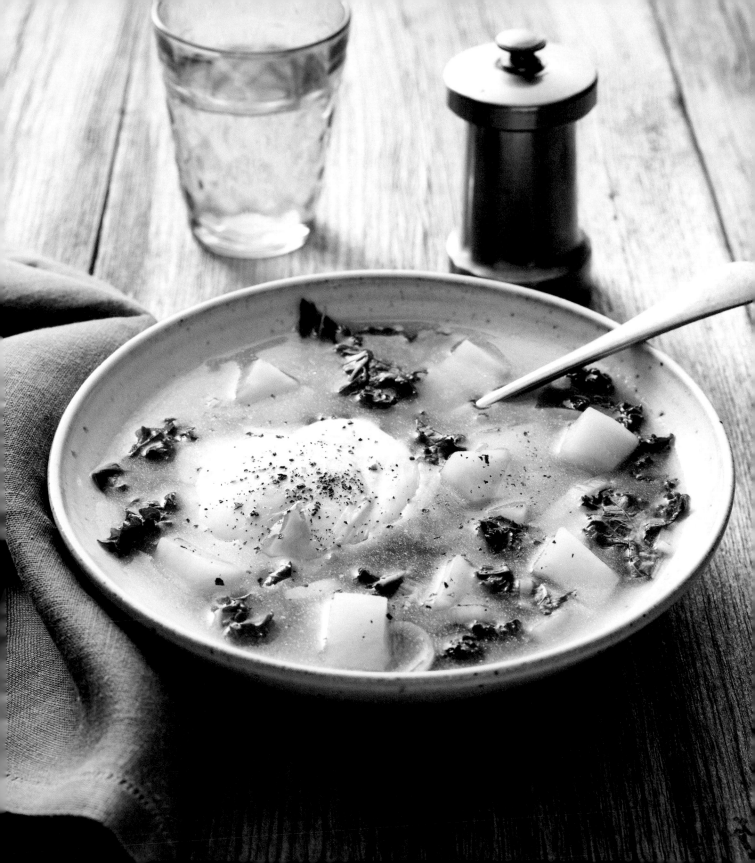

Fennel Soup with Spinach and Spicy Sausage

SERVES 4

FROM *Laura Miner of the Cook at Home Mom*

Fennel has a light licorice or anise flavor that comes through nicely in this soup, creating brightness in a hearty recipe. And the secret ingredient that makes it oh-so-creamy? Cauliflower!

PREP: 10 minutes	
COOK: 30 minutes	
TOTAL: 40 minutes	

1 pound Whole30-compliant spicy ground pork sausage (see Tip)

1 tablespoon extra-virgin olive oil

4 cups cauliflower florets

1 medium onion, coarsely chopped

3 stalks celery, coarsely chopped

1 fennel bulb, trimmed, cored, and coarsely chopped

2 cloves garlic, coarsely chopped

5 cups Whole30-compliant chicken broth or Chicken Bone Broth (page 280)

¼ teaspoon paprika

½ teaspoon black pepper

5 ounces fresh baby spinach leaves

IN a large heavy pot, brown the sausage over medium heat. Using a slotted spoon, transfer the sausage to a plate lined with paper towels to drain. Drain off any fat in the skillet.

HEAT the olive oil in the same pot over medium-high heat. Add the cauliflower, onion, celery, fennel, and garlic and cook, stirring occasionally, for 5 to 6 minutes. Stir in the broth, scraping up any browned bits on the bottom. Bring to a boil, reduce the heat, and simmer for 15 minutes.

CAREFULLY transfer the soup to a blender, in batches if necessary, and let cool briefly; blend until the soup is smooth and creamy. (Or use an immersion blender to blend the soup in the pot.) Return the soup to the pot and add the paprika and black pepper. Just before serving, stir the spinach and sausage into the soup.

TIP *To make your own spicy ground pork sausage, in a small bowl combine 1 tablespoon red pepper flakes, 2 teaspoons fennel seeds, 2 teaspoons garlic powder, 2 teaspoons dried oregano, 1 teaspoon paprika, 1 to 2 teaspoons salt, and 1 teaspoon black pepper. Use 1 tablespoon seasoning for each pound of ground pork. Store the seasoning in an airtight container up to 6 months.*

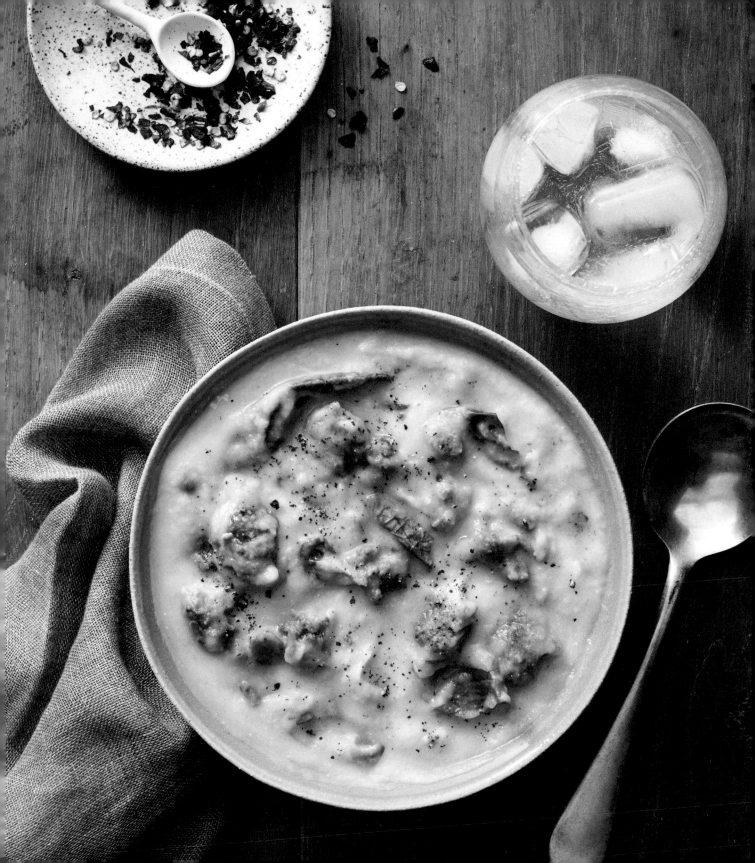

Asian Pork and Carrot-Noodle Bowls

SERVES 4

All you need to make the carrot noodles for this one-bowl meal flavored with ginger, garlic, toasted sesame oil, and spicy red pepper flakes is a vegetable peeler.

PREP: 15 minutes

COOK: 20 minutes

TOTAL: 35 minutes

FOR THE PORK

1 pound ground pork

2 teaspoons toasted sesame oil

2 green onions, sliced

2 teaspoons minced fresh ginger

2 cloves garlic, minced

⅛ teaspoon red pepper flakes

2 tablespoons coconut aminos

FOR THE CARROT NOODLES

4 large carrots, peeled

1 tablespoon Clarified Butter (page 283) or ghee

⅛ teaspoon salt

Chopped fresh cilantro

Lime wedges

MAKE THE PORK: In a large nonstick skillet, cook the pork over medium-high heat, breaking it up with a wooden spoon, until browned, about 10 minutes. Transfer to a bowl. Drain any fat from the skillet.

HEAT the sesame oil in the same skillet over medium heat. Add the green onions, ginger, garlic, and pepper flakes. Cook, stirring, until fragrant, 1 to 2 minutes. Stir in the pork and coconut aminos and heat through, about 1 minute.

MAKE THE CARROT NOODLES: Meanwhile, use a vegetable peeler to cut the carrots lengthwise into long, thin noodles. Heat the butter in a large skillet over medium heat. Add the carrot noodles and salt and cook, stirring occasionally, until just tender, 3 to 4 minutes.

SERVE the pork mixture on top of the carrot noodles. Top with cilantro and serve with lime wedges.

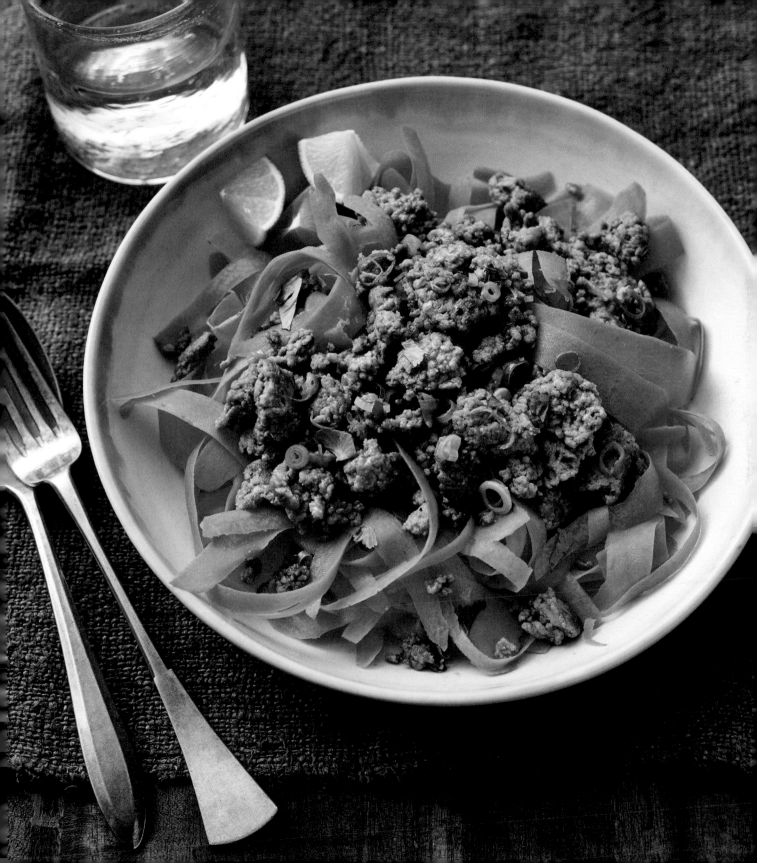

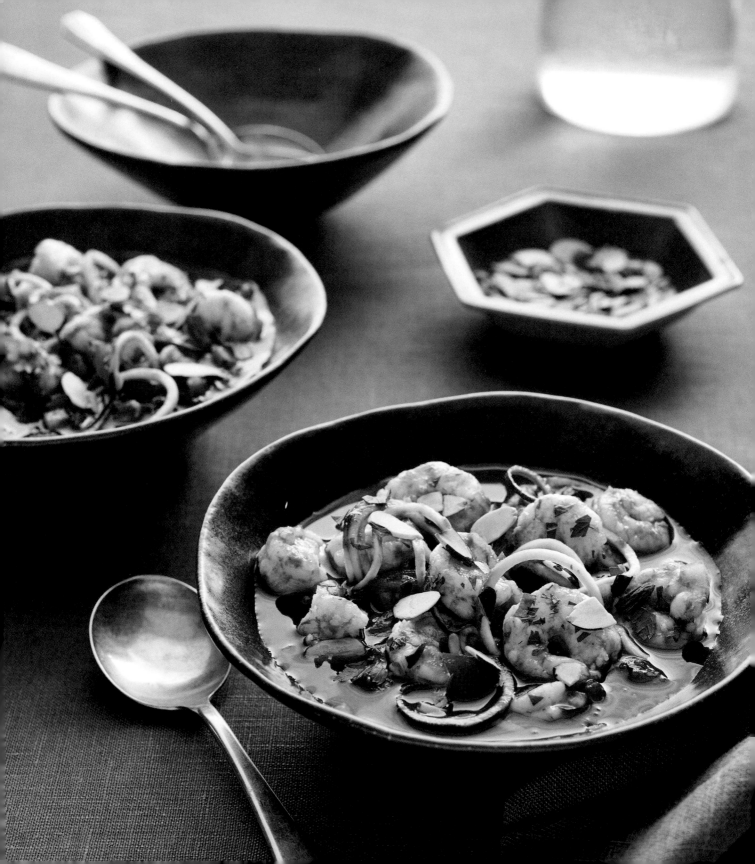

Gazpacho Noodle Soup

SERVES 4

This cool Mexican-style soup is super-refreshing on a hot day. Based on tomato juice and jarred salsa, it comes together in 5 minutes but does need to be chilled for a minimum of 2 hours. Make it in the morning and enjoy it for lunch or dinner.

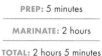

PREP: 5 minutes

MARINATE: 2 hours

TOTAL: 2 hours 5 minutes

1 package (16 ounces) very small cooked peeled deveined shrimp

1 package (10.7 ounces) zucchini noodles; or 2 small zucchini, spiralized and long noodles snipped

4 cups Whole30-compliant tomato juice or 100% vegetable juice

1½ cups fresh medium-hot salsa

¼ cup fresh lemon juice

¼ cup chopped fresh parsley and/or basil

⅓ cup sliced almonds, toasted (see Tip)

IN a large non-metal bowl, stir together the shrimp, zucchini, tomato juice, salsa, lemon juice, and half of the parsley. Cover and chill for 2 to 24 hours.

TO serve, top servings with the remaining parsley and almonds.

TIP *To toast almonds, place in a skillet over medium heat, stirring, until fragrant and lightly browned, about 2 minutes.*

Pork-Apple Meatball Noodle Bowls

SERVES 4

Two of the most familiar flavors of fall—sage and apple—come together in this hearty one-dish meal. We like Granny Smith apples for use in savory dishes because they are the tartest of all apple types.

PREP: 30 minutes
COOK: 20 minutes
TOTAL: 50 minutes

1 spaghetti squash (about 2 pounds)

5 tablespoons extra-virgin olive oil

½ cup minced shallots

½ Granny Smith apple, cored, peeled, and shredded

1 pound ground pork

1 large egg, lightly beaten

1 tablespoon minced fresh sage, plus 12 fresh sage leaves

¾ teaspoon salt

¼ teaspoon black pepper

1 cup Whole30-compliant chicken broth or Chicken Bone Broth (page 280)

2 teaspoons grated lemon zest

CUT the squash in half lengthwise and remove the seeds. Place the squash, cut sides down, in a 3-quart microwave-safe baking dish. Cover with plastic wrap, then pull back one corner to let the steam escape. Microwave until tender, 12 to 15 minutes.

MEANWHILE, heat 1 tablespoon of the olive oil in a large skillet over medium heat. Add the shallots and apple and cook, stirring occasionally, until tender, 3 to 5 minutes. Transfer to a large bowl. Reserve the skillet.

MIX the ground pork, egg, minced sage, ½ teaspoon of the salt, and the pepper into the apple mixture and shape into 20 (1-inch) meatballs.

IN the same large skillet, heat 1 tablespoon of the olive oil. Add the meatballs and cook, carefully turning occasionally, until the internal temperature is 160°F, about 10 minutes. Transfer the meatballs to a shallow bowl and cover with foil to keep warm. Add the broth to the hot skillet and scrape up any browned bits with a spatula. Add the broth to the meatballs.

WIPE out the large skillet, add 2 tablespoons of the olive oil, and heat over medium-high heat. Add the sage leaves and fry for 30 seconds, turning with tongs two or three times. Transfer the sage leaves to paper towels with a slotted spoon. (The leaves will crisp as they cool.)

USE forks to separate the squash into strands and place in a medium bowl. Add the remaining 1 tablespoon olive oil, the remaining ¼ teaspoon salt, and the lemon zest. Toss to combine.

DIVIDE the squash among 4 bowls. Add the meatballs and broth, top with the fried sage leaves, and serve.

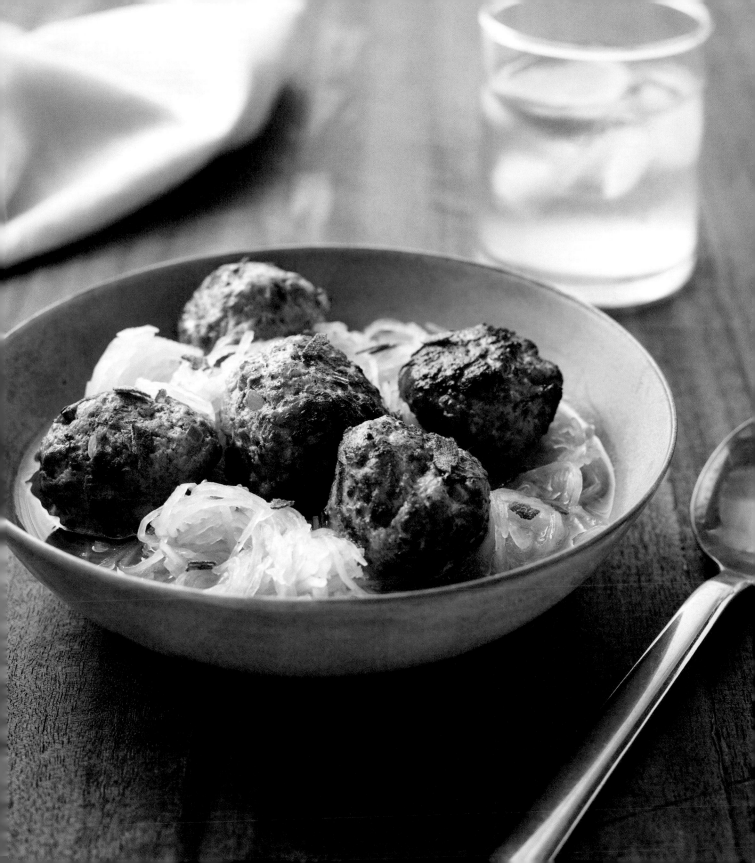

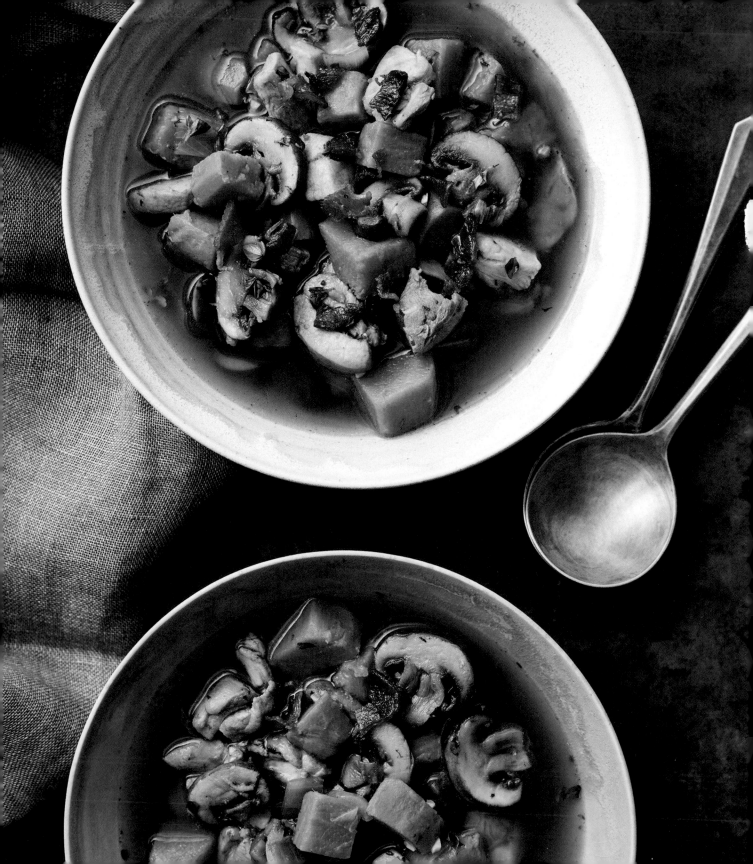

Chicken and Mushroom Soup

SERVES 4

A 3½-pound chicken will yield the 3 cups of coarsely chopped cooked meat you need for this soup. If you don't have leftover chicken in your refrigerator, look to a compliant rotisserie chicken from your grocery store.

PREP: 20 minutes

COOK: 25 minutes

TOTAL: 45 minutes

2 slices Whole30-compliant bacon, chopped

1 package (8 ounces) fresh cremini or button mushrooms, sliced

½ cup chopped onion

2 cloves garlic, minced

½ teaspoon salt

⅛ teaspoon red pepper flakes

4 cups Whole30-compliant chicken broth or Chicken Bone Broth (page 280)

3 medium sweet potatoes, peeled and chopped

3 cups coarsely chopped cooked chicken

2 teaspoons chopped fresh thyme

COOK the bacon in a large pot over medium heat, stirring frequently, until crisp, about 5 minutes. Transfer with a slotted spoon to paper towels to drain.

HEAT the bacon drippings in the pot over medium heat. Add the mushrooms, onion, garlic, salt, and pepper flakes and cook, stirring frequently, until the mushrooms are tender, 4 to 6 minutes. Stir in the broth and sweet potatoes. Bring to a boil then reduce the heat. Simmer, covered, until the sweet potatoes are tender, about 15 minutes.

ADD the chicken and thyme and heat through, about 1 minute. Top servings with the bacon.

Citrusy Fish Stew

SERVES 4

This is essentially a super-quick version of cioppino (chuh-PEE-noh), a stew created by Italian immigrant fisherman in San Francisco. It doesn't have a mix of fish and shellfish like traditional cioppino does, but the basic flavor notes—tomato, garlic, and fennel—are there.

PREP:	15 minutes
COOK:	10 minutes
TOTAL:	25 minutes

2 tablespoons extra-virgin olive oil

2 medium bulbs fennel, trimmed, cored, and coarsely chopped

1 medium red bell pepper, coarsely chopped

4 cloves garlic, chopped

2 teaspoons Whole30-compliant seafood seasoning

4 cups Whole30-compliant chicken broth or Chicken Bone Broth (page 280)

1 can (15 ounces) Whole30-compliant diced tomatoes, undrained

1 pound cod or other white fish fillets, cut into 1-inch pieces

Grated zest and juice of 1 tangerine (see Tip)

½ cup chopped fresh parsley (optional)

HEAT the olive oil in a large pot over medium heat. Add the fennel and bell pepper and cook, stirring occasionally, until just tender, about 5 minutes. Add the garlic and seafood seasoning and cook, stirring, for 1 minute. Add the broth and tomatoes and bring to a boil. Add the cod, reduce the heat, and simmer until the fish barely starts to flake when pulled apart, about 3 minutes. Remove from the heat. Stir in the juice and zest, and parsley, if desired, and serve.

TIP *If you can't find a tangerine, you can use a navel orange. You'll want 2 teaspoons zest and ¼ cup juice.*

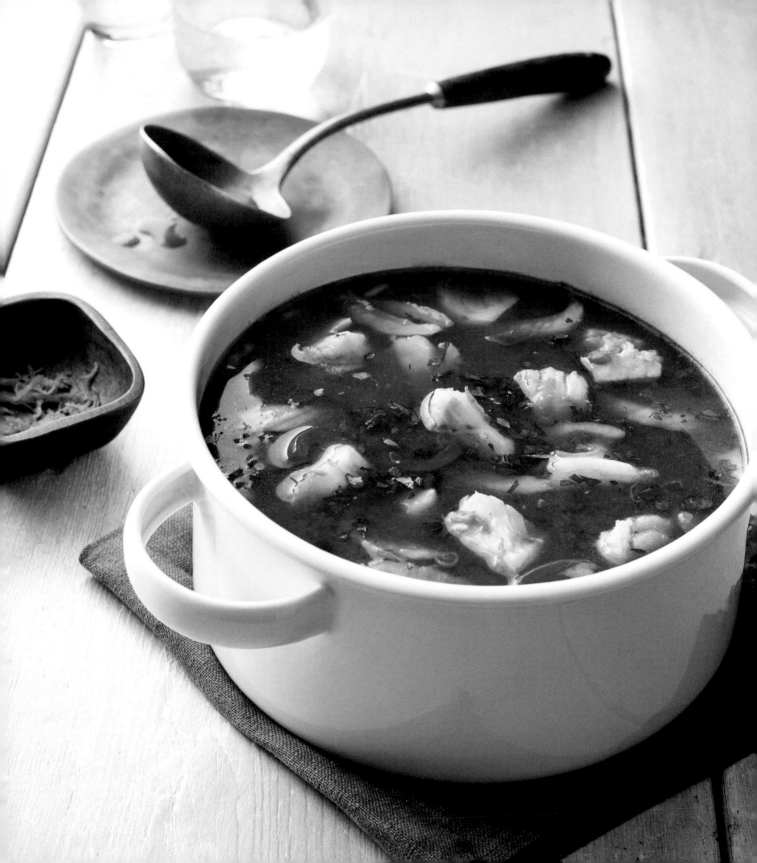

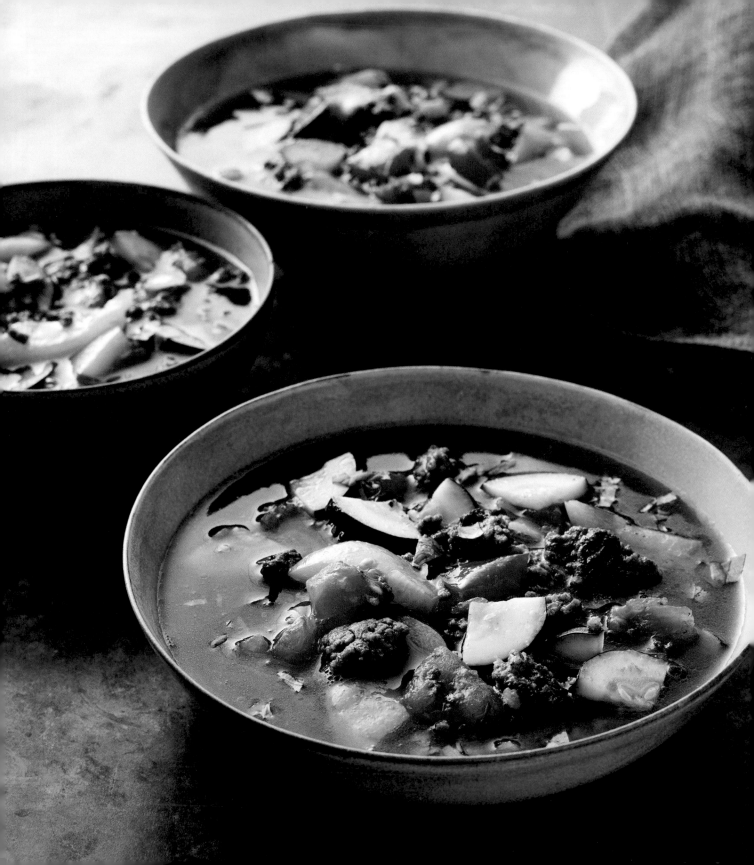

Italian Beef Soup

SERVES 4

This soup has very simple, clean flavors. If you like it a little spicier, use ¼ teaspoon of the red pepper flakes instead of the ⅛ teaspoon.

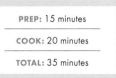

PREP: 15 minutes

COOK: 20 minutes

TOTAL: 35 minutes

1 pound ground beef

½ cup chopped onion

2 cloves garlic, minced

4 cups Whole30-compliant beef broth or Beef Bone Broth (page 280)

1 medium yellow or red bell pepper, chopped

1 medium zucchini, quartered lengthwise, then slice the quarters

1 teaspoon salt

¼ teaspoon black pepper

⅛ teaspoon red pepper flakes

3 medium Roma (plum) tomatoes, coarsely chopped

2 tablespoons chopped fresh basil

IN a large pot, cook the ground beef, onion, and garlic over medium heat, stirring to break up the meat, until the meat is browned, about 5 minutes. Drain off any fat.

STIR the broth, bell pepper, zucchini, salt, pepper, and pepper flakes into the pot and bring the soup to a boil. Reduce the heat and simmer until the vegetables are tender, 8 to 10 minutes. Add the tomatoes and cook until heated through, about 2 minutes more. Stir in the fresh basil and serve.

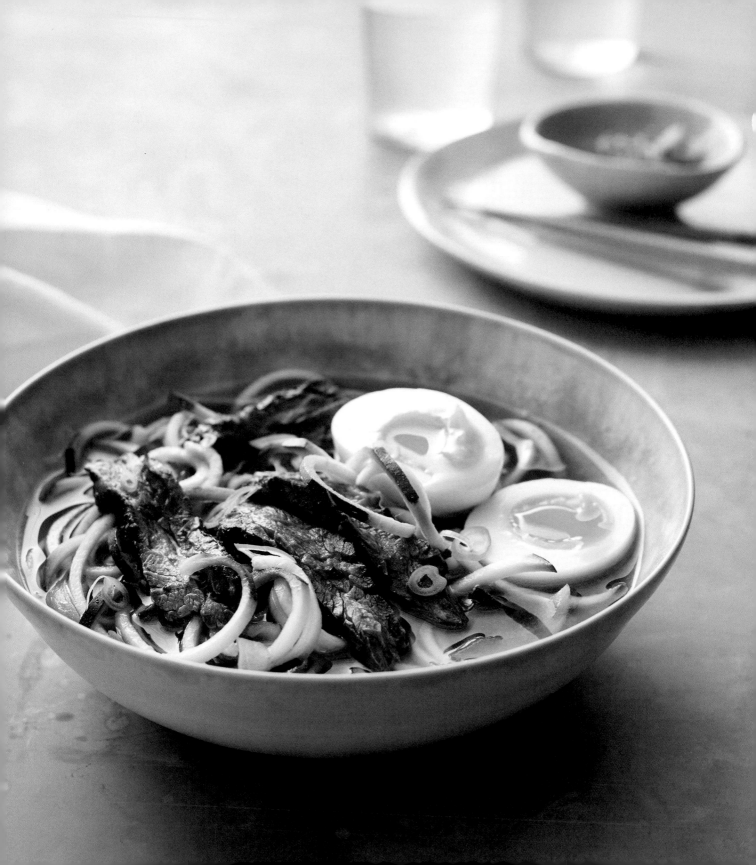

Flank Steak with Zucchini Noodle Ramen

SERVES 4

Marinate the steak for a minimum of 1 hour and up to 4 hours. Of course, the longer it sits in the marinade of olive oil, toasted sesame oil, garlic and ginger, the tastier it will be.

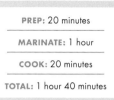

PREP: 20 minutes	
MARINATE: 1 hour	
COOK: 20 minutes	
TOTAL: 1 hour 40 minutes	

¼ cup extra-virgin olive oil

¼ cup sesame oil

4 cloves garlic, minced

4 teaspoons minced fresh ginger

2 teaspoons salt

½ teaspoon black pepper

1 pound beef skirt steak or scored flank steak

1 small onion, halved and thinly sliced

6 cups Whole30-compliant beef broth of Beef Bone Broth (page 280)

2 packages (10.7 ounces) zucchini noodles; or 3 medium zucchini, spiralized

4 large eggs, soft-cooked and halved (see Tip)

2 green onions, sliced

IN a small bowl, combine the olive oil, sesame oil, garlic, ginger, salt, and pepper. Spoon 2 tablespoons of the seasoned oil into a large resealable plastic bag. Set the remaining seasoned oil aside for the ramen. Add the steak to the bag; seal and turn to coat the steak. Marinate in the refrigerator, turning occasionally, for 1 to 4 hours.

PREHEAT the grill to medium (350° to 375°F). Remove the steak from the marinade and discard the marinade. Grill the steak over direct heat until the internal temperature is 145° to 150°F, 10 to 12 minutes for skirt steak, or 15 to 17 minutes for flank steak. Place the steak on a cutting board and let rest for 5 minutes before slicing.

MEANWHILE, in a large pot, heat the remaining seasoned oil over medium heat. Add the onion and cook, stirring, until tender, 3 to 4 minutes. Add the broth and bring to a boil. Reduce the heat to low, cover, and simmer for 10 minutes. Add the zucchini noodles and cook until the noodles are tender, 1 to 2 minutes.

LADLE the soup and noodles into bowls. Top with the sliced steak, halved eggs, and green onions and serve.

TIP *To make soft-cooked eggs, fill a large saucepan with 3 to 4 inches of water. Bring to a full rolling boil over high heat. Reduce the heat to a rapid simmer and gently lower the eggs into the water. Cook the eggs for 7 minutes. Remove the eggs with a slotted spoon and place in a bowl filled with ice and water.*

Salisbury Steak Meatball and Noodle Bowls

SERVES 4

Good old Salisbury steak—beef patties traditionally made with bread crumbs, onion, celery, and mustard and topped with a pan sauce—get a Whole30 makeover (and a new shape!) in this comfort-food recipe.

PREP:	15 minutes
COOK:	25 minutes
TOTAL:	40 minutes

FOR THE MEATBALLS

⅓ cup finely chopped red onion

⅓ cup finely chopped celery

1 large egg, lightly beaten

2 tablespoons almond flour

2 teaspoons Whole30-compliant coarse ground mustard

¼ teaspoon salt

¼ teaspoon black pepper

1 pound ground beef

1 tablespoon extra-virgin olive oil

1 cup Whole30-compliant beef broth or Beef Bone Broth (page 280)

FOR THE NOODLES

1 tablespoon extra-virgin olive oil

2 packages (10.7 ounces each) sweet potato noodles, or 2 medium sweet potatoes, peeled and spiralized

⅛ teaspoon salt

⅛ teaspoon black pepper

Chopped fresh parsley

FOR THE GRAVY

½ cup Whole30-compliant beef broth or Beef Bone Broth (page 280)

¼ cup Whole30-compliant tomato paste

1 tablespoon arrowroot powder

MAKE THE MEATBALLS: In a medium bowl, mix together the onion, celery, egg, almond flour, mustard, salt, and pepper. Add the beef and gently mix to combine. Shape into 16 meatballs.

IN a large skillet, heat the olive oil over medium heat. Add the meatballs and cook for 3 minutes. Gently turn the meatballs over and cook for 3 minutes more. Add the broth and bring to a boil. Reduce the heat and simmer, covered, until the internal temperature of the meatballs is 160°F, about 5 minutes more. Transfer the meatballs to a plate with a slotted spoon and cover to keep warm. (Reserve the cooking liquid in the skillet.)

MAKE THE NOODLES: Meanwhile, in another large skillet, heat the olive oil over medium-high heat. Add the sweet potato noodles and gently toss to coat. Cook, tossing occasionally, until the noodles are tender, 8 to 10 minutes. Season with the salt and pepper.

MAKE THE GRAVY: In a small bowl, whisk together the broth, tomato paste, and arrowroot. Whisk into the cooking liquid in the skillet and cook over medium-high heat, stirring, until the gravy is thickened, 1 to 2 minutes. Remove from the heat.

SERVE the meatballs on top of the noodles. Spoon the gravy over the top and sprinkle with parsley.

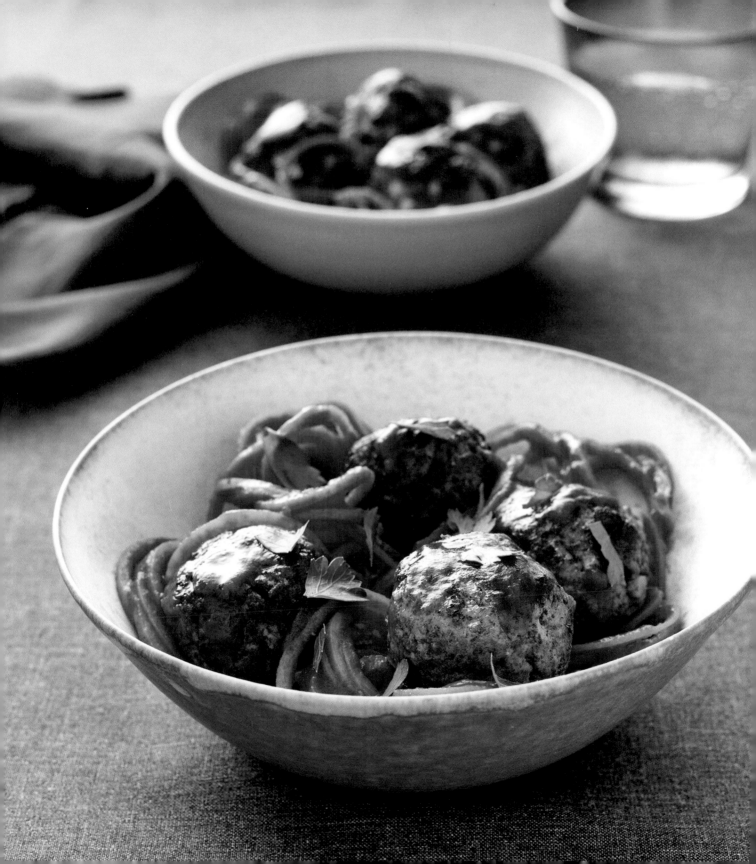

Quick Turkey Sausage and Sweet Potato Soup

SERVES 4

Most commercially available Italian sausage contains sugar or corn syrup (and often other no-nos), so although that is not a shortcut you can take, our fennel-and-garlic-flavored version comes together in minutes.

PREP: 10 minutes

COOK: 20 minutes

TOTAL: 30 minutes

1¼ pounds ground turkey

2 teaspoons fennel seeds, crushed

2 teaspoons ground paprika

4 cloves garlic, minced

1 tablespoon extra-virgin olive oil

4 cups Whole30-compliant chicken broth or Chicken Bone Broth (page 280)

1 package (16 ounces) frozen fire-roasted sweet potatoes

1 can (15 ounces) Whole30-compliant fire-roasted tomatoes with garlic

2 teaspoons Whole30-compliant Italian seasoning

½ cup chopped fresh basil

COMBINE the turkey, fennel seeds, paprika, and garlic in a large bowl. Use your hands to mix well.

HEAT the olive oil in a large pot over medium heat. Add the turkey and cook, stirring frequently, until lightly browned, 8 to 10 minutes. Add the broth, sweet potatoes, tomatoes, and Italian seasoning and bring to a boil. Reduce the heat and simmer, stirring occasionally, until the sweet potatoes are tender, about 10 minutes. Stir in the basil and serve.

Southwest Chicken Noodle Bowl

SERVES 4

Use a mix of sweet peppers—red, yellow, or orange—to make the most colorful bowls.

PREP: 15 minutes

COOK: 15 minutes

TOTAL: 30 minutes

1 pound boneless, skinless chicken breast halves, thinly sliced

1 tablespoon Whole30-compliant Southwest seasoning

2 tablespoons extra-virgin olive oil

4 cups Whole30-compliant chicken broth or Chicken Bone Broth (page 280)

1 large red and/or yellow bell pepper, chopped

4 green onions, trimmed and cut diagonally into 1-inch pieces

1 medium russet potato, peeled and spiralized

1 cup fresh Whole30-compliant salsa

2 tablespoons fresh lime juice

SPRINKLE the chicken all over with the Southwest seasoning. Heat 1 tablespoon of the olive oil in an extra-large skillet over medium-high heat. Add half the chicken and cook, stirring occasionally, until no longer pink on the outside, about 2 minutes (the chicken will not be cooked through). Transfer the chicken to a plate. Add the remaining olive oil and chicken to the skillet. Cook the chicken until no longer pink, 2 to 3 minutes. Return all of the chicken to the skillet.

ADD the broth and bring to a boil. Stir in the bell peppers, green onions, and potato noodles and return to a boil. Reduce the heat and simmer, stirring occasionally, until the vegetables are tender and the chicken is cooked through, 3 minutes. Gently stir in the salsa and lime juice and serve.

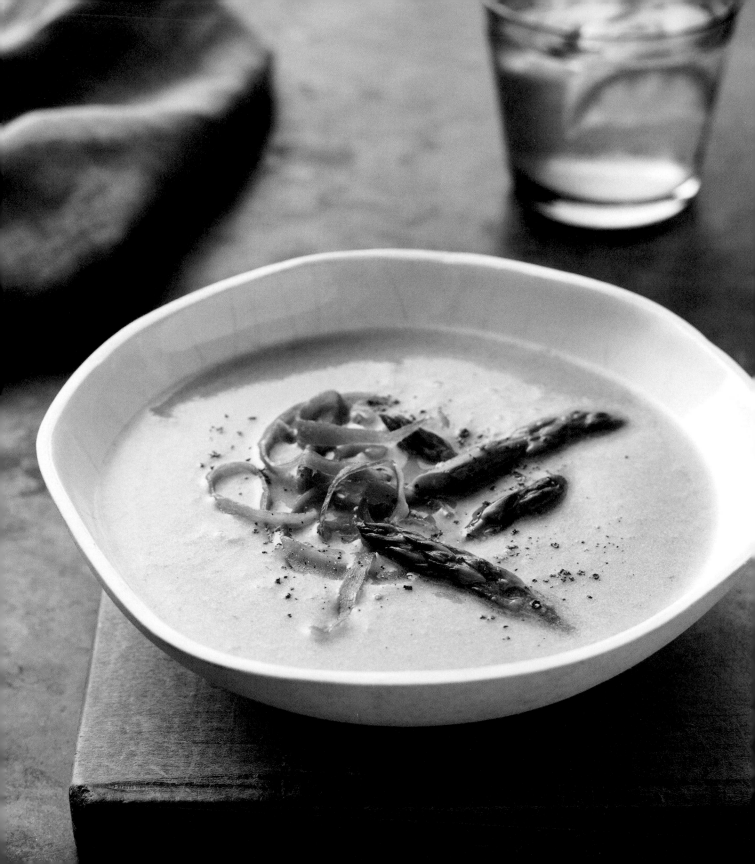

Asparagus Cream Soup

SERVES 4

This gorgeous pale green soup has spring written all over it. It's creamy and delicately flavored and topped with ribbons of prosciutto. If you're not a fan of tarragon—or can't find it—fresh basil makes a good substitute.

PREP: 25 minutes
COOK: 25 minutes
TOTAL: 50 minutes

2 tablespoons coconut oil

1 medium onion, chopped

2 bunches asparagus (about 2 pounds)

5 cups Whole30-compliant chicken broth or Chicken Bone Broth (page 280)

1 tablespoon chopped fresh tarragon

½ cup Whole30-compliant coconut milk (see Tip)

2 tablespoons fresh lemon juice

½ teaspoon salt

¼ teaspoon black pepper

2 slices Whole30-compliant prosciutto, rolled up and cut into thin ribbons

HEAT the coconut oil in a large pot over medium heat. Add the onion and cook, stirring occasionally, until tender, about 5 minutes.

MEANWHILE, cut the tips off the asparagus and set aside. Cut the asparagus stalks into 1-inch pieces, discarding any woody ends. Add the stalk pieces, broth, and tarragon to the onion and bring to a boil. Reduce the heat to low and cook for 15 minutes. Place the asparagus tips in a metal steamer and lower into the broth mixture. Cook, uncovered, just until tender, about 4 minutes. Carefully remove the strainer and run the tips under cold water; set aside. Remove the pot from the heat and stir in the coconut milk and lemon juice.

CAREFULLY transfer the soup in batches to a blender, in batches if necessary, and let cool briefly; pulse a few times, then blend until smooth. (Or use an immersion blender to blend the soup directly in the pot.) Season with salt and pepper. Top servings with the asparagus tips and prosciutto ribbons.

TIPS *Canned coconut milk separates in the can with the cream rising to the top. Be sure to whisk the coconut milk well before measuring.*

Serve this velvety soup with perfectly cooked chicken breasts: Lightly pound 4 boneless, skinless chicken breasts chicken (about 6 ounces each) to ¼-inch thickness with a meat mallet. Sprinkle the chicken with salt and coarsely ground black pepper. Heat 2 tablespoons extra-virgin olive oil in a large heavy skillet over medium-high heat. Reduce the heat to medium and add the chicken. Cook until the internal temperature is 165°F, turning once, 5 to 6 minutes.

Southwest "Breakfast for Dinner" Bowls

SERVES 4

In your pre-Whole30 days, "breakfast for dinner" might have meant pancakes or waffles swimming in maple syrup. Now it's these savory bowls of sausage, sweet potato, green peppers, and fried eggs topped with salsa. We promise you will feel so much better when you go to bed!

PREP: 25 minutes

COOK: 25 minutes

TOTAL: 50 minutes

2 tablespoons coconut oil

1 package (12 to 14 ounces) Whole30-compliant smoked kielbasa or Polish beef sausage, thinly sliced crosswise

1 medium sweet potato, peeled, halved lengthwise, and thinly sliced crosswise

1 small green bell pepper, cut into strips

1 package (16 ounces) cauliflower crumbles, or 4 cups raw cauliflower rice (see page 75)

2 green onions, thinly sliced

1 tablespoon Clarified Butter (page 283) or ghee

4 large eggs

¼ teaspoon salt

⅛ to ¼ teaspoon black pepper

¾ cup Whole30-compliant salsa

HEAT 1 tablespoon of the coconut oil in a large skillet over medium heat. Add the kielbasa and sweet potato, cover, and cook, stirring occasionally, for 5 minutes. Uncover and cook, stirring occasionally, until the potato is tender and the kielbasa is browned, about 5 minutes.

MEANWHILE, heat the remaining 1 tablespoon coconut oil in a large nonstick skillet over medium heat. Add the bell pepper and cook, stirring occasionally, for 4 minutes. Add the cauliflower crumbles and green onions and cook, stirring occasionally, until the pepper is just tender and the cauliflower is heated through, 4 to 6 minutes more.

SPOON the sausage and potatoes and the cauliflower into shallow bowls. Cover with foil to keep warm.

HEAT the butter in the nonstick skillet over medium heat. Break the eggs into the skillet and sprinkle with the salt and black pepper. Reduce the heat to medium-low. Cook the eggs until the whites are completely set and the yolks start to thicken, 2 to 3 minutes. Carefully turn the eggs over. Cook until the yolks are to desired doneness, 1 to 1½ minutes more.

UNCOVER the bowls and place an egg on top. Spoon the salsa on top and serve.

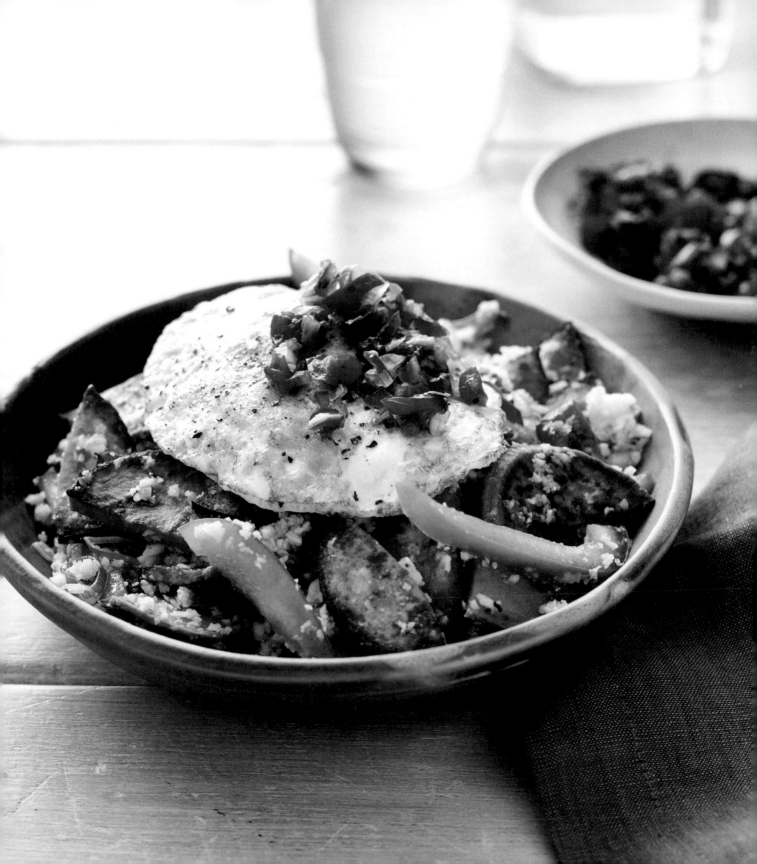

Creamy Broccoli-Kale Soup

SERVES 4

Two of the most nutritious green vegetables—one cruciferous, one leafy—come together in this superfood soup!

PREP: 15 minutes	
COOK: 15 minutes	
TOTAL: 30 minutes	

1 tablespoon extra-virgin olive oil

2 leeks, white parts only, cut into 1-inch pieces

2 cloves garlic, minced

1 pound broccoli, trimmed and coarsely chopped (about 4 cups)

1 bunch kale, stalks removed, leaves chopped

½ teaspoon salt

⅛ teaspoon red pepper flakes

5 cups Whole30-compliant chicken broth or Chicken Bone Broth (page 280)

1 can (13.5 ounces) Whole30-compliant coconut milk

IN a large pot, heat the olive oil over medium heat. Add the leeks and garlic and cook, stirring frequently, until the leeks are softened, 3 to 5 minutes.

STIR in the broccoli, kale, salt, pepper flakes, and broth. Bring to a boil. Reduce the heat to low. Cover and simmer, stirring occasionally, until the broccoli is tender, about 10 minutes. Add 1 cup of the coconut milk and cook until heated through, about 1 minute.

CAREFULLY transfer the soup to a blender, in batches if necessary, and let cool briefly; pulse a few times, then blend until smooth and return to the pot. (Or use an immersion blender and blend directly in the pot.) Top servings of the soup with a swirl of the remaining coconut milk.

TIP *A delicious protein to serve with this creamy soup is herbes de Provence steaks: Preheat the grill to medium (375°F to 400°F). Brush 4 (1-inch-thick) boneless ribeye steaks with 1 tablespoon extra-virgin olive oil. In a small bowl, combine 1 tablespoon herbes de Provence (crushed) and ½ teaspoon each salt and black pepper. Sprinkle the seasoning over both sides of the steaks and rub in with your fingers. Grill the steaks over direct heat, turning once, 10 to 12 minutes for medium rare (145°F) or 12 to 15 minutes for medium (160°F). Remove the steaks from the grill and let stand, covered, for 5 minutes.*

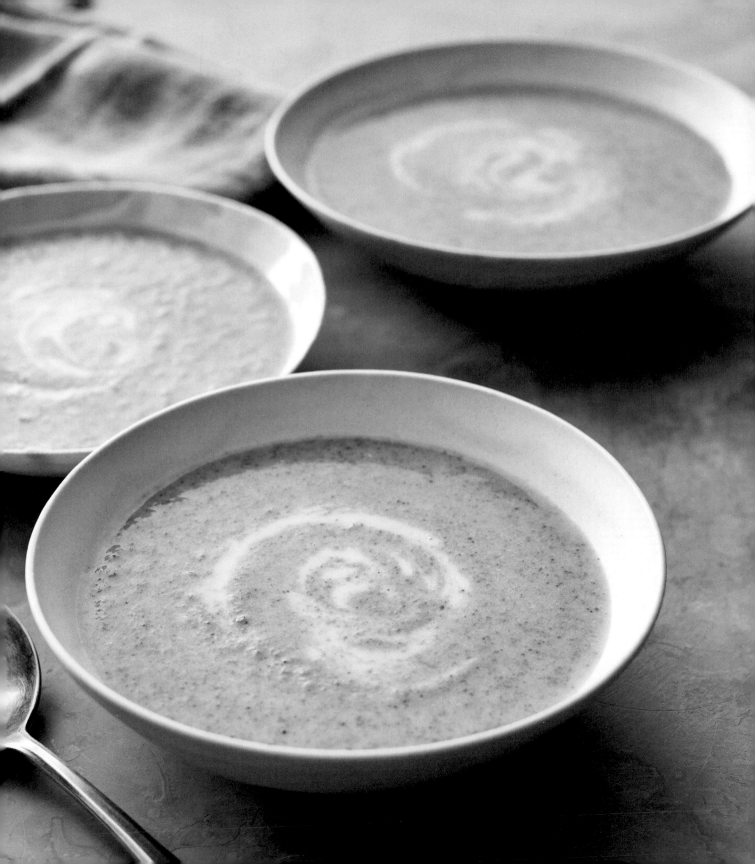

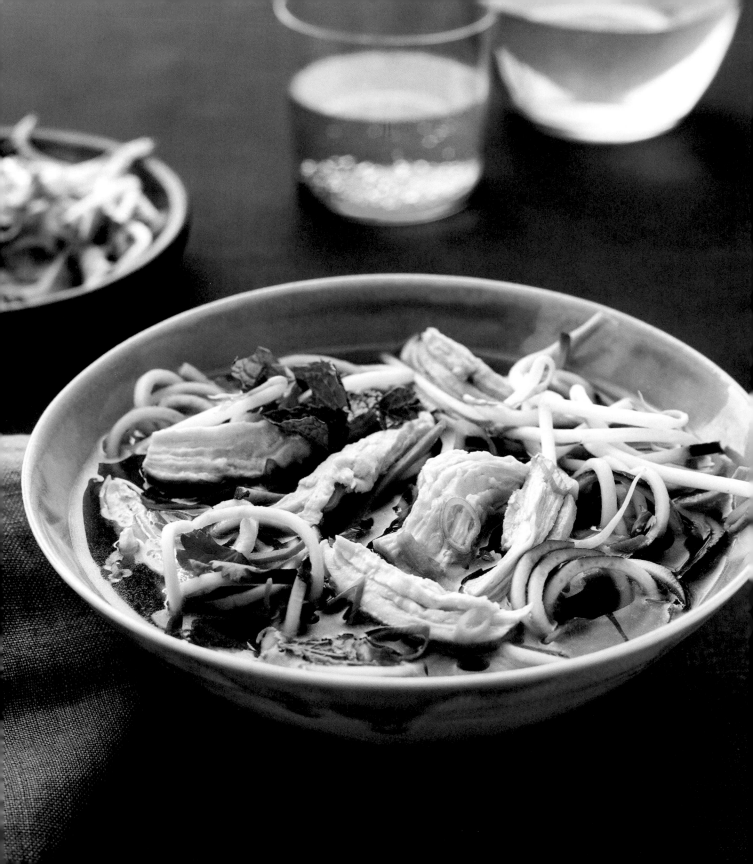

Chicken Zoodle Pho

SERVES 2

The Vietnamese noodle soup called pho (pronounced FUH) has enthusiastically been adopted into the American diet. The traditional soup takes hours to cook and contains rice noodles. This light, fresh, and fast Whole30 version featuring zucchini noodles has the same soul-soothing effect but takes just 30 minutes to put on the table.

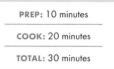

PREP: 10 minutes

COOK: 20 minutes

TOTAL: 30 minutes

1 tablespoon coconut oil

1 large boneless, skinless chicken breast (about 8 ounces)

2 cups Whole30-compliant chicken broth or Chicken Bone Broth (page 280)

1 tablespoon minced fresh ginger

2 teaspoons Red Boat fish sauce

⅛ to ¼ teaspoon red pepper flakes

1½ cups packaged zucchini noodles; or 1 small zucchini, spiralized

½ cup packaged shredded carrots or 1 medium carrot, shredded

¼ cup sliced green onions

2 tablespoons chopped fresh cilantro, plus more for garnish if desired

½ cup fresh bean sprouts

2 tablespoons chopped fresh mint

HEAT the coconut oil in a large saucepan over medium-high heat. Add the chicken and cook, turning once, until well-browned on both sides, 6 to 8 minutes. (The chicken will not be cooked through at this point.) Remove the pan from the heat. Carefully add the broth, ginger, fish sauce, and pepper flakes. Return to the heat and bring to a boil. Reduce the heat and simmer, covered, until the internal temperature of the chicken is 165°F, 5 to 6 minutes. Transfer the chicken to a cutting board to cool slightly.

ADD the zucchini noodles and carrots to the hot broth. Cook over medium-high heat until the vegetables are crisp-tender, 1 to 2 minutes.

USING two forks, coarsely shred the chicken. Add the chicken back to the pan and gently stir in the green onions and cilantro. Top servings with bean sprouts, mint, and additional cilantro if using.

Ratatouille Stew with Seared Scallops

SERVES 4

The key to getting a nicely browned crust on seared scallops is to ensure the scallops are perfectly dry when they go into the hot pan and to not move them before it's time to turn them.

PREP: 20 minutes

COOK: 30 minutes

TOTAL: 50 minutes

3 tablespoons extra-virgin olive oil

1 cup sliced fresh cremini or button mushrooms

1 medium onion, chopped

3 cups cubed eggplant, peeled if desired

1 yellow or orange bell pepper, cut into thin bite-size strips

1 small zucchini, trimmed, halved lengthwise, and cut crosswise into ¼-inch-thick half-moons

4 cloves garlic, minced

1 cup Whole30-compliant vegetable broth

1 large (6 ounces) Yukon Gold potato, scrubbed and cut into 1-inch pieces

2 sprigs fresh rosemary

½ teaspoon coarse salt

½ teaspoon black pepper

1 can (28 ounces) Whole30-compliant diced tomatoes, undrained

12 fresh or thawed frozen sea scallops (about 18 ounces total)

1 tablespoon minced fresh thyme

IN a 4- to 6-quart pot, heat 1 tablespoon of the olive oil over medium-high heat. Add the mushrooms and onion and cook, stirring occasionally, for 2 to 3 minutes. Add 1 tablespoon of the remaining olive oil, the eggplant, bell pepper, zucchini, and garlic. Cook, stirring occasionally, for 3 minutes more. Add the broth, potato, rosemary, ¼ teaspoon of the salt, and ¼ teaspoon of the black pepper and bring to a boil. Reduce the heat and simmer, covered, until the potato is just tender, 10 to 12 minutes.

ADD the tomatoes. Cook, uncovered, until the stew is thickened to desired consistency, 8 to 10 minutes more.

MEANWHILE, sprinkle the scallops with the remaining ¼ teaspoon salt and ¼ teaspoon black pepper. In a large skillet, heat the remaining 1 tablespoon olive oil over medium-high heat. Add the scallops and cook, turning once halfway through cooking, until opaque, 4 to 6 minutes.

STIR the fresh thyme into the stew. Top each serving with 3 scallops and serve.

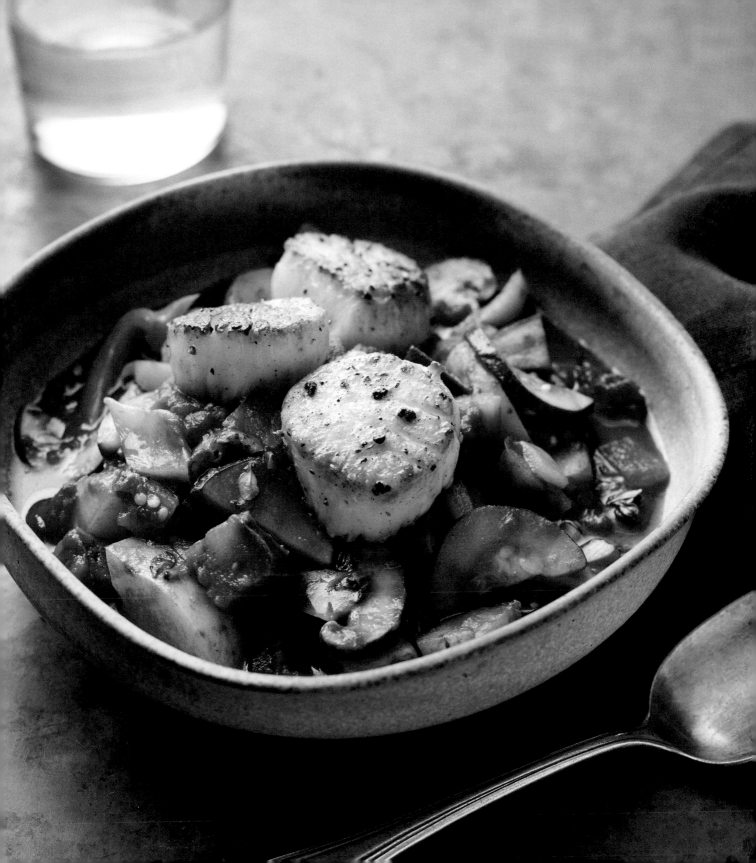

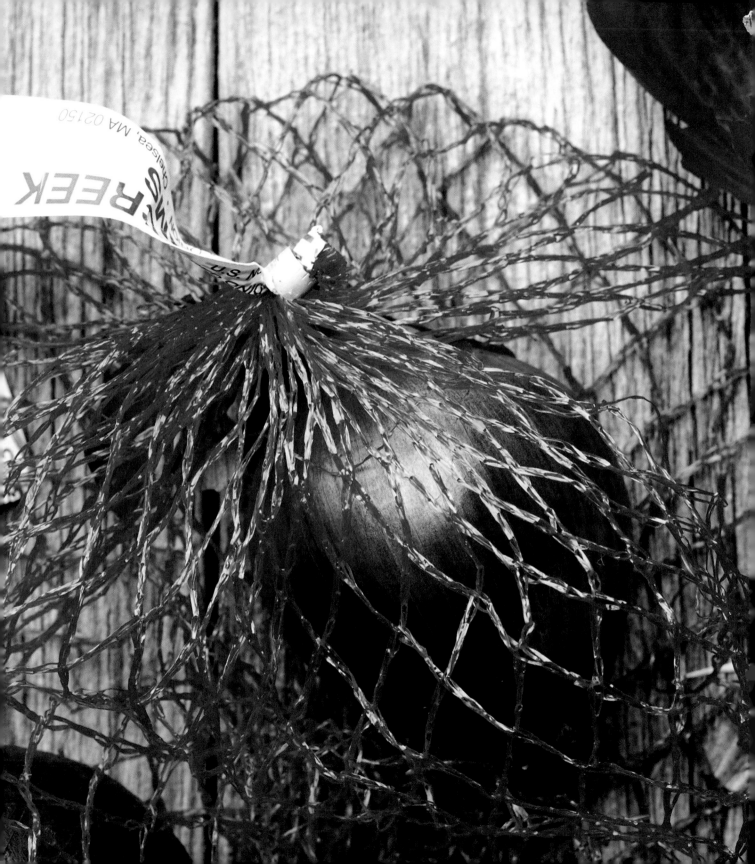

CHAPTER 5

STIR-AND-GO SLOW-COOKER RECIPES

Slow-Cooker Moroccan Chicken

SERVES 4 WITH LEFTOVERS

FROM *Dana Monsees of Real Food with Dana*

I'm big on bold flavors with simple ingredients and easy prep. And if you can make it a one-pot meal? Even better. This is one of my favorite recipes to make at the beginning of the week so I can have it for grab-and-go lunches on top of cauliflower rice! Be warned: Jealous stares from co-workers will definitely be coming your way!

PREP: 25 minutes

SLOW COOK: 6 hours (low)

TOTAL: 6 hours 30 minutes

FOR THE MARINADE

½ cup loosely packed fresh cilantro

2 tablespoons extra-virgin olive oil

2 teaspoons minced garlic

2 teaspoons minced fresh ginger

2 teaspoons paprika

1 teaspoon salt

1 teaspoon ground cinnamon

½ teaspoon turmeric

½ teaspoon ground cumin

½ teaspoon ground cardamom

1 large yellow onion, chopped

1½ pounds boneless, skinless chicken thighs

1½ pounds sweet potatoes, peeled and cut into 1-inch cubes

6 tablespoons chopped dates or sulfite-free raisins

2 bags (12 ounces each) frozen riced cauliflower, or about 6 cups raw cauliflower rice (see page 75), cooked

⅓ cup chopped fresh cilantro

⅓ cup slivered almonds, toasted (see Tip)

MAKE THE MARINADE: In a food processor or blender, combine all the marinade ingredients and process or blend until almost a smooth paste.

PLACE the onion in the bottom of a 3½- or 4-quart slow cooker. Pierce the chicken a few times with a fork. Place the chicken in a medium bowl and coat with all but 2 tablespoons of the marinade.

TRANSFER the chicken to the slow cooker. In the same bowl, toss the sweet potatoes with the remaining 2 tablespoons marinade. Scatter the sweet potatoes and the dates over the chicken.

COVER and cook on low for 6 to 7 hours. Remove the chicken and shred with two forks. Return the chicken to the slow cooker and gently stir to combine.

SERVE the chicken, vegetables, and cooking liquid over the cauliflower rice. Sprinkle with cilantro and almonds and serve.

TIP *To toast slivered almonds, heat them in a skillet over medium heat, stirring, until fragrant and lightly browned, about 2 minutes.*

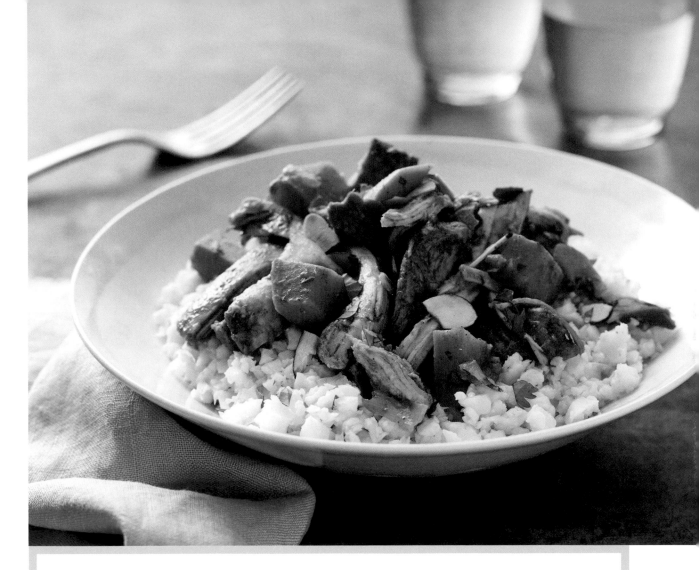

Dana Monsees

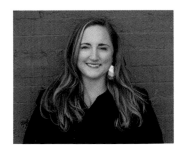

Dana Monsees is the founder of Real Food with Dana, a nutrition and lifestyle blog designed to help you thrive with real food and a paleo lifestyle—one delicious meal at a time. Dana's personal health journey as an athlete with celiac disease, thyroid problems, and adrenal fatigue sparked her passion for helping others through nutrition. In 2013, the Whole30 program totally transformed her eating habits and relationship with food—and she's never looked back. Dana works as a health and nutrition coach, swim coach, and is a soon-to-be nutritionist.

Steamed Cod with Spicy Roasted Tomato–Fennel Sauce

SERVES 4

While the vegetables can be cooked for up to 7 hours on low or 4 hours on high, the fish is added to the cooker just about 30 minutes before the end of cooking time. That's all it needs to get perfectly done.

PREP: 10 minutes

SLOW COOK: 6 hours (low) or 3 hours (high)

TOTAL: 6 hours 40 minutes

2 medium fennel bulbs

1 fresh serrano chile pepper, finely chopped

2 cloves garlic, minced

1½ teaspoons dried basil

1 teaspoon fennel seeds

1 can (28 ounces) Whole30-compliant fire-roasted diced tomatoes

4 cod fillets (5 to 6 ounces each)

1 tablespoon extra-virgin olive oil

½ teaspoon salt

½ teaspoon black pepper

4 slices Whole30-compliant bacon, crisp-cooked and crumbled

TRIM the fennel bulbs, reserving some of the feathery tops (fronds). Core the bulbs and then chop. In a 4- to 6-quart slow cooker, combine the fennel, serrano chile, garlic, basil, and fennel seeds. Add the tomatoes. Cover and cook on low for 6 to 7 hours or on high for 3 to 4 hours.

TURN the slow cooker to high setting if using low setting. Place the fillets on top of the sauce, spacing them evenly. Drizzle the fillets with the olive oil and then sprinkle with the salt and black pepper. Cover and cook until the fish just barely starts to break apart when pulled apart with a fork, 30 to 40 minutes longer. Top servings with bacon and chopped fennel fronds.

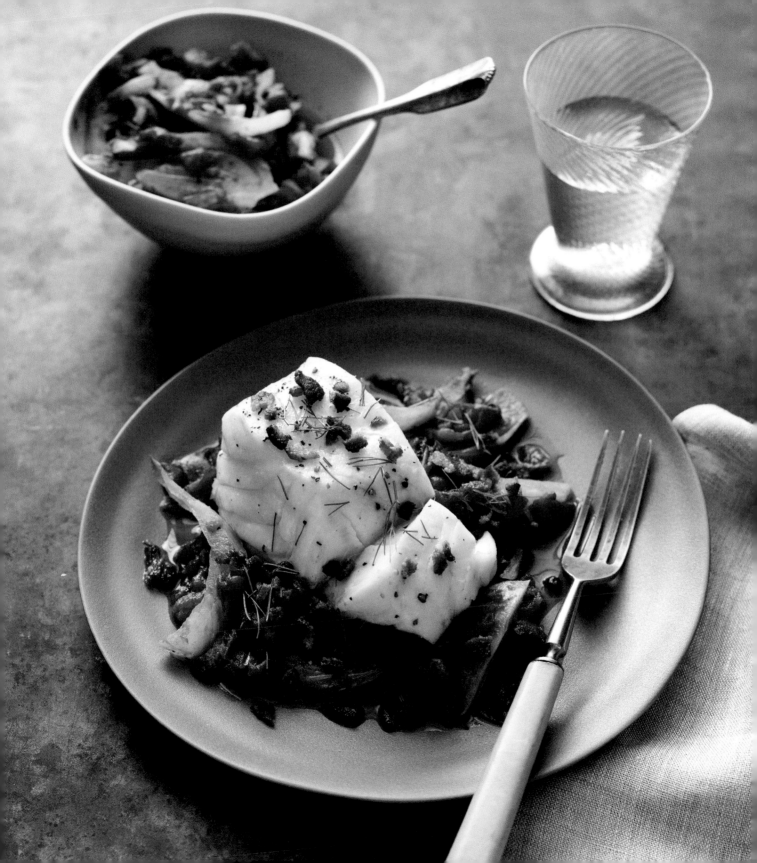

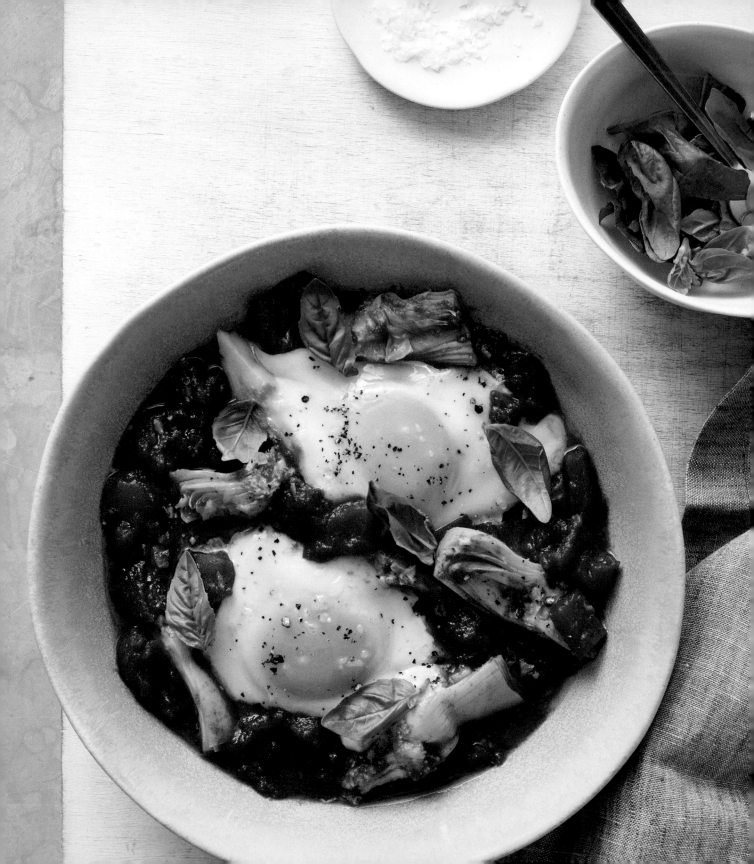

Slow-Cooker Shakshuka with Artichoke Hearts

SERVES 2 TO 3

This dish of eggs poached in a nicely spiced tomato sauce is a classic Israeli breakfast—but it's terrific for dinner too. Serve it with a big green salad.

PREP: 10 minutes

SLOW COOK: 6 hours (low)
or 3 hours (high)

TOTAL: 6 hours 40 minutes

1 can (28 ounces) Whole30-compliant whole tomatoes, coarsely chopped with can juices

1 red bell pepper, chopped

3 cloves garlic, minced

1½ teaspoons dried oregano

1 teaspoon ground cumin

½ teaspoon smoked paprika

½ teaspoon salt

½ teaspoon black pepper

1 can (14 ounces) Whole30-compliant artichoke hearts, drained

6 large eggs

Fresh basil

COMBINE the tomatoes, bell pepper, garlic, oregano, cumin, paprika, salt, and black pepper in a 5- to 6-quart slow cooker. Cover and cook on low for 6 to 7 hours or on high for 3 to 4 hours.

TURN the slow cooker to high if using the low setting. Stir in the artichokes. Using the back of a spoon, make 6 indents in the sauce. Crack an egg into each indent. Cover and cook until egg whites are set, about 30 minutes longer. Top servings with basil and additional black pepper.

Slow-Cooker Apple-Cider Pulled Pork

SERVES 6 TO 8

FROM *Kelly Smith of The Nourishing Home*

This recipe yields a heaping mound of melt-in-your-mouth pulled pork. Serve it with a side of homemade coleslaw, sandwich it between two sweet potato slices for tasty sliders, or pile it on spuds to create fully loaded baked potatoes. The possibilities for creating quick and easy meals are virtually endless!

PREP: 10 minutes

SLOW COOK: 6 hours (low) or 8 hours (high)

TOTAL: 6 hours 20 minutes

FOR THE RUB

1 tablespoon salt

1½ teaspoons smoked paprika

1½ teaspoons garlic powder

½ teaspoon chili powder

½ teaspoon ground ginger

½ teaspoon black pepper

4 pounds boneless pork butt

1 large sweet onion, sliced

1½ cups unsweetened, unfiltered apple cider

MAKE THE RUB: Combine all the seasonings in a small bowl. Sprinkle the rub over the pork and rub it in with your fingers.

ARRANGE the onion slices on the bottom of a 6-quart slow cooker. If necessary, cut the pork to fit in the cooker then place on top of the onions. Add the apple cider. Cover and cook on low for 8 to 10 hours or on high for 6 to 7 hours.

CAREFULLY transfer the meat to a large platter and allow it to rest for a few minutes. Strain the cooking liquid through a fine-mesh strainer into a large bowl. Place 1 cup of the liquid back into the slow cooker; discard the remaining liquid and the onion.

USING two forks, shred the meat. Return the meat to the slow cooker and toss with the cooking liquid. Season to taste with additional salt and pepper, if desired.

Kelly Smith

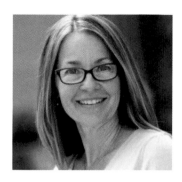

Kelly Smith loves sharing her passion for grain-free, whole-food cooking and meal planning with others. She is a cookbook author and founder of The Nourishing Home, a popular grain-free lifestyle blog dedicated to sharing delicious whole-food recipes, meal plans, cooking tips, and encouragement. With a passion for masterfully transforming everyday comfort foods into delicious grain-free creations, Kelly is on a mission to help individuals and families live a healthier, more nourished life.

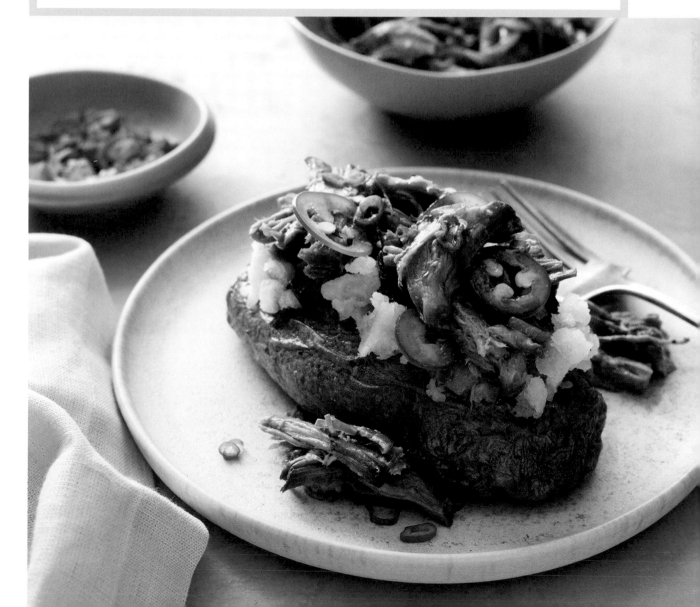

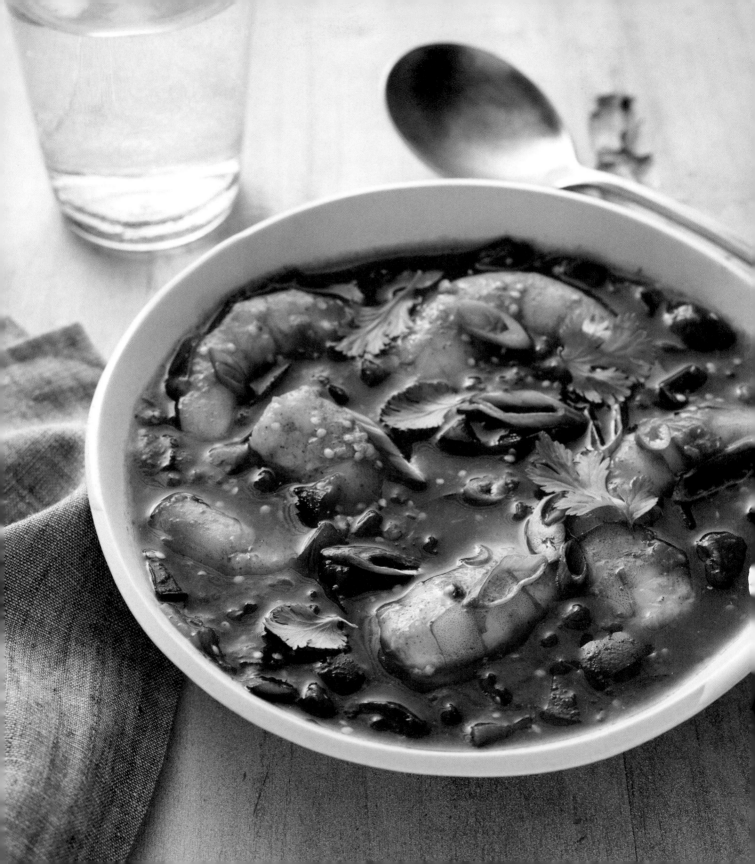

Shrimp–Salsa Verde Soup

SERVES 4

Tomatillos have a bright, lemony-apple flavor that pairs nicely with the richness of the shrimp. Fresh tomatillos have a sticky film under their crinkly husk. After removing the husk, just give them a quick rinse under cool water to remove it.

PREP: 20 minutes
SLOW COOK: 6 hours (low) or 3 hours (high)
TOTAL: 6 hours 50 minutes

1 pound tomatillos, husked and chopped

2 poblano chile peppers, seeded and chopped

½ cup fresh pineapple juice

2 tablespoons Whole30-compliant taco seasoning

1½ pounds peeled and deveined jumbo shrimp (see Tip)

Chopped fresh cilantro

Sliced green onions

Whole30 Sriracha (page 274) or Whole30-compliant hot sauce

COMBINE the tomatillos, poblanos, pineapple juice, and taco seasoning in a 3½-quart slow cooker. Cover and cook on low for 6 to 7 hours or on high for 3 to 4 hours.

TURN the slow cooker to high if using the low setting. Stir in the shrimp. Cover and cook until the shrimp are opaque, 30 to 40 minutes longer. Serve topped with cilantro, sliced green onions, and Sriracha.

TIP *To make this soup even easier, use cooked shrimp in place of the fresh shrimp: After cooking the tomatillos, peppers, pineapple juice, and taco seasoning, turn off the slow cooker, stir in the cooked shrimp, and let sit for 2 to 3 minutes. The shrimp will heat through in the hot soup without additional cooking.*

Slow-Cooker Chicken Chile Verde

SERVES 4

FROM *Jessica Beacom and Stacy Hassing of The Real Food Dietitians*

It hardly gets any easier than this recipe. Look for a salsa verde without preservatives or added sugars—we like Trader Joe's salsa verde because it's just tomatillos, green chiles, water, onions, jalapeños, salt, and spices. Throw in the optional jalapeño if you like more spice! Serve over cooked cauliflower rice (see page 75) or tuck into lettuce wraps.

PREP: 10 minutes

SLOW COOK: 4 hours (low)

TOTAL: 4 hours 20 minutes

1 ½ pounds boneless, skinless chicken thighs

1 jar (12-ounce) Whole30-compliant salsa verde

2 cans (4 ounces each) Whole30-compliant fire-roasted green chiles

½ teaspoon ground cumin

½ teaspoon dried oregano

1 small jalapeño, sliced (optional)

Chopped fresh cilantro and/or diced avocado

Lime wedges

PLACE the chicken in a 3½- or 4-quart slow cooker.

IN a small bowl, combine the salsa, green chiles, cumin, and oregano. Pour over the chicken. Cook on low for 4 hours.

USING a slotted spoon, transfer the chicken to a cutting board and let cool slightly. Use two forks to shred the chicken; return to the slow cooker and toss with the sauce.

TRANSFER to a serving dish and top with sliced jalapeño (if desired), cilantro, and/or avocado. Serve with lime wedges.

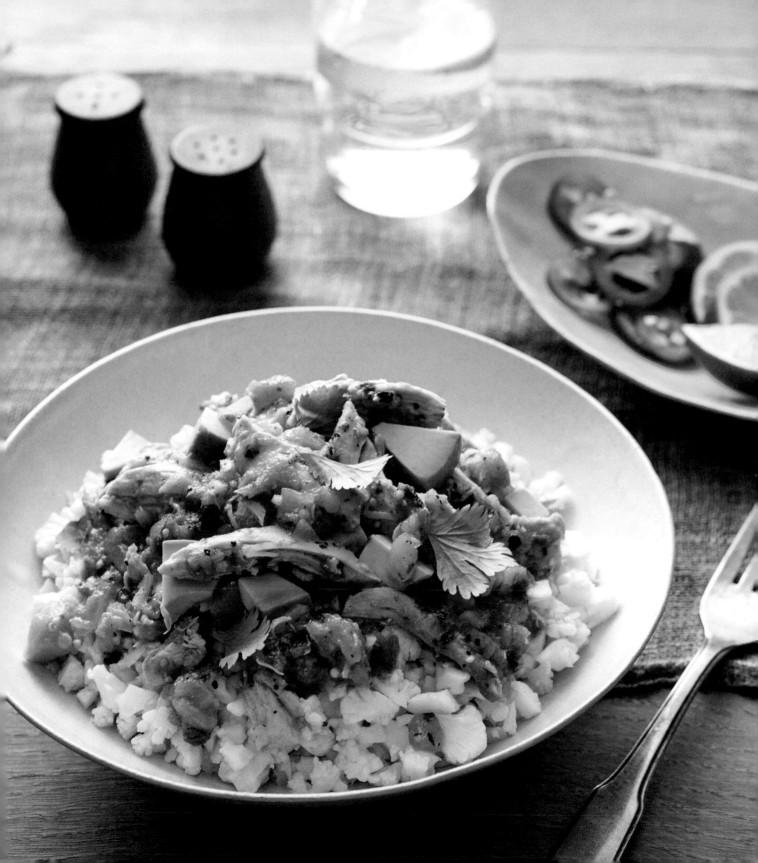

Pork Tacos with Sweet Potato Mash

SERVES 6

The slow cooker is the ideal tool for cooking what is essentially carnitas—braised Mexican-style pork shoulder. Long, moist cooking turns what starts out as a tough cut into fork-tender meat that is easily shredded for use in tacos.

> PREP: 20 minutes
>
> SLOW COOK: 8 hours (low) or 4 hours (high)
>
> TOTAL: 8 hours 25 minutes

FOR THE PORK

2 teaspoons cumin seeds, toasted (see Tip)

1 teaspoon dried oregano

¼ teaspoon cayenne pepper

1½ teaspoons coarse salt

2 pounds boneless pork shoulder roast, cut into 3 pieces

1 orange, cut into quarters

1 medium yellow onion, cut into wedges

FOR THE SWEET POTATO MASH

1 tablespoon extra-virgin olive oil

¼ cup minced onion

1 clove garlic, minced

1 teaspoon cumin seeds, toasted

¼ teaspoon smoked paprika

¼ teaspoon salt

1 can (15 ounces) Whole30-compliant sweet potato puree

Butterhead lettuce leaves

Snipped fresh cilantro

Lime wedges

Quick-Toasted Cumin and Pineapple Taco Sauce (page 275), optional

MAKE THE PORK: In a small bowl, combine the cumin seeds, oregano, cayenne, and salt. Sprinkle the rub all over the pork and rub it in with your fingers. Place the meat in a 3½- or 4-quart slow cooker. Squeeze the orange quarters over the meat then add them to the slow cooker. Place the onion wedges on top of the meat. Cover and cook on low for 8 to 10 hours or on high for 4 to 5 hours.

REMOVE the meat from the slow cooker; discard the cooking liquid. Cool the meat slightly then use two forks to shred.

MAKE THE SWEET POTATO MASH: Meanwhile, in a medium skillet, heat the olive oil over medium heat. Add the onion and garlic and cook, stirring, for about 1 minute. Add the cumin seeds, paprika, and salt, and then the sweet potato puree. Cook, stirring, until heated through, 1 to 2 minutes.

FOR each taco, place some of the sweet potato mash on a lettuce leaf. Top with the shredded pork and cilantro. Serve with lime wedges and, if desired, the taco sauce.

TIP *To toast cumin seeds, heat in a dry skillet over medium heat until fragrant and lightly browned, about 2 minutes.*

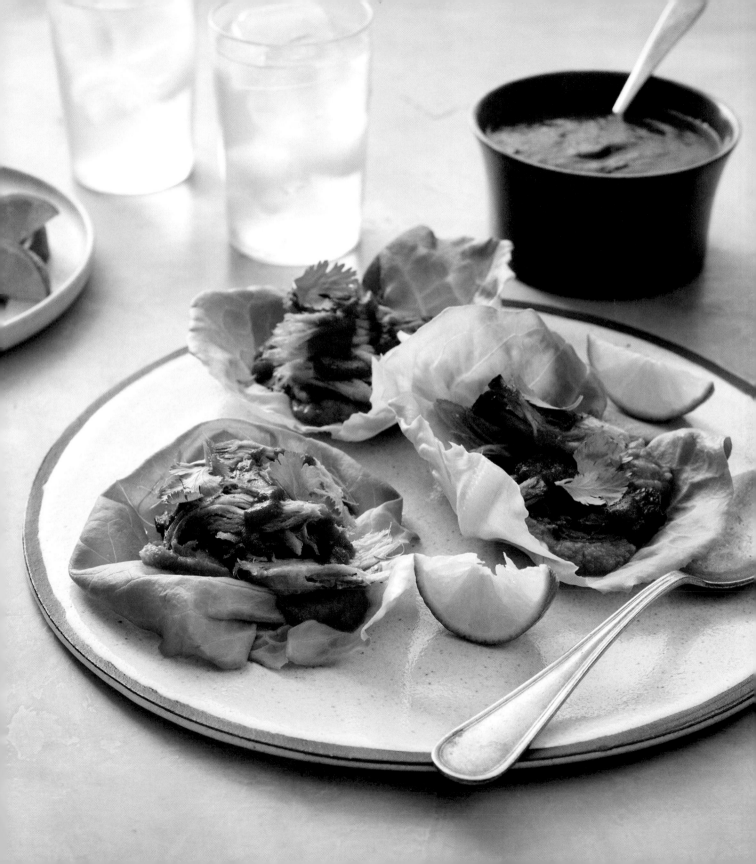

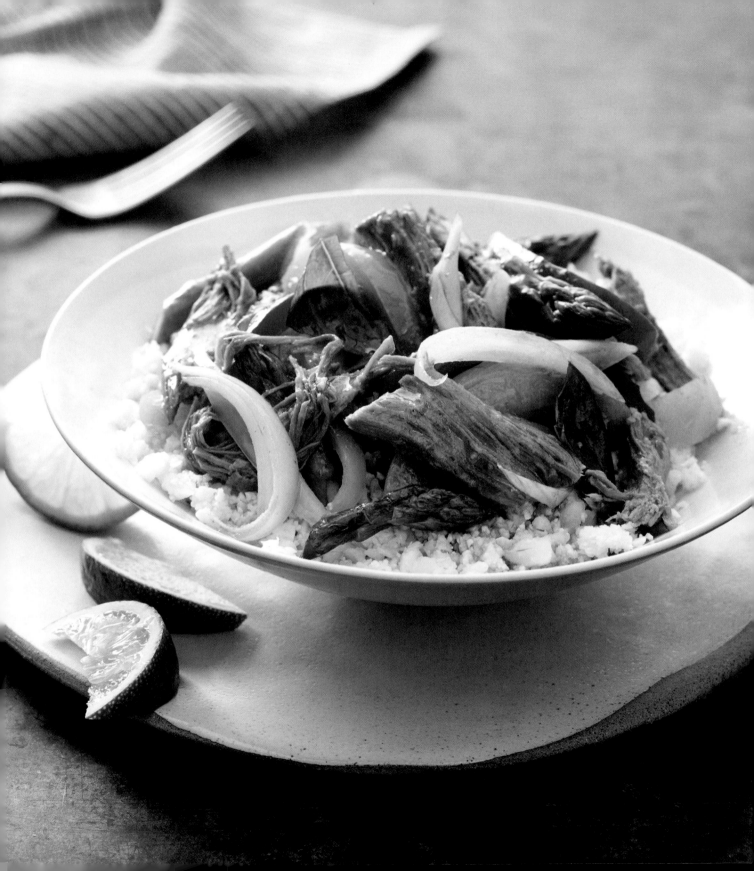

Green Curry Pork with Asparagus

SERVES 4 TO 6

If you can find pork stew meat that's already been cut up in your supermarket meat department, it cuts the prep time and mess on this Thai-inspired stew to nearly nothing.

<table>
<tr><td>PREP: 15 minutes</td></tr>
<tr><td>SLOW COOK: 7 hours (low) or 3½ hours (high)</td></tr>
<tr><td>TOTAL: 7 hours 30 minutes</td></tr>
</table>

1½ to 2 pounds boneless pork shoulder, cut into 2-inch cubes

3 medium red, yellow, and/or green bell peppers, sliced, or 3 cups frozen sliced bell peppers, thawed slightly

1 medium onion, cut into ½-inch wedges

1 cup Whole30-compliant chicken broth or Chicken Bone Broth (page 280)

¼ cup Whole30-compliant green curry paste

1 pound asparagus, cut into 1- to 2-inch pieces

1 can (14 ounces) full-fat Whole30-compliant coconut milk

1 cup sliced fresh basil leaves

1 bag (12 ounces) frozen riced cauliflower, cooked according to package directions; or 3 cups cauliflower rice (see page 75), cooked (optional)

Lime wedges (optional)

COMBINE the pork, bell peppers, onion, broth, and curry paste in a 4- to 5-quart slow cooker. Cover and cook on low for 7 to 8 hours or on high for 3½ to 4 hours.

TURN the slow cooker to high if using the low setting. Stir in the asparagus. Cover and cook until the asparagus is crisp-tender, 15 to 20 minutes. Stir in the coconut milk and basil. Serve the stew over the cauliflower rice and with lime wedges, if desired.

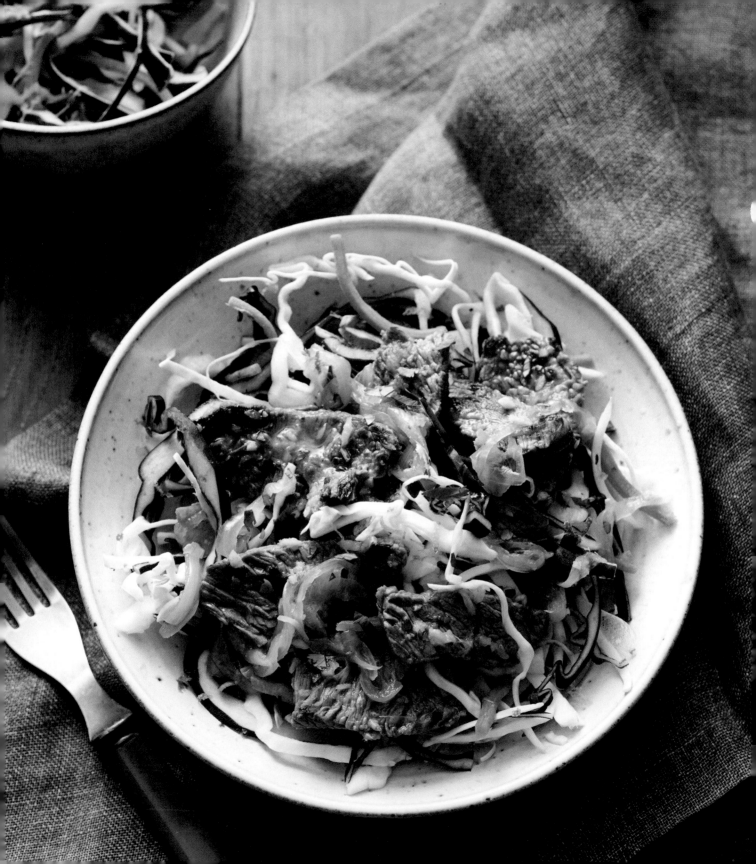

Garlicky Pepper Beef with Crunchy Cabbage

SERVES 4

When we say "garlicky," we're talking five cloves of minced garlic! If you're a fan of "the stinking rose," you'll love this dish. A generous dose of black pepper gives it subtle heat.

PREP: 10 minutes

SLOW COOK: 6 hours (low) or 3 hours (high)

TOTAL: 6 hours 15 minutes

1½ pounds beef stir-fry strips

2 cups thinly sliced onions

5 cloves garlic, minced

1 tablespoon minced fresh ginger

½ cup Whole30-compliant beef broth or Beef Bone Broth (page 280)

2 teaspoons Red Boat fish sauce

1 teaspoon black pepper

1 bag (14 ounces) packaged coleslaw mix (shredded cabbage and carrots)

½ teaspoon grated lime zest

1 tablespoon lime juice

Chopped fresh cilantro and/or basil (optional)

COMBINE the beef, onions, garlic, ginger, broth, fish sauce, and ½ teaspoon of the black pepper in a 3½- to 4-quart slow cooker. Cover and cook on low for 6 to 7 hours or on high for 3 to 4 hours.

JUST before serving, stir in the remaining ½ teaspoon black pepper, the coleslaw mix, and the lime zest and juice. Top each serving with cilantro and/or basil, if desired.

Cuban Beef with Peppers and Onions

SERVES 4

The flavors of this slow-cooked beef roast are the same as those in classic Cuban mojo sauce—cumin, oregano, orange, and lime.

> **PREP:** 10 minutes
>
> **SLOW COOK:** 8 hours (low) or 4 hours (high)
>
> **TOTAL:** 8 hours 20 minutes

3 cloves garlic, minced

2 teaspoons dried oregano

1 teaspoon ground cumin

1 teaspoon salt

½ teaspoon black pepper

1 boneless beef chuck roast (2 pounds)

2 large red bell peppers, seeded, cored, and sliced

2 medium yellow onions, cut into 6 wedges each

¼ cup orange juice

¼ cup lime juice

1 avocado, halved, pitted, peeled, and sliced

IN a small bowl, combine the garlic, oregano, cumin, salt, and black pepper. Rub the spice mixture onto both sides of the roast.

IN a 3½- or 4-quart slow cooker, layer the peppers and onions. Pour the juices over the vegetables. Place the roast on the vegetables. Cover and cook on low for 8 to 10 hours or on high for 4 to 5 hours.

USING a slotted spoon, transfer the meat to a cutting board. Using a slotted spoon, remove the peppers and onions and set aside. Strain the cooking liquid and set aside. Use two forks to shred the meat; return to the slow cooker. Stir in the onions, peppers, and ½ cup of the cooking liquid. Serve the meat and vegetables with the avocado.

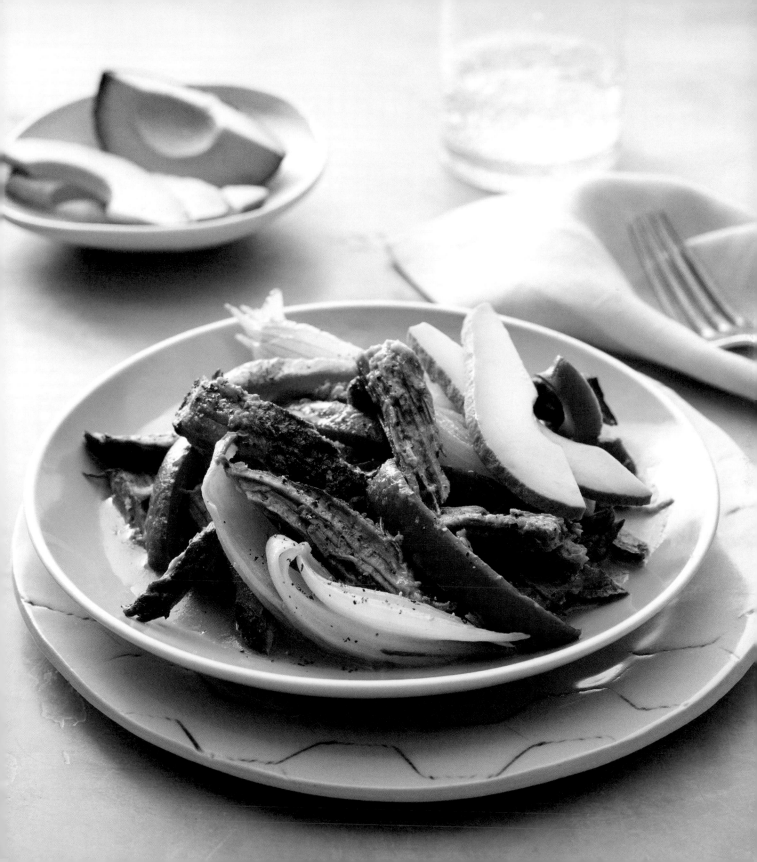

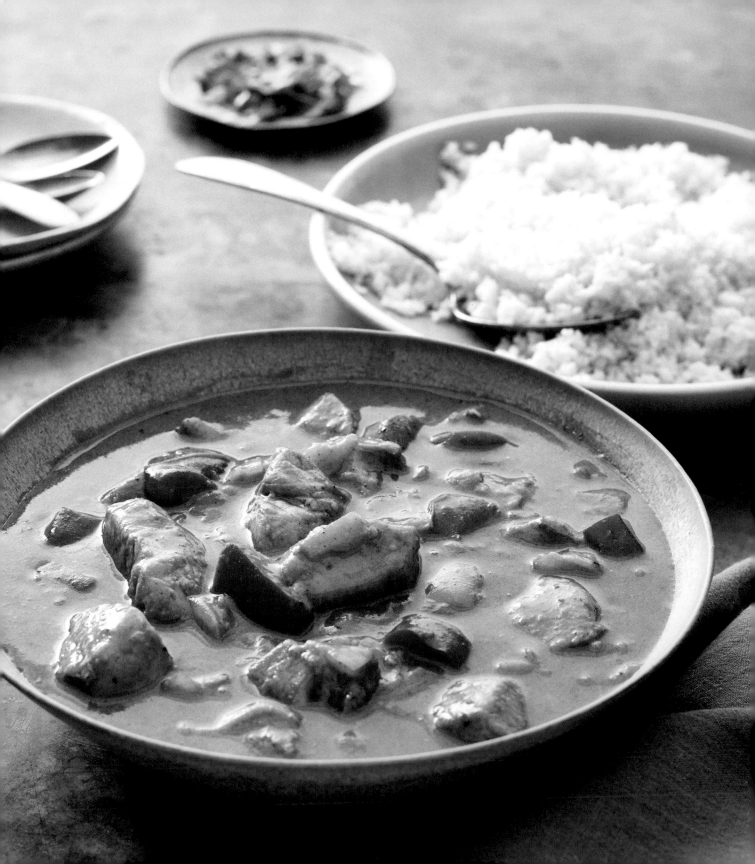

Chicken Tikka Masala with Cauliflower Rice

SERVES 4

Coconut milk stands in for the yogurt in this Whole30 version of the popular Indian dish. We think it makes it even better! Garam masala is not hot—but it is a complex blend of ground spices that typically includes black and white pepper, cloves, cinnamon, mace, cardamom, bay leaf, and cumin.

PREP: 15 minutes
SLOW COOK: 7 hours (low) or 4 hours (high)
TOTAL: 7 hours 30 minutes

1 to 1½ pounds boneless, skinless chicken breasts, cut into 1-inch pieces

1 large red bell pepper, seeded, cored, and cut into 1-inch pieces

½ medium onion, chopped

2 cloves garlic, minced

1 tablespoon minced fresh ginger

3 tablespoons Whole30-compliant tomato paste

1 tablespoon Whole30-compliant garam masala

1 tablespoon Whole30-compliant mild curry powder

½ teaspoon salt

½ teaspoon black pepper

1 cup Whole30-compliant full-fat coconut milk (see Tip)

1 tablespoon fresh lemon juice

1 bag (16-ounce) cauliflower crumbles, or 4 cups raw cauliflower rice (see page 75), cooked

Snipped fresh cilantro, optional

IN a 3- to 4½-quart slow cooker, combine the chicken, bell pepper, onion, garlic, ginger, tomato paste, garam masala, curry powder, salt, and black pepper. Cover and cook on low for 7 to 8 hours or on high for 4 hours.

STIR in the coconut milk and lemon juice. Cook until heated through, about 15 minutes.

SERVE the chicken masala over the cauliflower rice and top with cilantro, if desired.

TIP *Canned coconut milk separates in the can with the cream rising to the top. Be sure to whisk the coconut milk well before measuring.*

Slow-Cooker Pork Chili

SERVES 4

Pork chili is most often made with salsa verde, or green sauce, based on tomatillos. This red-sauced pork chili made with tomatoes and chili powder is a delicious twist on that tradition.

PREP: 15 minutes

SLOW COOK: 8 hours (low) or 4 hours (high)

TOTAL: 8 hours 20 minutes

2 pounds boneless pork shoulder, trimmed and cut into 2-inch chunks

1 medium onion, chopped

1 medium jalapeño, seeded and chopped

3 cloves garlic, minced

1 can (28 ounces) Whole30-compliant diced tomatoes, undrained

1 cup Whole30-compliant chicken broth or Chicken Bone Broth (page 280)

2 tablespoons chili powder

1 teaspoon ground cumin

1 teaspoon salt

¼ teaspoon black pepper

Chopped fresh cilantro

Sliced avocado

Sliced jalapeño

IN a 4- or 5-quart slow cooker, combine the pork, onion, jalapeño, garlic, tomatoes, broth, chili powder, cumin, salt, and black pepper. Cover and cook on low for 8 to 10 hours or on high for 4 to 5 hours.

USING two forks, shred the pork in the slow cooker. Serve the chili topped with cilantro, avocado, and jalapeño.

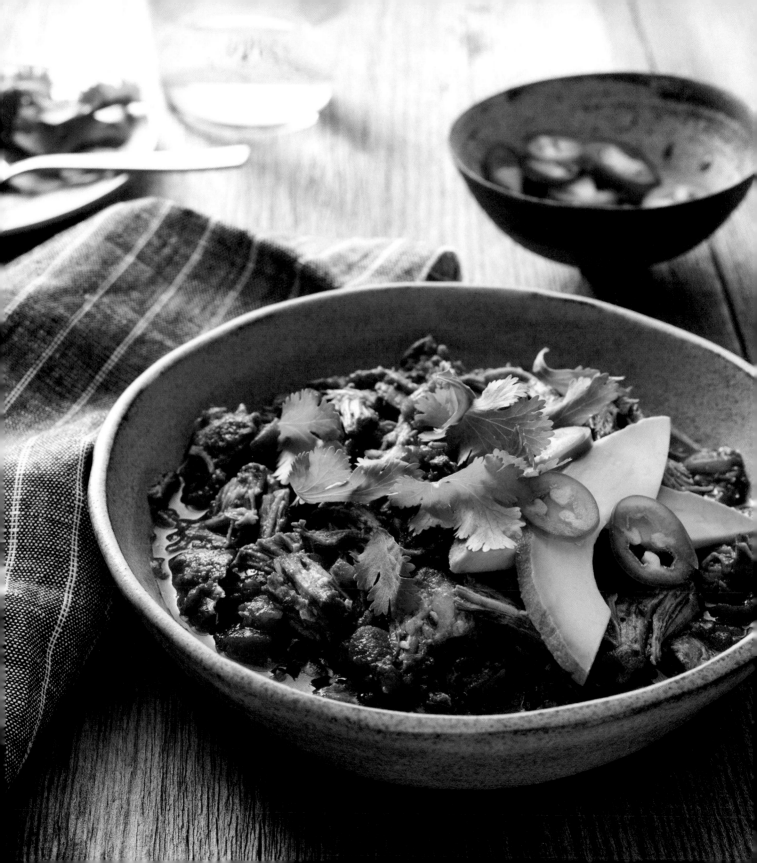

Cilantro-Lime Chicken

SERVES 4

A quartered lime, cilantro, and garlic placed in the cavity of the chicken infuse the meat with wonderful flavor as it cooks. A quick trip under the broiler browns up the skin beautifully.

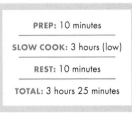

PREP: 10 minutes	
SLOW COOK: 3 hours (low)	
REST: 10 minutes	
TOTAL: 3 hours 25 minutes	

1 lime, quartered

¼ cup roughly chopped fresh cilantro

3 cloves garlic, peeled and smashed

1 whole chicken (3 to 3½ pounds)

1 tablespoon extra-virgin olive oil

1 teaspoon grated lime zest

1½ teaspoons fresh lime juice

½ teaspoon salt

¼ teaspoon black pepper

2 large onions, cut into large wedges

Chopped fresh cilantro (optional)

Lime wedges (optional)

PLACE the quartered lime, cilantro, and garlic in the cavity of the chicken. In a small bowl, combine the olive oil, lime zest and juice, salt, and pepper. Rub the mixture all over the chicken. Tie the legs together with cotton kitchen string.

PLACE the onion wedges in the bottom of a 5- to 6-quart slow cooker. Place the chicken, breast side up, on top of the onions. Cover and cook on high for 3 to 4 hours, until the chicken is no longer pink and a thermometer registers 170°F when inserted into a thigh.

CAREFULLY remove the chicken from the slow cooker and place in an ovenproof 9x13-inch pan. With a slotted spoon, remove the onion from the cooking liquid and place next to the chicken. Discard the cooking liquid. Let the chicken cool for 10 minutes.

CUT the string and remove and discard the lime, cilantro, and garlic from the cavity. Turn the oven to broil. Brown the chicken under the broiler until the skin is golden brown and crispy, 4 to 5 minutes. Serve with chopped cilantro and lime wedges, if desired.

TIP *The chicken can also be shredded or chopped and used in recipes that call for cooked chicken. This recipe makes 3 to 3½ cups shredded or chopped chicken.*

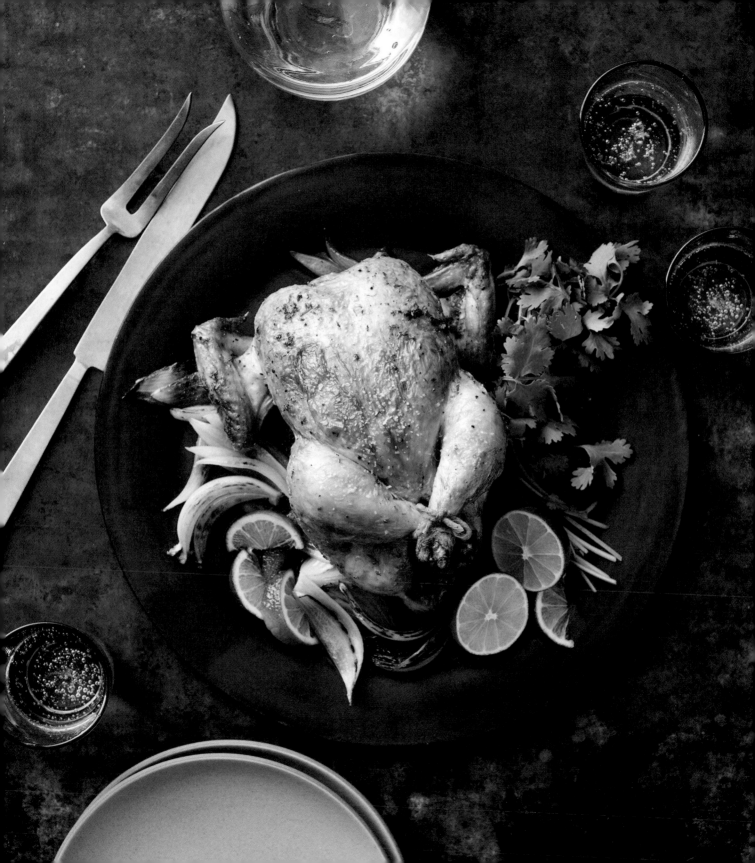

Shredded Barbecue Chicken on Sweet Potato "Buns"

SERVES 4

These knife-and-fork open-face sandwiches feature the flavors of a classic Southern-style BBQ sandwich without the high sugar and carb content—and with nutrient-rich sweet potatoes.

PREP: 20 minutes

SLOW COOK: 3 hours 20 minutes (high)

TOTAL: 3 hours 40 minutes

FOR THE CHICKEN

2 tablespoons Clarified Butter (page 283) or ghee, melted

2 cloves garlic, minced

2 teaspoons Whole30-compliant hot sauce

½ teaspoon salt

¼ teaspoon black pepper

1½ pounds boneless, skinless chicken thighs

1 cup Whole30-compliant barbecue sauce

FOR THE SWEET POTATO BUNS

2 large sweet potatoes (about 3 pounds; see Tip), peeled

2 tablespoons extra-virgin olive oil

¼ teaspoon salt

⅓ cup thinly sliced green onions

MAKE THE CHICKEN: In a 3½- or 4-quart slow cooker, stir together the butter, garlic, hot sauce, salt, and pepper. Add the chicken and turn to coat the pieces. Cover and cook on high for 3 to 4 hours.

TRANSFER the chicken to a cutting board and discard the cooking liquid. Shred the chicken with two forks then return to the slow cooker. Stir the barbecue sauce into the chicken. Cover and cook on high until heated through, about 10 minutes.

MAKE THE SWEET POTATO BUNS: Meanwhile, preheat the oven to 400°F. Line a large baking sheet with parchment paper. Cut six ½-inch-thick rounds from the widest portion of each sweet potato. In a large bowl, toss the sweet potato rounds with the olive oil and salt and place in a single layer on the pan. Bake until the potatoes are tender, about 20 minutes.

SERVE the barbecue chicken on sweet potato buns and top with green onions.

TIPS *Choose sweet potatoes that are round in the middle to cut the best rounds for the buns.*

You will have ends from each sweet potato that are too small to use for the rounds, but don't throw them away! Simply chop and cook with olive oil, salt, and black pepper in a skillet for an easy side dish the next day.

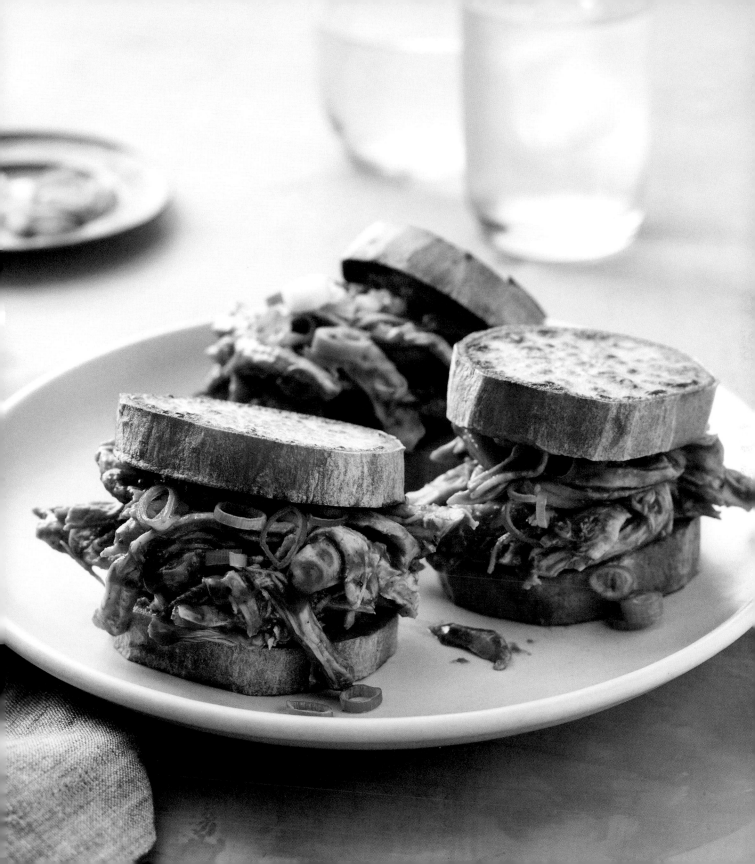

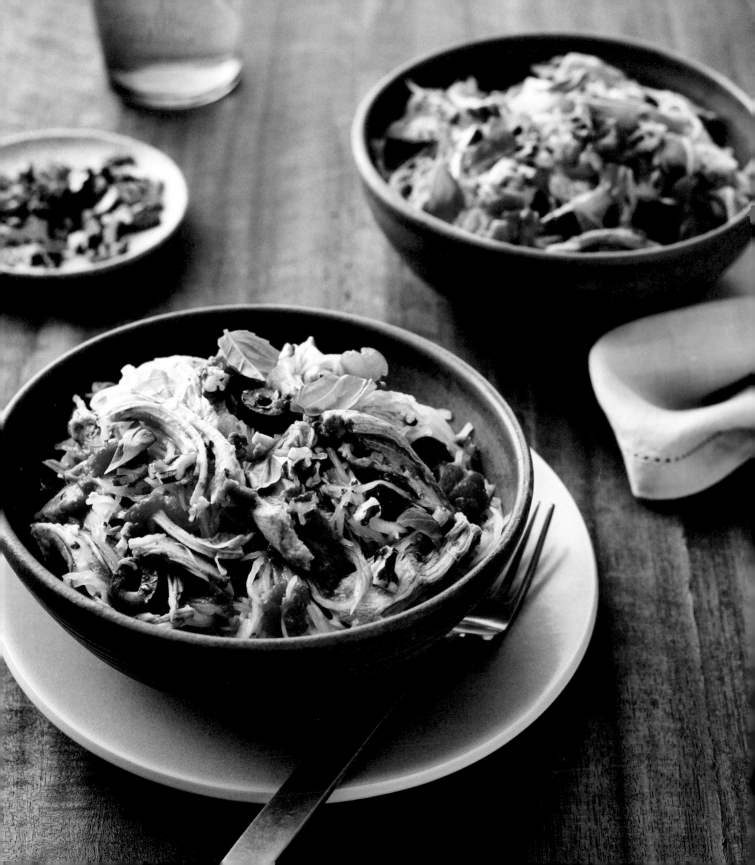

Spaghetti Squash with Chicken, Kalamata Olives, and Tomatoes

SERVES 4

Kalamata olives are magical. They add rich, briny flavor to any food they touch, including this saucy squash-and-chicken dish. A topping of toasted pecans and fresh basil adds flavor and crunch.

> **PREP:** 15 minutes
>
> **SLOW COOK:** 8 hours (low) or 4 hours (high)
>
> **TOTAL:** 8 hours 45 minutes

1 cup Whole30-compliant chicken broth or Chicken Bone Broth (page 280)

1 can (14.5 ounces) Whole30-compliant diced tomatoes, drained

1 tablespoon chopped fresh oregano

2 cloves garlic, sliced

1 teaspoon salt

¼ teaspoon black pepper

1 spaghetti squash (about 2½ pounds)

1½ to 2 pounds boneless, skinless chicken thighs

¼ cup sliced kalamata olives

⅓ cup chopped pecans, toasted (see Tip)

Chopped fresh basil

IN a 5- to 6-quart slow cooker, combine the broth, tomatoes, oregano, garlic, salt, and pepper. Cut the squash in half lengthwise and remove the seeds. Place the squash, cut sides down, in the slow cooker. Place the chicken around the squash. Cover and cook on low for 8 to 9 hours or on high for 4 to 5 hours.

REMOVE the squash and chicken from the slow cooker, leaving the cooking liquid in the cooker. Let the squash and chicken cool for 5 minutes. Use forks to separate the squash into strands and to shred the chicken. Discard the squash shell.

TURN the slow cooker to high if using the low setting. Return the squash and chicken to the slow cooker and stir in the olives. Cover and cook until heated through, about 25 minutes longer. Top servings with the pecans and basil.

TIP *To toast pecans, heat in a skillet over medium heat, stirring, until fragrant and lightly browned, about 2 minutes.*

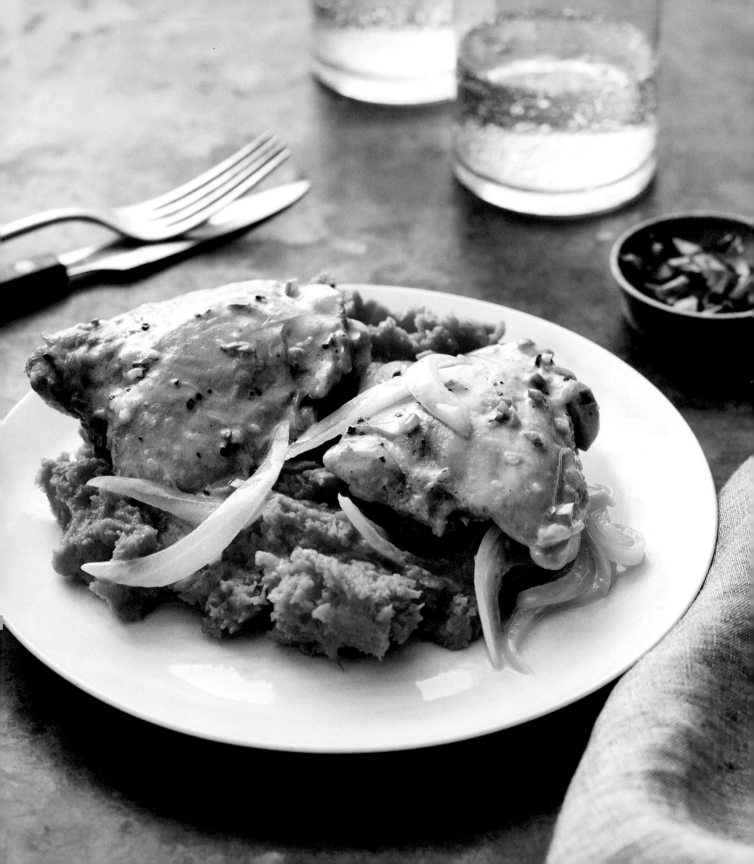

Chicken Adobo with Mashed Sweet Potatoes

SERVES 2

When chicken is braised or cooked in liquid, it's best to remove the skin. Dry heat—such as that in an oven—creates crispy and appealing skin but moist heat does not.

PREP: 20 minutes

SLOW COOK: 6 hours (low) or 3 hours (high)

TOTAL: 6 hours 20 minutes

1 cup Whole30-compliant coconut milk (see Tip)

2 tablespoons coconut aminos

1 tablespoon minced fresh ginger

1 jalapeño, seeded and finely chopped

½ teaspoon salt

¼ teaspoon black pepper

1½ to 2 pounds skinless bone-in chicken thighs

1 large onion, cut into thin wedges

1 bag (12 ounces) frozen roasted sweet potato chunks

1 teaspoon arrowroot powder

Chopped fresh cilantro

IN a small bowl, mix together the coconut milk, coconut aminos, ginger, jalapeño, salt, and pepper. Place the chicken and onion in a 4- to 5-quart slow cooker. Pour the coconut milk mixture over the chicken. Cover and cook on low for 6 to 7 hours or on high for 3 to 3½ hours.

MEANWHILE, prepare the sweet potatoes according to package directions. In a large bowl, mash the cooked potatoes with a potato masher to the desired consistency.

PLACE the chicken and onion on a plate and cover to keep warm. Pour the cooking liquid from the slow cooker into a small saucepan. In a small bowl, whisk together the arrowroot powder and 2 teaspoons cold water and add to the cooking liquid. Bring to a boil over medium heat, stirring occasionally, then boil for 1 minute, stirring constantly until thickened. Serve the gravy over the chicken and mashed potatoes and sprinkle with cilantro.

TIP *Canned coconut milk separates in the can with the cream rising to the top. Be sure to whisk the coconut milk well before measuring.*

Balsamic Chicken

SERVES 4

The balsamic vinegar not only gives this dish wonderful flavor but the acid in it also tenderizes the chicken as it cooks.

PREP: 10 minutes

SLOW COOK: 3 hours (low)

TOTAL: 3 hours 10 minutes

1 ¼ **pounds boneless, skinless chicken breasts**

2 **medium shallots, thinly sliced**

2 **cloves garlic, minced**

1 **tablespoon extra-virgin olive oil**

½ **teaspoon Italian seasoning**

¼ **teaspoon salt**

⅛ **teaspoon red pepper flakes**

¼ **cup apple cider**

2 **tablespoons balsamic vinegar**

2 **Roma (plum) tomatoes, chopped**

2 **tablespoons chopped fresh parsley**

IN a 3½- or 4-quart slow cooker, combine the chicken, shallots, garlic, olive oil, Italian seasoning, salt, and pepper flakes. Turn the chicken to coat. Pour the cider and vinegar over the chicken. Cover and cook on low for 3 to 4 hours.

TRANSFER the chicken to a serving platter. Strain the cooking liquid. Top the chicken with the tomatoes and parsley. Drizzle with additional balsamic vinegar and the cooking liquid and serve.

Bolognese Sauce with Bacon and Pearl Onions

SERVES 4 WITH LEFTOVERS

Just a handful of ingredients create a rich, thick, and hearty Italian-style sauce for zucchini noodles. The bacon gives it a nice smoky flavor.

PREP: 10 minutes

SLOW COOK: 7 hours (low) or 4 hours (high)

TOTAL: 7 hours 10 minutes

1½ pounds ground beef

2 slices Whole30-compliant bacon, chopped

1 teaspoon dried oregano, crushed

1 bay leaf

1 jar (25 ounces) Whole30-compliant roasted garlic pasta sauce

¼ cup Whole30-compliant beef broth or Beef Bone Broth (page 280)

1 bag (14.4 ounces) frozen pearl onions

Hot cooked zucchini noodles (see Tip; optional)

IN a 3½- or 4-quart slow cooker, crumble the beef with a spatula. Top with the bacon, oregano, and bay leaf. Cover with the pasta sauce and broth, then top with the onions. Cover and cook on low for 7 to 8 hours or on high for 4 to 4½ hours.

IF necessary, use a spoon to skim fat from the top of the sauce and discard. Remove and discard the bay leaf. Stir the sauce before serving. If desired, serve over cooked zucchini noodles.

TIP *Cook zucchini noodles in a skillet with small amount of hot olive oil over medium heat. Toss noodles lightly with tongs and cook until just tender, 5 to 7 minutes.*

Creamy Curried Butternut Squash– Shrimp Soup

SERVES 4

Jarred red curry paste gives this sweet and creamy soup complex flavor and a touch of heat. Adding the shrimp at the end of the cooking time prevents them from overcooking and turning rubbery.

PREP: 10 minutes
COOK: 5 hours (low) or 2½ hours (high)
TOTAL: 5 hours 30 minutes

2 bags (10 ounces each) frozen diced butternut squash

2 cups Whole30-compliant chicken broth or Chicken Bone Broth (page 280)

1 tablespoon Clarified Butter (page 283) or ghee

½ teaspoon salt

1 can (13.5 ounces) Whole30-compliant coconut milk (see Tip)

3 tablespoons red curry paste

1 pound peeled and deveined medium shrimp

Snipped fresh basil

IN a 3½- or 4-quart slow cooker, combine the squash, broth, butter, and salt. Cover and cook on low for 5 to 7 hours or on high for 2½ to 3½ hours.

STIR the coconut milk and curry paste into the slow cooker. Carefully transfer the soup to a blender, in batches if necessary, and let cool briefly; blend until smooth. (Or use an immersion blender and blend in the cooker.)

TURN the slow cooker to high if using the low setting. Return the soup to the cooker and add the shrimp. Cover and cook for 20 minutes. Top with basil and serve.

TO use cooked shrimp instead of raw, add the shrimp to the pureed soup. Cover, and let stand for 1 to 2 minutes, or until heated through.

TIP *Canned coconut milk separates in the can with the cream rising to the top. Be sure to whisk the coconut milk well before measuring.*

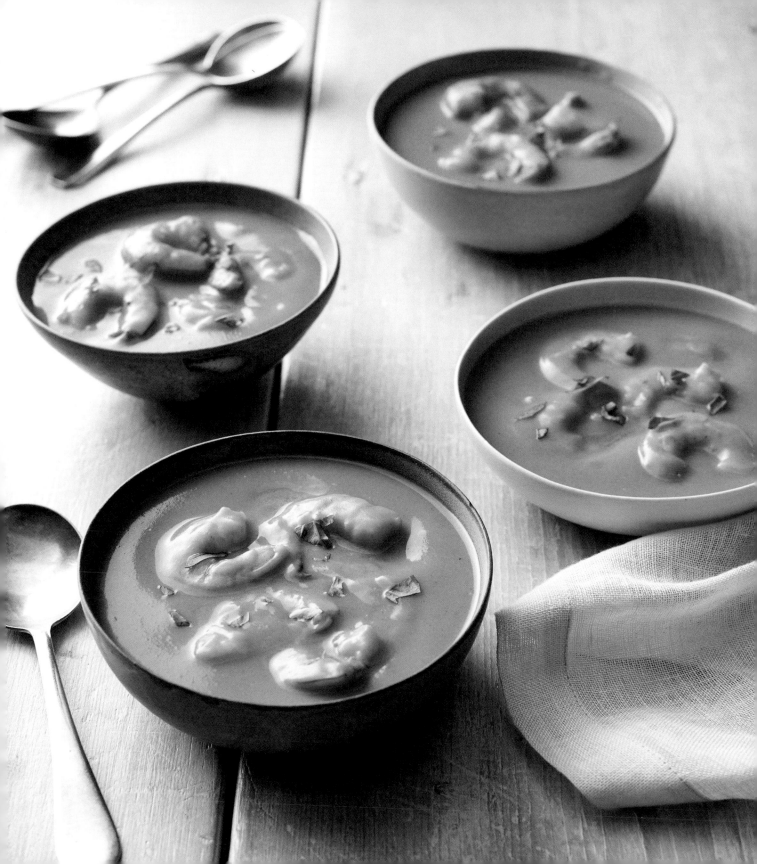

Buffalo Chicken Dip

SERVES 4

FROM *Dana Monsees of Real Food with Dana*

Football season is probably my favorite time of the year. Not only because I grew up going to games with my family, but because the food is amazing and can easily be made Whole30-friendly! Like this Buffalo dip, made without pounds of cheese but still as creamy as the traditional dip and even more delicious. Serve with cut-up vegetables, or you can even spoon it over baked sweet potatoes.

PREP: 10 minutes

SLOW COOK: 2 hours (low)

TOTAL: 2 hours 10 minutes

4 cups chopped or shredded cooked chicken breast

½ cup Whole30-compliant mayonnaise or Basic Mayonnaise (page 281)

½ cup Whole30-compliant hot sauce

½ cup Whole30-compliant ranch dressing or Whole30 Ranch Dressing (page 282)

¼ cup chopped fresh chives

¼ cup chopped fresh cilantro

Bell pepper wedges, romaine lettuce leaves, carrot sticks, and/or celery sticks, or other vegetables for serving

IN a 3½ or 4-quart slow cooker, combine the chicken, mayonnaise, hot sauce, dressing, chives, and cilantro. Cover and cook for 2 hours on low (see Tip).

SERVE the dip with cut-up vegetables.

TIP *If you don't have time to slow cook the dip, you can bake it instead: Preheat the oven to 350°F. Combine the chicken mixture in a 1½-quart baking dish, cover, and bake for 25 minutes. Remove the cover and bake until bubbling around the edges, 5 to 10 minutes longer.*

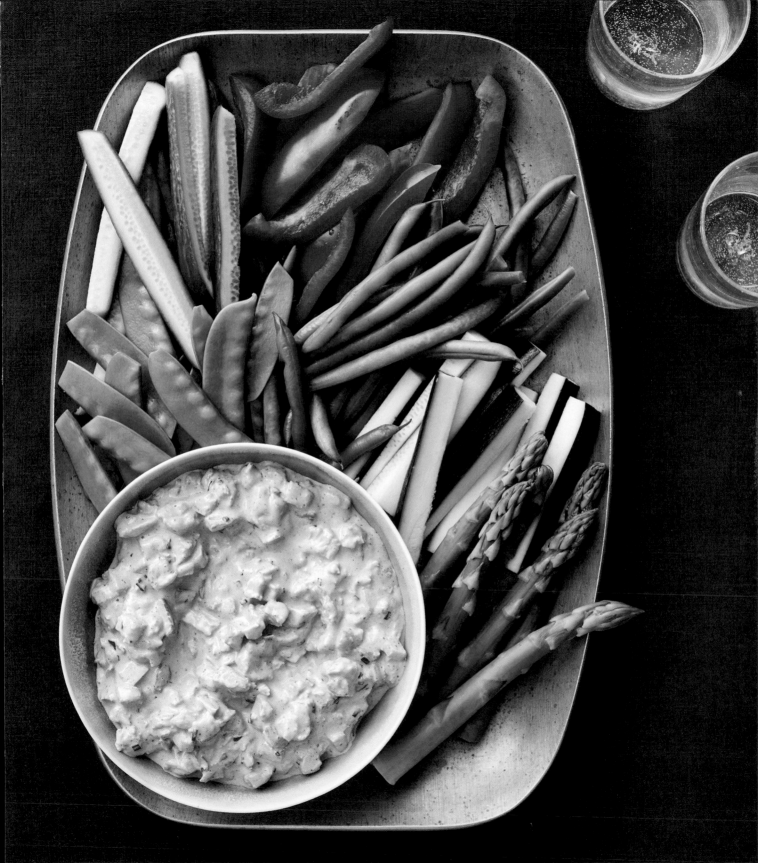

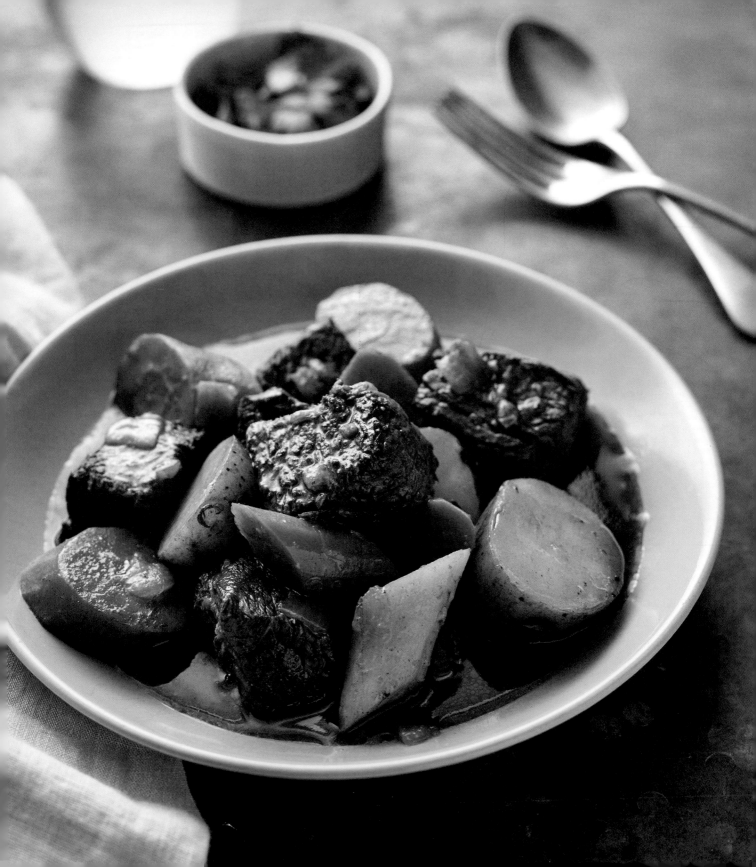

Balsamic Beef Roast and Root Vegetables

SERVES 4 WITH LEFTOVERS

Although it's not a necessity—and it does add a few minutes to your prep time—browning meat before it goes into the slow cooker adds flavor to the finished dish. Browning caramelizes the natural sugars in the surface of the meat, which imparts a richness you won't get without it. But if time is short, you can skip it!

> **PREP:** 30 minutes
>
> **SLOW COOK:** 5½ hours (low) or 3 hours (high)
>
> **TOTAL:** 6 hours

1 tablespoon coconut oil

1½ to 2 pounds boneless chuck roast or bottom round, cut into 1½-inch cubes

Salt

Black pepper

1 pound large carrots, peeled and cut into 1-inch pieces

1 pound parsnips, peeled and cut into ½-inch pieces

1 pound small red potatoes, halved

1 medium onion, chopped

1 clove garlic, minced

2 cups Whole30-compliant beef broth or Beef Bone Broth (page 280)

¼ cup balsamic vinegar

2 teaspoons Whole30-compliant dried Italian seasoning

Chopped fresh parsley (optional)

HEAT the coconut oil in a large heavy skillet over medium-high heat. Season the beef lightly with salt and pepper. Add the beef to the skillet and cook, stirring occasionally, until browned on all sides, about 5 minutes. Place the beef in a 5- to 6-quart slow cooker with the carrots, parsnips, and potatoes.

ADD the onion to the same skillet and add additional coconut oil if needed. Cook, stirring frequently, until the onion is soft, 4 to 5 minutes. Add the garlic and cook, stirring, until fragrant, about 30 seconds. Add the broth, vinegar, and Italian seasoning and stir to scrape up any brown bits on the bottom of the skillet. Transfer to the slow cooker.

COVER and cook on low for 5½ to 6 hours or on high for 3 hours. Top servings with parsley, if desired.

Sweet and Spicy Vegetable-Pork Stew

SERVES 4

The sweetness in this North-African style stew spiced with paprika, cumin, ginger, cayenne, and cloves comes from golden raisins (sometimes called sultanas). Be sure to look for those that don't contain sulfites.

PREP: 20 minutes
SLOW COOK: 8 hours (low) or 4 hours (high)
TOTAL: 8 hours 20 minutes

1 ¼ to 1 ½ pounds boneless pork shoulder, fat trimmed, cut into 1-inch pieces

1 tablespoon paprika

1 teaspoon coarse salt

1 teaspoon ground cumin

½ teaspoon ground ginger

¼ to ½ teaspoon cayenne pepper

⅛ teaspoon ground cloves

1 butternut squash (1 pound), peeled, seeded, and cut into 1-inch pieces (about 1 ½ cups)

1 medium rutabaga, peeled and cut into 1-inch pieces (about 2 cups)

2 stalks celery, cut crosswise into ½-inch-thick pieces

1 medium red onion, chopped

2 cups Whole30-compliant chicken broth or Chicken Bone Broth (page 280)

¼ cup unsulfured golden raisins

Chopped green onions or fresh chives

PLACE the pork in a 3½- or 4-quart slow cooker In a small bowl, stir together the paprika, salt, cumin, ginger, cayenne pepper, and cloves. Sprinkle over the meat and toss to coat. Add the squash to the slow cooker along with the rutabaga, celery, onion, and broth. Cover and cook on low for 8 to 9 hours or on high for 4 to 4½ hours.

STIR the raisins into the stew just before serving. Top with chopped green onions or chives.

Chili Con Carne

SERVES 4

Chili made with ground beef evolved out of this more traditional and authentic chili, which is made with chunks of beef cooked low and slow until they are fork-tender. The cayenne adds just a touch of heat while the ground chipotle chili pepper—made from dried, smoked jalapeños—imparts some heat and a subtle smokiness.

PREP: 30 minutes

SLOW COOK: 9 hours (low) or 4½ hours (high)

TOTAL: 9 hours 30 minutes

1 pound boneless beef chuck roast, trimmed and cut into 1-inch pieces

1 medium red onion, peeled

1 can (28 ounces) Whole30-compliant crushed tomatoes, undrained

1 cup Whole30-compliant beef broth or Beef Bone Broth (page 280)

1 small red bell pepper, seeded, cored, and chopped

1 medium poblano pepper, chopped

3 cloves garlic, minced

2 tablespoons chili powder

½ teaspoon ground cumin

¼ teaspoon cayenne pepper or ground chipotle chili pepper

Salt

¼ teaspoon black pepper

1 jalapeño, seeded (if desired) and thinly sliced

¼ cup cider vinegar

¼ cup chopped fresh cilantro

PLACE the beef in a 3½- or 4-quart slow cooker. Cut enough of the red onion into thin slivers to make ⅓ cup. Place the slivers in a small bowl and set aside. Chop the remaining red onion and add to the slow cooker along with the tomatoes, broth, bell pepper, poblano, garlic, chili powder, cumin, cayenne pepper, ¼ teaspoon salt, and the black pepper. Cover and cook on low for 9 to 10 hours or on high for 4½ to 5 hours.

MEANWHILE, add the jalapeño, vinegar, and ⅛ teaspoon salt to the slivered red onion. Toss to combine. Using a spoon, press the vegetables into the vinegar. Cover and let stand while the chili cooks.

DRAIN the onion mixture and serve on top of the chili. Sprinkle with the cilantro.

Coconut-Curry Chicken Drumsticks

SERVES 4

The popularity of low-carb diets such as Whole30 has inspired food companies to come up with compliant convenience products—such as the frozen riced cauliflower and broccoli on which this saucy chicken dish is served. It makes doing a Whole30 just that much easier!

> **PREP:** 15 minutes
>
> **SLOW COOK:** 5 hours (low) or 3 hours (high)
>
> **TOTAL:** 5 hours 25 minutes

2 medium tomatoes, cored and cut into wedges

2 medium carrots, peeled and thinly sliced

1 small red bell pepper, seeded, cored, and coarsely chopped

1 small onion, coarsely chopped

4 cloves garlic, sliced

1 tablespoon curry powder

½ teaspoon salt

¼ to ½ teaspoon red pepper flakes

8 skinless chicken drumsticks (1½ to 2 pounds total)

1 cup canned Whole30-compliant coconut milk (see Tip)

1 package (12 ounces) frozen riced cauliflower and broccoli

1 tablespoon coconut oil

¼ cup roasted and salted pumpkin seed kernels (pepitas)

IN a 3½- or 4-quart slow cooker, combine the tomatoes, carrots, bell pepper, onion, garlic, curry powder, salt, and pepper flakes. Arrange the chicken on top of the vegetables. Cover and cook on low for 5 to 6 hours or on high for 3 to 4 hours.

PLACE the chicken on a plate and cover with foil to keep warm. Add the coconut milk to the slow cooker with the vegetables and let the mixture cool briefly. Transfer to a blender, in batches if necessary, blend until smooth, and return to the cooker. (Or blend with an immersion blender in the cooker.) Return the chicken to the slow cooker and toss gently with tongs to coat.

MEANWHILE, prepare the cauliflower and broccoli according to package directions using the coconut oil.

SERVE the sauce over the drumsticks and cauliflower-broccoli rice. Sprinkle with the pepitas.

TIP *Canned coconut milk separates in the can with the cream rising to the top. Make sure to whisk the coconut milk well before measuring.*

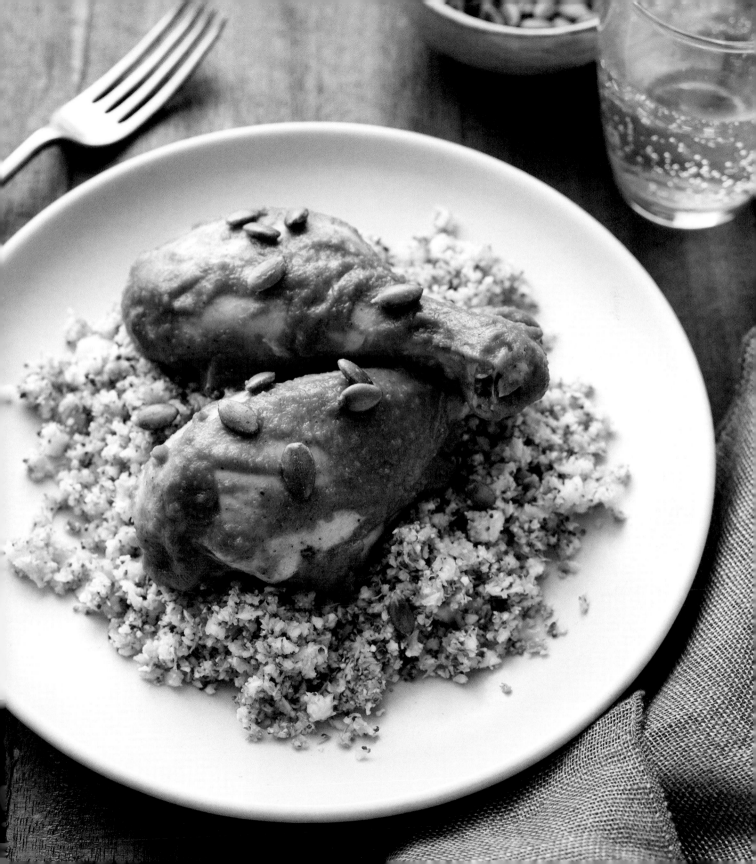

CHAPTER 6

SIMPLE
SIDES

Baked Brussels Sprouts with Tahini

SERVES 2

FROM *Scott Gooding of The Scott Gooding Project*

I was never a huge fan of Brussels sprouts growing up, but I feel this is a familiar story among friends of my generation. It seems these days it's widely accepted that if the sprouts are cooked in the right way, they can be a big crowd-pleaser!

PREP: 10 minutes

ROAST: 10 minutes

TOTAL: 20 minutes

2 cups Brussels sprouts, trimmed and halved (or quartered if large)

2 tablespoons Clarified Butter (page 283) or ghee, melted

1 teaspoon paprika

½ to 1 teaspoon red pepper flakes

¼ teaspoon salt

¼ black pepper

2 teaspoons fresh lemon juice

2 tablespoons Whole30-compliant tahini

PREHEAT the oven to 400°F. Line a baking sheet with parchment paper.

COMBINE the Brussels sprouts, butter, paprika, pepper flakes, salt, and black pepper in a large bowl. Place the Brussels sprouts in a single layer on the pan.

ROAST the Brussels sprouts, stirring once halfway through cooking, until the outer leaves are crispy and lightly browned, 8 to 10 minutes. Drizzle the lemon juice over the Brussels sprouts and serve with the tahini for dipping.

Chile-Lime Roasted Sweet Potatoes

SERVES 4

These nicely spicy sweet potatoes get a kick-start by being partially cooked in the microwave—then they're finished off in the high, dry heat of the oven.

PREP: 5 minutes

ROAST: 20 minutes

TOTAL: 25 minutes

1 bag (16 ounces) frozen cubed sweet potatoes (see Tip)

2 tablespoons coconut oil, melted

½ jalapeño, seeded and finely chopped; or ¼ to ½ teaspoon chipotle powder

1 teaspoon ground cumin

½ teaspoon salt

Lime wedges

PREHEAT the oven to 450°F. Line a large baking sheet with parchment paper.

PLACE the sweet potatoes in a medium bowl, cover with microwave-safe plastic wrap, and pull back a small section of the plastic wrap so the steam can escape. Microwave on high for 2 minutes.

ADD the coconut oil, jalapeño, cumin, and salt and toss to coat. Place the sweet potatoes on the pan and roast, stirring once halfway through, until golden, about 20 minutes. Serve with the lime wedges.

TIP *You can also use 1 pound peeled and cubed fresh sweet potatoes.*

Veggie Confetti Cauli-Rice

SERVES 5

FROM *Kelly Smith of The Nourishing Home*

What a beautiful rainbow of flavorful veggies! This simple, colorful dish comes together quickly and is a delicious complement to any meal. It also easily transforms into a tasty one-skillet meal by tossing in some leftover meat, poultry, or seafood.

PREP: 10 minutes

COOK: 10 minutes

TOTAL: 20 minutes

3 tablespoons Clarified Butter (page 283) or ghee

½ cup finely diced yellow onion

½ cup finely diced cremini mushrooms

¼ cup finely diced carrot

¼ cup finely diced red bell pepper

¼ cup finely diced zucchini

¾ teaspoon salt

½ teaspoon dried parsley

½ teaspoon garlic powder

¼ teaspoon black pepper

1 package (16 ounces) cauliflower crumbles, or 4 cups raw cauliflower rice (see page 75)

⅓ cup Whole30-compliant chicken broth or Chicken Bone Broth (page 280)

HEAT the butter in a large skillet over medium heat. Add the onion, mushrooms, carrot, bell pepper, and zucchini. Cook, stirring occasionally, until the vegetables begin to soften, about 5 minutes.

ADD the salt, parsley, garlic powder, and black pepper and cook, stirring, until combined. Stir in the cauliflower. Cook, stirring occasionally, until the cauliflower begins to soften, 2 to 3 minutes. Add the broth and cook, covered, until the cauliflower is just tender, about 2 minutes. Fluff with a fork and serve.

Quick Beet and Cabbage Salad

SERVES 4

Beets provide sweetness and red cabbage contributes crunch to this vibrantly purple-red salad studded with dried dark sweet cherries and roasted salted sunflower seeds.

PREP: 10 minutes

TOTAL: 10 minutes

1 package (8 ounces) refrigerated cooked baby beets; or 1 can (15 ounces) whole beets, drained

1 bag (10 ounces) shredded red cabbage

⅓ cup finely chopped shallot

½ cup Whole30-compliant dried dark sweet cherries, chopped

¼ cup roasted salted sunflower seeds

¼ cup chopped fresh parsley

3 tablespoons red wine vinegar

1 tablespoon balsamic vinegar

¼ cup extra-virgin olive oil

¼ teaspoon salt

¼ teaspoon black pepper

SLICE the beets and cut into thin strips. Combine the beets, cabbage, shallot, cherries, sunflower seeds, and parsley in a large bowl. Drizzle with both of the vinegars and toss to coat. Drizzle with the olive oil, sprinkle with the salt and black pepper, and toss again. Serve immediately or store in an airtight container in the refrigerator for up to 24 hours.

Lemon-Dill Parsnips

SERVES 4

Parsnips look like white carrots but have a less sweet, nuttier flavor. They're at peak season in the fall. Serve these roasted roots with beef or pork roast.

PREP: 20 minutes

ROAST: 20 minutes

TOTAL: 40 minutes

2 pounds parsnips, peeled and cut into 3 x ¼-inch matchsticks

3 tablespoons extra-virgin olive oil

3 cloves garlic, thinly sliced

½ teaspoon salt

⅛ teaspoon black pepper

2 tablespoons fresh lemon juice

2 teaspoons snipped fresh dill or ½ teaspoon dried dill

PREHEAT the oven to 425°F.

COMBINE the parsnips, olive oil, garlic, salt, and pepper in a large bowl and toss to coat. Place the parsnips in an even layer on two baking sheets.

ROAST, uncovered, stirring twice, until the parsnips are tender and starting to brown, 20 to 30 minutes. Drizzle with the lemon juice and sprinkle with the dill; toss to coat and serve.

Hasselback Zucchini with Gremolata

SERVES 4

Hasselback potatoes are a Swedish invention—a whole potato into which thin, accordion-like cuts are made almost all of the way through to the bottom of the potato. The potato is then brushed with butter, seasoned, and roasted. As it bakes, the slices separate and get browned and crisp in the oven. The same idea is applied here to zucchini!

PREP: 10 minutes

ROAST: 25 minutes

TOTAL: 35 minutes

4 small zucchini

2 tablespoons extra-virgin olive oil

2 cloves garlic, minced

1 teaspoon grated lemon zest

2 tablespoons finely chopped fresh basil

½ teaspoon salt

PREHEAT the oven to 425°F. Line a baking sheet with foil.

ARRANGE two chopsticks or wooden spoons lengthwise on opposite sides of one zucchini. Cut the zucchini crosswise into ¼-inch-thick slices, stopping when the knife reaches the chopsticks to prevent slicing all the way through. Carefully fan the slices slightly. Repeat with the remaining zucchini. Place the zucchini on the pan.

IN a small bowl, combine the olive oil, garlic, lemon zest, basil, and salt. Carefully spoon the gremolata between the zucchini slices and over the tops.

ROAST the zucchini just until tender, 25 to 30 minutes.

Herbed Celery Root Fries with Lemon Aioli

SERVES 2

Celery root—also called celeriac—is a root vegetable that has an incredibly homely exterior—gnarly brown skin with straggly roots. But it has a wonderfully crisp, juicy texture and flavor that's a mild mix of celery and parsley. It can be shredded and eaten as a salad or cooked—as it is here.

PREP: 20 minutes

ROAST: 25 minutes

TOTAL: 45 minutes

1 celery root without top (1 pound)

3 tablespoons extra-virgin olive oil

2 teaspoons fines herbes, Whole30-compliant Italian seasoning, or herbes de Provence

½ teaspoon salt

½ teaspoon black pepper

½ cup Whole30-compliant mayonnaise or Basic Mayonnaise (page 281)

½ teaspoon grated lemon zest

1 tablespoon fresh lemon juice

1 clove garlic, minced

PREHEAT the oven to 450°F.

USE a small sharp knife or a vegetable peeler to remove the tough skin from the celery root. Cut the root into ½-inch-thick fries. Place the fries in a large bowl, drizzle with the olive oil, and sprinkle with the fines herbes, salt, and black pepper. Toss to coat.

PLACE the fries in an even layer on a large baking sheet. Roast, stirring once, until tender and golden, about 25 minutes.

MEANWHILE, for the aioli, combine the mayonnaise, lemon zest and juice, and garlic in a small bowl. Serve the fries immediately with the aioli.

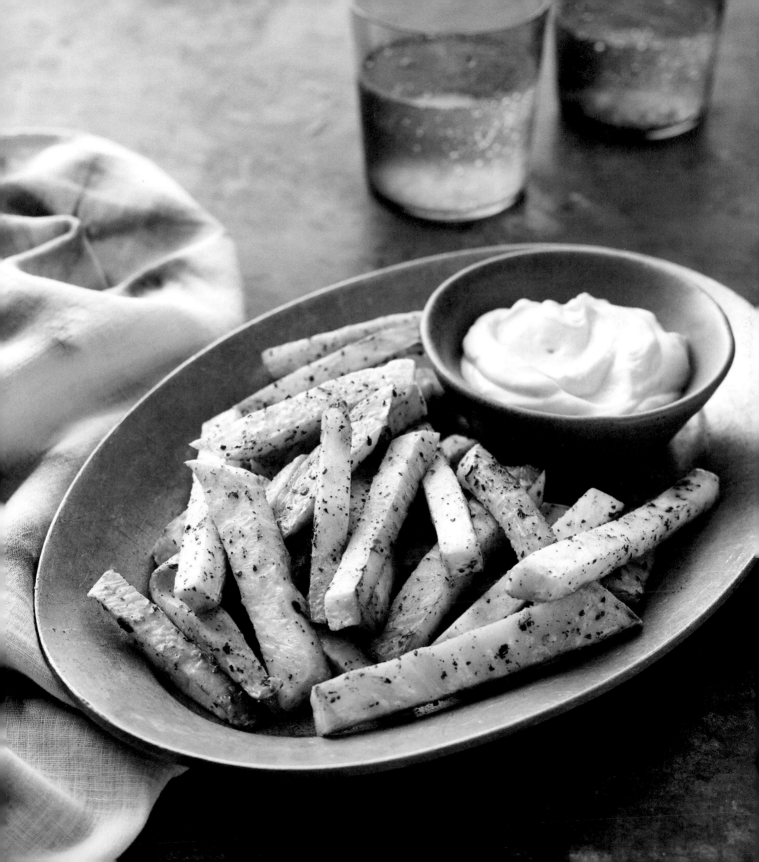

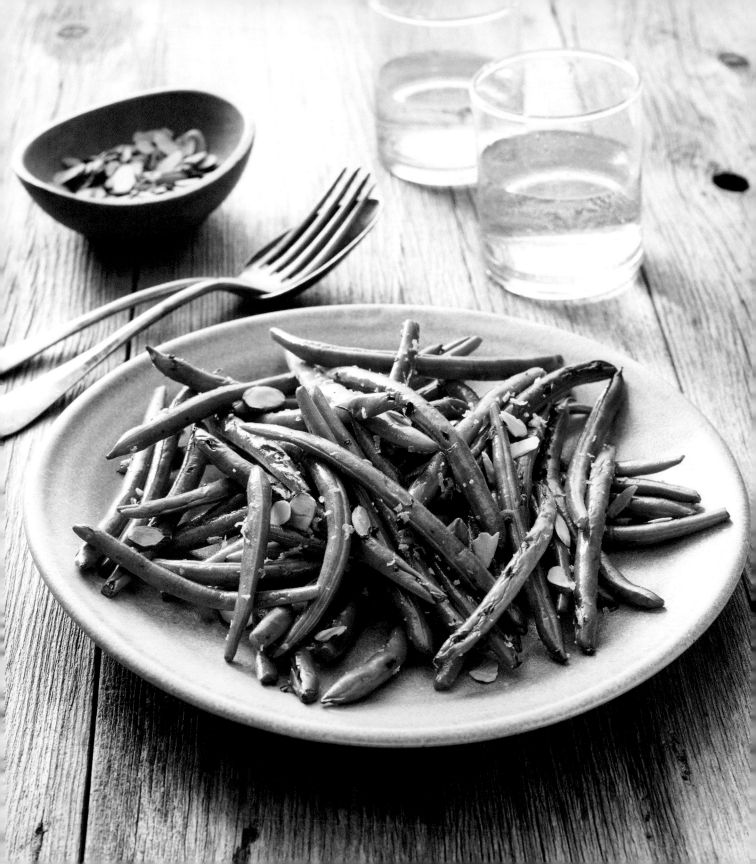

Blistered Green Beans with Toasted Almonds

SERVES 4

"Blistering" simply means you're cooking a vegetable in hot oil until brown spots begin to appear. It's a sign that the natural sugars in the vegetable are concentrating and caramelizing. Don't be tempted to stir the beans before about 2 minutes—they need a little time to char.

PREP: 5 minutes

COOK: 8 minutes

TOTAL: 15 minutes

1 tablespoon coconut oil

1 pound fresh green beans, trimmed (see Tip)

1 teaspoon grated lemon zest

1 to 2 teaspoons fresh lemon juice

¼ teaspoon salt

¼ teaspoon black pepper

¼ cup sliced almonds, toasted (see Tip)

HEAT the coconut oil in a large skillet over medium-high heat. Add the green beans and cook, without stirring, until the beans begin to blister, about 2 minutes. Stir and continue to cook, stirring occasionally, until crisp-tender and blistered in spots, 5 to 6 minutes.

REMOVE the skillet from the heat and stir in the lemon zest and juice, salt, and black pepper. Sprinkle with the almonds and serve.

TIPS *To trim green beans, cut or snap off the stem end.*
To toast sliced almonds, place in a skillet and heat until fragrant and lightly browned, about 1 minute.

Sautéed Sugar Snap Peas

SERVES 2

Sugar snap peas are allowed on the Whole30 because they are far more pod than bean. So while they are technically a legume, the green plant matter is good for you. Cook these just briefly so they stay bright green and crunchy.

PREP:	5 minutes
COOK:	5 minutes
TOTAL:	10 minutes

1 tablespoon Clarified Butter (page 283) or ghee

2 tablespoons finely chopped shallot

1 teaspoon minced fresh ginger

⅛ teaspoon red pepper flakes

1 bag (8 ounces) fresh stringless sugar snap peas

2 teaspoons coconut aminos

HEAT the butter in a medium skillet over medium heat. Add the shallot, ginger, and pepper flakes and cook, stirring, until fragrant, about 1 minute. Add the sugar snap peas and cook until crisp-tender, 3 to 5 minutes longer. Stir in the coconut aminos and serve.

Italian Roasted Whole Cauliflower

SERVES 4

You have probably roasted cauliflower florets before, but have you ever roasted a whole head? This makes an impressive side to serve to company. Slivers of garlic are tucked into the grooves on the partially baked cauliflower to infuse it with flavor as it bakes.

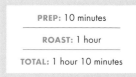

PREP: 10 minutes

ROAST: 1 hour

TOTAL: 1 hour 10 minutes

1 medium head cauliflower

½ cup water

2 tablespoons extra-virgin olive oil

½ teaspoon salt

¼ teaspoon black pepper

3 cloves garlic, thinly sliced

2 tablespoons chopped fresh basil and/or parsley

2 teaspoons chopped fresh oregano

PREHEAT the oven to 400°F.

TRIM the leaves and about 1 inch of the core from the cauliflower, leaving the head intact. Place the cauliflower, stem side down, in an 8 x 8-inch square baking dish. Add the water to the dish and cover tightly with foil. Roast for 30 minutes.

REMOVE the foil. Brush the cauliflower with the olive oil and sprinkle with the salt and black pepper. Insert the garlic slices between the grooves on the cauliflower. Roast the cauliflower, uncovered, until a sharp knife easily pierces through to the core, about 30 minutes longer.

IN a small bowl, combine the basil and oregano. Cut the cauliflower into wedges, sprinkle with the fresh herbs, and serve.

Cauliflower–Sweet Potato Mash

SERVES 4

This quick mash couldn't be simpler to make. It's wonderful with grilled steak or pork chops.

PREP: 5 minutes	
COOK: 15 minutes	
TOTAL: 20 minutes	

1 pound sweet potatoes, peeled and chopped

3 cups cauliflower florets

2 cloves garlic, peeled

3 tablespoons Clarified Butter (page 283) or ghee

½ teaspoon salt

¼ teaspoon black pepper

PLACE the sweet potatoes, cauliflower, and garlic in a large saucepan, add enough water to cover, and bring to a boil. Reduce the heat, cover, and simmer until the vegetables are tender, 12 to 15 minutes. Drain.

USING a potato masher, mash the vegetables until desired consistency. Stir in the butter, salt, and pepper and serve.

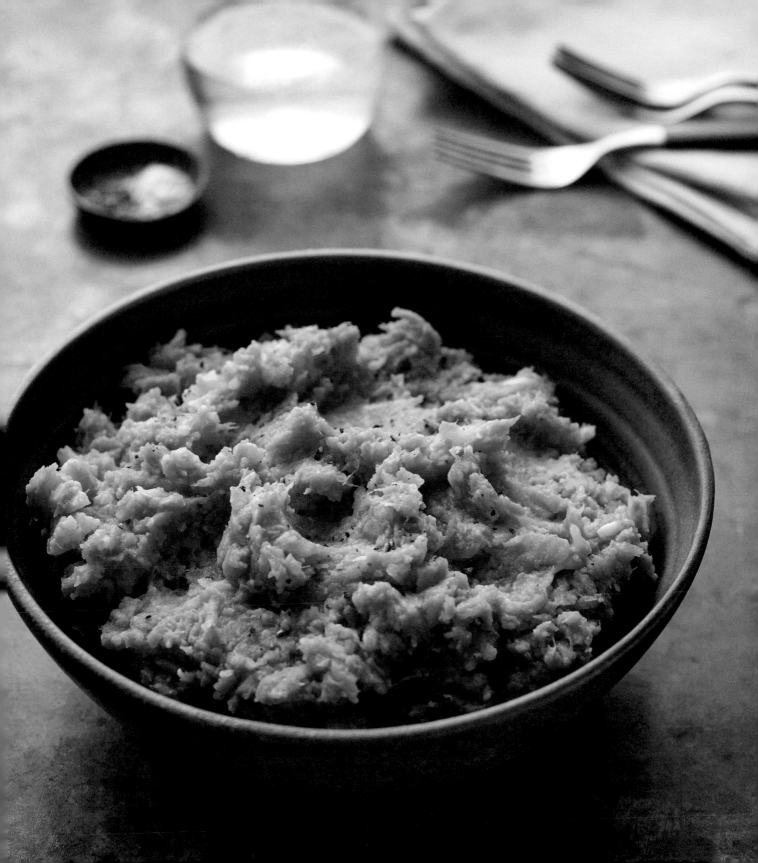

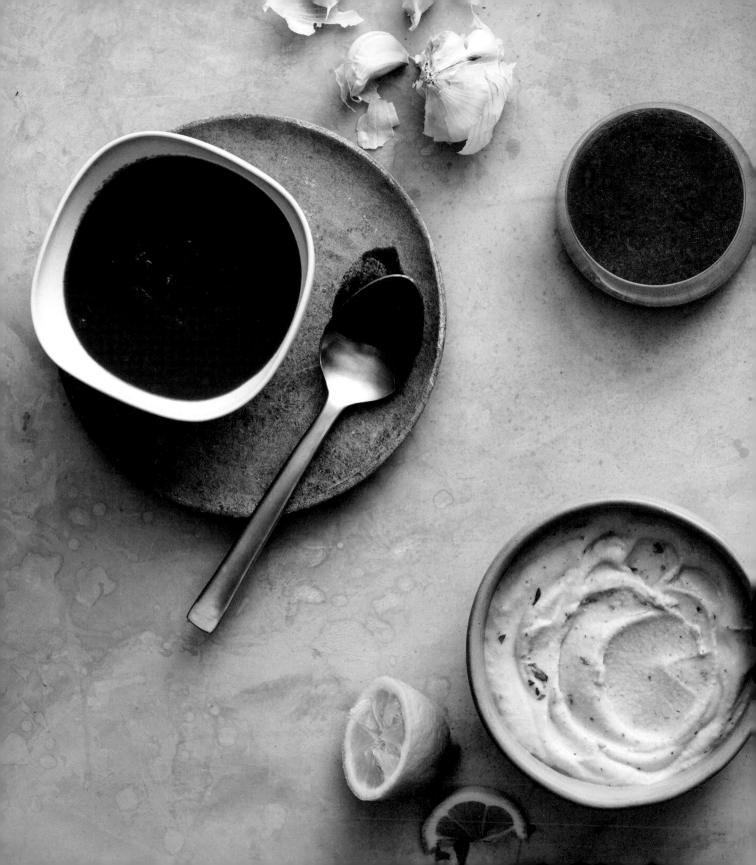

CHAPTER 7

SAUCES AND DRESSINGS

Whole30 Sriracha

MAKES 1½ CUPS

This spicy condiment has been all the rage for years now, but the bottled stuff contains sugar. This totally compliant version gets a touch of sweetness from a single dried date—so go crazy with it!

PREP: 15 minutes   **COOK:** 10 minutes   **TOTAL:** 25 minutes

1 pound Fresno chile peppers, stemmed, seeded, and roughly chopped

5 cloves garlic, smashed and peeled

2 tablespoons cider vinegar

2 tablespoons tomato paste

1 medium dried Medjool date, pitted

2 tablespoons Red Boat fish sauce

½ teaspoon salt

IN a high-power blender (see Tip), combine all the ingredients and process until smooth.

TRANSFER to a small saucepan and bring to a boil. Reduce the heat and simmer, stirring occasionally, for 10 minutes. Taste the sauce and adjust for salt. If the sauce is too thick, add water, 1 tablespoon at a time, until it reaches the desired consistency. Let cool.

USE immediately, or store in an airtight container in the refrigerator for up to 1 week.

TIP *If using a regular blender, chop the peppers into smaller pieces and mince the garlic for a smoother consistency.*

Roasted Garlic Chimichurri

MAKES 1¼ CUPS

Traditional Argentinean chimichurri gets a touch of acidity and briny flavor from red wine vinegar. In this roasted-garlic adaptation, it comes from capers. It's perfection on a grilled steak.

PREP: 10 minutes   **COOK:** 10 minutes   **TOTAL:** 20 minutes

2 bulbs garlic, separated into cloves but not peeled

1 cup packed fresh parsley

1 cup packed fresh basil

¾ cup extra-virgin olive oil

2 teaspoons grated lemon zest

1 tablespoon capers, drained

½ teaspoon salt

IN a cast-iron skillet or other heavy skillet, roast the garlic cloves over medium heat, removing small cloves as they soften, until the skins are toasted and cloves have softened, 10 to 15 minutes. Cool slightly, then remove and discard the skins.

PLACE the cloves in a food processor. Add the parsley, basil, olive oil, lemon zest, capers, and salt and process until nearly smooth.

USE immediately, or store in an airtight container in the refrigerator for up to 24 hours.

Quick-Toasted Cumin and Pineapple Taco Sauce

MAKES 2 CUPS

There's likely to be corn syrup and/or sugar and modified cornstarch in typical taco sauce. This totally fresh take on taco sauce can be made in less than 30 minutes and it's so much better!

PREP: 5 minutes   **COOK:** 20 minutes   **TOTAL:** 25 minutes

1 teaspoon cumin seeds

1 tablespoon extra-virgin olive oil

3 tablespoons finely chopped onion

1 tablespoon chili powder

1 can (15 ounces) Whole30-compliant tomato sauce

3 tablespoons pineapple juice

½ teaspoon salt

1 to 2 teaspoons Whole30-compliant hot sauce

TOAST the cumin seeds in a small heavy saucepan over medium heat until fragrant, about 2 minutes. Transfer to a mortar and pestle, spice grinder, or a cutting board and coarsely crush, grind, or chop the seeds.

HEAT the oil in the saucepan over medium heat. Add the onion and cook, stirring occasionally, until softened and beginning to brown, about 5 minutes. Stir in the cumin seeds and chili powder and cook, stirring, for 1 minute. Stir in the tomato sauce, pineapple juice, and salt. Bring to a boil, then reduce the heat and simmer, uncovered, for 10 minutes. Stir in the hot sauce.

USE immediately, or store in an airtight container in the refrigerator for up to 1 week.

Quick Blender Green Goddess Dressing

MAKES 1 CUP

Rich, creamy and a beautiful shade of pale green, this herby dressing is flavored with garlic, parsley, chives, lemon, and the signature ingredient in classic Green Goddess: tarragon. Use it to dress sturdy greens, as a dip for veggies—even as a drizzle for grilled chicken or shrimp.

PREP: 10 minutes   **TOTAL:** 10 minutes

½ avocado, pitted and peeled

¼ cup minced fresh parsley

¼ cup fresh lemon juice

2 tablespoons Whole30-compliant mayonnaise or Basic Mayonnaise (page 281)

2 tablespoons extra-virgin olive oil

1 tablespoon snipped fresh chives

2 to 3 teaspoons minced fresh tarragon

2 cloves garlic, minced

½ teaspoon salt

⅛ teaspoon black pepper

IN a blender or food processor, combine all the ingredients. Cover and blend or process until smooth.

USE immediately or place in an airtight container and store in the refrigerator for up to 24 hours.

Curried Sunflower Seed Sauce

MAKES 1 CUP

Be sure to look for sulfite-free dried apricots to make this sauce. Most commercial apricots are treated with sulfite as a preservative to maintain their bright color—but it's not something you want to be ingesting. Unsulfured apricots are available in the health-food sections of most supermarkets and at whole-foods stores. As an added bonus, we think they taste even better than the treated ones.

PREP: 5 minutes   **COOK:** 5 minutes   **TOTAL:** 10 minutes

⅓ cup sunflower seed butter

3 tablespoons coconut aminos

1 tablespoon sesame oil or coconut oil

1 tablespoon finely chopped sulfite-free dried apricot

½ to 1 teaspoon curry powder, to taste

1 clove garlic, minced

WHISK together ¼ cup water, the sunflower seed butter, coconut aminos, sesame oil, apricot, curry powder, and garlic in a small saucepan. Cook over medium-low heat, stirring, until bubbly and the sauce is smooth except for the fruit and garlic pieces, 5 minutes.

USE immediately or cool to room temperature and store in an airtight container in the refrigerator for up to 4 days.

Cauliflower-Cashew Alfredo Sauce

MAKES 2 CUPS

This rich and creamy sauce is absolutely amazing—and super kid-friendly. Toss lightly sautéed zucchini noodles with the warm sauce and top with cooked chicken or shrimp. So yummy!

PREP: 15 minutes   **COOK:** 15 minutes   **TOTAL:** 30 minutes

1 cup chopped raw cashews

4 or 5 cloves garlic, chopped

2 tablespoons Clarified Butter (page 283) or ghee

1 cup cauliflower florets

2 teaspoons fresh lemon juice

1 teaspoon salt

½ teaspoon black pepper

Chopped fresh parsley and/or basil (optional)

PLACE the cashews in a small bowl and add enough boiling water to cover. Let stand for 10 minutes. Drain and rinse.

IN a large skillet, cook the garlic in the butter over medium heat, stirring, until softened, about 2 minutes. Add the drained cashews, cauliflower, and 1 cup water. Increase the heat and bring to a simmer. Cover, reduce the heat, and simmer until the cauliflower is very tender, about 8 minutes.

TRANSFER the cauliflower mixture to a blender and add the lemon juice, salt, and black pepper. Let cool briefly and then blend until smooth, 2 to 3 minutes. Stir in the fresh parsley and/or basil, if desired.

USE immediately, or store in an airtight container in the refrigerator for up to 24 hours.

Asian Citrus Dressing

MAKES 1 CUP

Look for light or untoasted sesame oil to make this gingery dressing. Toasted sesame oil would overpower the other flavors.

PREP: 5 minutes **COOK:** 10 minutes **TOTAL:** 15 minutes

2 tablespoons coconut oil

2 tablespoons minced fresh ginger

4 cloves garlic, minced

⅔ cup fresh orange juice

⅓ cup coconut aminos

¼ cup cider vinegar

2 teaspoons sesame oil (not toasted)

HEAT the coconut oil in a medium skillet over medium heat. Add the ginger and garlic and cook, stirring, for 1 minute. Add the orange juice, coconut aminos, and vinegar. Bring to a boil, then reduce the heat and simmer for 5 minutes. Remove from the heat and add the sesame oil.

USE immediately, or store in an airtight container in the refrigerator for up to 1 week.

Apple-Mustard Vinaigrette

MAKES 1¼ CUPS

The classic flavors of this French-style vinaigrette—cider vinegar, Dijon mustard, garlic, and thyme—go with so many different things. At its most basic, it is wonderful on a mixed-greens salad. Whisk the olive oil in very slowly to emulsify and thicken it so it will stay combined and not separate.

PREP: 10 minutes **TOTAL:** 10 minutes

3 tablespoons cider vinegar

2 tablespoons apple cider

2 teaspoons Whole30-compliant Dijon or whole-grain mustard

1 clove garlic, minced

1 teaspoon chopped fresh thyme

½ teaspoon salt

¼ teaspoon black pepper

¾ cup extra-virgin olive oil

IN a small bowl, combine the vinegar, cider, mustard, garlic, thyme, salt, and pepper. While whisking, drizzle in the olive oil until blended.

USE immediately, or store in an airtight container in the refrigerator for up to 3 days.

Almond Satay Sauce

MAKES 1½ CUPS

This sauce has all of the flavors of traditional Indonesian-style peanut sauce—without the legume. Thread thin slices of sliced chicken breast on metal skewers (or wood skewers that have been soaked in water for 30 minutes), then broil or grill. Serve the chicken with this sauce.

PREP: 10 minutes   **TOTAL:** 10 minutes

½ cup almond butter

½ cup Whole30-compliant coconut milk (see Tip)

2 tablespoons coconut aminos

1 tablespoon fresh lime juice

1 tablespoon minced fresh ginger

1 teaspoon Red Boat fish sauce

1 clove garlic, minced

IN a blender or food processor, combine all the ingredients. Cover and blend or process until smooth.

USE immediately, or store in an airtight container in the refrigerator for up to 5 days.

TIP *Canned coconut milk separates in the can with the cream rising to the top. Be sure to whisk the coconut milk well before measuring.*

Everyday Whole30 Salad Dressing

MAKES 1¼ CUPS

FROM *Anya Kaats of Anya's Eats*

PREP: 5 minutes   **TOTAL:** 5 minutes

1 cup coconut aminos

1 tablespoon fresh lemon juice

1 tablespoon Whole30-compliant spicy brown mustard

2 cloves garlic, crushed

¼ teaspoon salt

¼ teaspoon black pepper

IN a blender, combine all the ingredients. Cover and blend until fully combined and frothy.

USE immediately, or store in an airtight container in the refrigerator for up to 1 week.

CHAPTER 8

BASICS

Chicken Bone Broth

MAKES 1 GALLON

PREP: 15 minutes   COOK: 12 hours   TOTAL: 12 hours

Carcass from a roasted 3- to 4-pound chicken

2 carrots, roughly chopped

3 stalks celery, roughly chopped

2 onions, roughly chopped

5 or 6 sprigs fresh parsley

1 sprig fresh thyme

2 tablespoons cider vinegar

10 whole black peppercorns

1 teaspoon salt

COMBINE all the ingredients in a large stockpot, add water to cover, and bring to a boil over high heat. Cover, reduce the heat to low, and simmer for 12 to 24 hours without stirring. (You can also do this in a slow cooker: Set the cooker to high until the water comes to a boil, then turn the temperature down to low and simmer for 12 to 24 hours.)

STRAIN the broth through a fine-mesh strainer set over a large bowl or clean pot. Discard the solids. Transfer the broth to multiple containers to speed up cooling—don't freeze or refrigerate the broth while it's hot! Allow the broth to sit in the fridge, uncovered, for several hours, until the fat rises to the top and hardens. Scrape off the fat with a spoon and discard it.

REFRIGERATE the broth in airtight containers for 3 to 4 days or freeze for up to 6 months.

TIP *A properly prepared chicken broth might look a little jiggly when cold. That's just the gelatin from the collagen in the bones. When ready to use the broth, gently heat it and it will return to a liquid state.*

Beef Bone Broth

MAKES 1 GALLON

PREP: 15 minutes   COOK: 12 hours   TOTAL: 12 hours

3 to 4 pounds beef bones

2 carrots, roughly chopped

3 stalks celery, roughly chopped

2 onions, roughly chopped

5 or 6 sprigs fresh parsley

1 sprig fresh thyme

2 tablespoons cider vinegar

10 whole black peppercorns

1 teaspoon salt

COMBINE all the ingredients in a large stockpot, add water to cover, and bring to a boil over high heat. Cover, reduce the heat to low, and simmer for 12 to 24 hours without stirring. (You can also do this in a slow cooker: Set the cooker to high until the water comes to a boil, then turn the temperature down to low and simmer for 12 to 24 hours.)

STRAIN the broth through a fine-mesh strainer set over a large bowl or clean pot. Discard the solids. Transfer the broth to multiple containers to speed up cooling—don't freeze or refrigerate the broth while it's hot! Allow the broth to sit in the fridge, uncovered, for several hours, until the fat rises to the top and hardens. Scrape off the fat with a spoon and discard it.

REFRIGERATE the broth in airtight containers for 3 to 4 days or freeze for up to 6 months.

TIP *A properly prepared beef broth will look solid but jiggly when cold—think "meat Jell-O." That's just the gelatin from the collagen in the bones. When ready to use the broth, gently heat it and it will return to a liquid state.*

Basic Mayonnaise

MAKES 1½ CUPS

PREP: 10 minutes TOTAL: 10 minutes

1¼ cups light olive oil

1 large egg (see Tip)

½ teaspoon dry mustard

½ teaspoon salt

Juice of ½ lemon

PLACE ¼ cup of the olive oil, the egg, mustard, and salt in a blender, food processor, or mixing bowl. Blend, process, or mix thoroughly. While the food processor or blender is running (or while mixing in a bowl with an immersion blender), slowly drizzle in the remaining 1 cup olive oil until the mayonnaise has emulsified. Add the lemon juice and blend on low or stir to incorporate.

TIP *The key to this emulsion is making sure all the ingredients are at room temperature. Leave your egg out on the counter for an hour, or let it sit in a bowl of hot water for 5 minutes before mixing. Keep one lemon on the counter at all times for the express purpose of making mayo—trust us, you'll be making a lot of this. The slower you add the oil, the thicker and creamer the emulsion will be. You can slowly pour the oil by hand out of a spouted measuring cup, or use a plastic squeeze bottle to slowly drizzle it into the bowl, food processor, or blender. If you're using an immersion blender, pump the stick up and down a few times toward the end to whip some air into the mixture, making it even fluffier.*

Egg-Free Mayonnaise

MAKES 1¼ CUPS

PREP: 10 minutes TOTAL: 10 minutes

½ cup coconut butter, slightly warmed

½ cup warm water

¼ cup light olive oil

2 cloves garlic, peeled

1 tablespoon fresh lemon juice
(optional; see Tip)

¼ teaspoon salt

PLACE all the ingredients in a food processor or blender and blend on high until the mixture thickens, 1 to 2 minutes.

TIP *If you plan on using this egg-free mayo as a base for dressings and sauces, skip the lemon juice. You then have a neutral flavor base to which you can add any kind of acid (like a citrus juice or vinegar) based on the dressing or sauce you select.*

Whole30 Ranch Dressing

MAKES 1½ CUPS

PREP: 10   **CHILL:** 1 hour   **TOTAL:** 1 hour, 10 minutes

1 cup Whole30-compliant mayonnaise or Basic Mayonnaise (page 281)

½ cup Whole30-compliant coconut milk

1 small clove garlic, minced

½ teaspoon onion powder

¼ teaspoon black pepper

1 tablespoon finely chopped fresh dill

1 tablespoon finely chopped chives

2 teaspoons fresh lemon juice

IN a medium bowl, whisk together all the ingredients. Cover with plastic wrap and refrigerate for 1 hour.

USE immediately, or store in an airtight container in the refrigerator for up to 1 week.

Whole30 Ketchup

MAKES 1 CUP

Don't expect the familiar Heinz 57 from this recipe. Grocery store ketchup is thick and sweet thanks to sugar—nearly 4 grams per tablespoon. In fact, Heinz uses both high-fructose corn syrup and corn syrup to sweeten their paste. We could use date paste to make our ketchup sugary, but that's not really in line with the spirit of the Whole30. This ketchup will have a lighter vinegar flavor; different but still delicious on eggs, burgers, and baked potato fries.

PREP: 5 minutes   **COOK:** 10 minutes   **TOTAL:** 15 minutes

1 cup Whole30-compliant tomato paste

½ cup apple cider

½ cup cider vinegar

1 teaspoon garlic powder

½ teaspoon salt

⅛ teaspoon ground cloves (optional)

HEAT a medium saucepan over medium heat. Add the tomato paste, apple cider, and vinegar. Stir to combine and let the mixture come to a simmer, but do not allow it to boil. Add the garlic powder, salt, and cloves (if using) and cook, stirring frequently to prevent scorching—you may need to turn the heat down to low or simmer here—until the ketchup has thickened enough to evenly coat the back of a spoon, 5 to 8 minutes. Remove from the heat and allow to cool.

SERVE when cool, or store in an airtight container in the refrigerator for up to 2 weeks.

Clarified Butter

MAKES 1½ CUPS

Plain old butter isn't allowed on the Whole30 because it contains traces of milk proteins, which may be problematic for dairy-sensitive individuals. Clarifying butter is the technique of simmering butter slowly at a low temperature to separate the milk solids from the pure butterfat. The end result is a delicious, pure, dairy-free fat, perfect for flavoring dishes or cooking (even on high heat).

You'll also see ghee suggested in the recipes—ghee is just a different form of clarified butter. To make ghee, simply simmer the butter longer, until the milk proteins begin to brown, clump, and drift to the bottom of the pan. Ghee has a sweeter, nuttier flavor than clarified butter. You can also purchase pastured organic ghee online.

While it's not part of our official Whole30 rules, we always encourage you to look for pastured organic butter when making your own clarified butter or ghee. Common brands available at health food stores nationwide include Straus, Kerrygold, Kalona SuperNatural, and Organic Valley.

PREP: 5 minutes   **COOK:** 20 minutes   **TOTAL:** 25 minutes

1 pound (4 sticks) unsalted butter

CUT the butter into 1-inch cubes. In a small pot or saucepan, melt the butter over medium-low heat and let it come to a simmer without stirring. As the butter simmers, foamy white dairy solids will rise to the surface. With a spoon or ladle, gently skim the dairy solids off the top and discard, leaving just the pure clarified butter in the pan.

ONCE you've removed the majority of the milk solids, strain the butter through cheesecloth into a glass storage jar, discarding the milk solids and cheesecloth when you are done. Allow the butter to cool before storing.

CLARIFIED butter can be stored in the refrigerator for up to 6 months or at room temperature for up to 3 months. (With the milk solids removed, clarified butter is shelf-stable for a longer period of time than regular butter.)

Simple Cauliflower Rice

SERVES 2 (2 CUPS EACH)

This rice is very subtly flavored with just a little bit of onion (and a little parsley, if you like) so it is adaptable to many dishes and flavor profiles. You can serve it as is or stir in additional herbs, seasonings, chopped toasted nuts, or dried fruits.

PREP: 15 minutes   **COOK:** 15 minutes   **TOTAL:** 30 minutes

---

1 large head cauliflower, cut into florets

3 tablespoons Clarified Butter (page 283) or ghee

½ onion, finely chopped

½ cup Chicken Bone Broth (page 280) or Whole30-compliant chicken broth

1½ teaspoons minced fresh parsley (optional)

½ teaspoon salt

¼ teaspoon black pepper

PLACE half the cauliflower in a food processor and pulse until they have broken down to a rice-like consistency, 15 to 20 pulses. (Don't overcrowd the cauliflower in the food processor, and don't over-pulse or the "rice" will get mushy.) Transfer to a bowl and rice the remaining cauliflower.

IN a large skillet, melt the butter over medium heat and swirl to coat the bottom of the pan. When the butter is hot, add the onion and cook, stirring, until translucent, 2 to 3 minutes.

ADD the riced cauliflower to the skillet and mix thoroughly to combine with the onion. Add the broth, cover the pan, and steam the cauliflower for 10 to 12 minutes, until tender but not mushy or wet.

REMOVE the pan from the heat and mix in the parsley, if using. Season with salt and pepper.

WHOLE30 RESOURCES

This first part of this resources section includes websites, cookbooks, and social media feeds we really like, from people with whom I have developed a close personal and professional relationship. They're smart, talented people who are Whole30 experts in their own right. They've done the program, offer specific resources for your Whole30 success, and really get the spirit and intention of the Whole30.

Not everything in these websites, cookbooks, and social media feeds is Whole30 compliant, but you already knew that, right? They don't eat Whole30 all the time, and as I explain in *Food Freedom Forever*, neither will you. I'm just pointing this out because you have to read website content, recipes, and social media hashtags just as carefully as you have to read labels. Anybody on the Internet can say a meal or ingredient is "#Whole30" or "Whole30 compliant," but it's your job to determine whether that's actually true.

Unless it's coming from me (the Whole30 website, my books, or our social media feeds), don't take any label of "Whole30 compliant" at face value. Use your critical thinking skills, read your labels/ingredients/recipes carefully, and make your own educated decision about whether the item in question really is "Whole30."

Websites

Whole30
whole30.com

The official home of the Whole30 program. This is where you'll find our free Whole30 Forum, all our free downloads, Whole30 Approved products and affiliates, and more Whole30-related articles than you could possibly hope to read in thirty days. Spend lots of time exploring here before, during, and after your Whole30—this is the very heart of our community.

Facebook: whole30

Instagram: @whole30, @whole30recipes, @whole30approved

Twitter: @whole30

Snapchat: whole30

Ziing: Whole30

YouTube: whole30

Pinterest: @whole30

Well Fed: Melissa Joulwan
meljoulwan.com

Not only is Melissa Joulwan the author of three Whole30-friendly cookbooks (*Well Fed, Well Fed 2,* and *Well Fed Weeknights*) and a Whole30 Certified Coach, she's also a brilliant food, fitness, health, and lifestyle blogger with hundreds of Whole30-compliant recipes, meal plans, and resources freely available on her site.

Facebook: MelJoulwan

Instagram: @meljoulwan

Twitter: @meljoulwan

Pinterest: meljoulwan

Nom Nom Paleo: Michelle Tam

nomnompaleo.com

Since 2010, Michelle Tam has been religiously taking pictures of her Whole30 meals and sharing her Whole30 meal plans and recipes. She also penned the *New York Times* best-selling cookbook *Nom Nom Paleo* and the new *Ready or Not*, both of which feature a large number of Whole30-friendly meals.

Facebook: nomnompaleo

Instagram: @nomnompaleo

Twitter: @nomnompaleo

Pinterest: nomnompaleo

Snapchat: michitam

Danielle Walker's Against All Grain

againstallgrain.com

Danielle Walker is a *New York Times* best-selling author and photographer who shares her grain-free and gluten-free recipes on her blog and in her cookbooks, *Against All Grain*, *Meals Made Simple*, and *Celebrations*. With her acquired culinary skills, love for food, and deeply touching personal story, she is a go-to source for those suffering from all types of diseases and allergies.

Facebook: AgainstAllGrain

Instagram: @againstallgrain

Twitter: @againstallgrain

Youtube: AgainstAllGrain

Pinterest: @Againstallgrain

Sustainable Dish: Diana Rodgers

sustainabledish.com

Diana Rodgers, RD, LDN, NTP, is a real-food registered dietitian and Whole30 Certified Coach living on a working organic farm. She is the author of *The Homegrown Paleo Cookbook* and *Paleo Lunches and Breakfasts on the Go* and hosts the *Sustainable Dish* podcast. She speaks internationally about nutrition, the environmental impact of our food choices, and animal welfare, and fully embraces the Whole30 philosophy in her practice.

Facebook: sustainabledish

Instagram: @sustainabledish

Twitter: @sustainabledish

The Whole Smiths: Michelle Smith

thewholesmiths.com

Michelle Smith is passionate about eating real food and creating a sustainable food system that everyone can enjoy for many years to come. Her recipes focus on minimally processed and sustainable foods that are easy to prepare, taste great, and make us feel good again.

Facebook: thewholesmiths

Instagram: @thewholesmiths

Twitter: @thewholesmiths

Snapchat: @thewholesmiths

Pinterest: thewholesmiths

Cookbooks

There are only three books in which 100 percent of the recipes featured are Whole30 approved. You're reading one of them right now—the others are *The Whole30: The 30-Day Guide to Total Health and Food Freedom* and *The Whole30 Cookbook*.

> ### The "How-To" for the Whole30
> Although *The Whole30* features more than 100 delicious and totally compliant recipes, it's more than just a cookbook—it's a complete Whole30 handbook, start to finish, including planning and preparation tips, an extensive FAQ, and Whole30 kitchen basics. If you're loving the recipes in *The Whole30 Fast & Easy* but want a game plan to help you maximize your Whole30 success, *The Whole30* is all you'll need.

However, there are other cookbooks that feature delicious, Whole30-compliant recipes or recipes that could easily be adapted to our Whole30 program. In fact, once you gain experience with the program, you'll be able to take just about *any* cookbook and make it Whole30 friendly. Until then, we'll give you a few cookbooks that include many Whole30-compliant recipes. You'll still need to be on the lookout for noncompliant ingredients, however, and save the baked goods, desserts, and "treat" sections for life after your Whole30.

The Whole30 Cookbook
by Melissa Hartwig

More than 150 totally compliant recipes to help you prepare delicious, healthy meals during your Whole30 and beyond.

Well Fed, Well Fed 2, *and* Well Fed Weeknights
by Melissa Joulwan

Hundreds of mouth-watering recipes and meal ideas from every corner of the world, plus time-saving meal prep and cooking tutorials.

Nom Nom Paleo: Food for Humans *and* Ready or Not: 150+ Make-Ahead, Make-Over, and Make-Now Recipes
by Michelle Tam and Henry Fong

Whether you're a planner or an improviser, these cookbooks feature family-friendly recipes and step-by-step instructional photographs for everything from make-ahead feasts to lightning-fast leftover makeovers.

Against All Grain, Meals Made Simple, *and* Celebrations
by Danielle Walker

Grain-free, dairy-free, and Whole30-friendly, Danielle provides family-friendly meals, quick and easy dinners, and complete holiday and special event menus in these three best-selling cookbooks.

Paleo Breakfasts and Lunches on the Go *and* The Homegrown Paleo Cookbook
by Diana Rodgers

You'll find healthy "on-the-go" packable meals (no sandwiches in sight) in *Paleo Breakfasts and Lunches on the Go*; and 100 delicious farm-to-table recipes and a complete guide to growing your own healthy food in *The Homegrown Paleo Cookbook*.

The Frugal Paleo Cookbook
by Ciarra Hannah

This cookbook features nearly 100 recipes, and combines great taste with a budget-conscious approach.

The Performance Paleo Cookbook
by Stephanie Gaudreau

This specialized book (part fueling strategies, part cookbook) delivers 100 delicious, nutrient-packed recipes specially designed to deliver a better performance in your sport or the gym.

The Paleo Foodie Cookbook *and* The Paleo Slow Cooker
by Arsy Vartanian

With nearly 250 healthy everyday meals, these cookbooks feature delicious, creative dishes, with plenty of grocery shopping and cooking tips for the budding real-food chef.

Whole30 Inspiration

Our special guest contributors to *Whole30 Fast and Easy* have gorgeous websites and social media feeds with hundreds of Whole30-compliant recipes, meal planning strategies, kitchen tips, and lifestyle guidance to keep you happy and healthy long after your Whole30 journey is over. Note, not everything they create is Whole30-friendly; read your recipes carefully, and save sweets and treats for your food freedom.

Real Food with Dana: Dana Monsees
realfoodwithdana.com

Dana Monsees offers a nutrition and lifestyle blog designed to help you thrive with real food and a paleo lifestyle one delicious meal at a time.

Facebook: realfoodwithdana

Instagram: @realfoodwithdana

Pinterest: realfoodwdana

Anya's Eats: Anya Kaats
anyaseats.com

Anya Kaats is a San Diego-based blogger, health coach, and professional marketer for natural product brands.

Facebook: anyaseats

Instagram: @anyas_eats

Pinterest: anyas_eats

The Scott Gooding Project: Scott Gooding
scottgoodingproject.com

Scott Gooding is an Australian chef and thought leader, encouraging and inspiring people to cook real food at home for themselves and their loved ones.

Facebook: scottgoodingproject

Instagram: @scottgoodingproject

The Real Food Dietitians:
Jessica Beacom, RDN, and
Stacie Hassing, RDN, LD

therealfoodrds.com

Jessica Beacom and Stacie Hassing are Registered Dietitian Nutritionists (RDN) and Whole30 Certified Coaches who create gluten-free and Whole30-friendly recipes designed to be big on taste and short on ingredients.

Facebook: therealfoodrds

Instagram: @therealfoodrds

Twitter: @therealfoodrds

Pinterest: therealfoodrds

The Nourishing Home: Kelly Smith

thenourishinghome.com

Kelly Smith is a cookbook author and blogger who shares delicious grain-free whole-food recipes, meal plans, cooking tips, and encouragement.

Facebook: TheNourishingHome

Instagram: @TheNourishingHome

Pinterest: NourishingHome

I Heart Umami: ChihYu Smith

iheartumami.com

ChihYu Smith is the founder of *Cook Once Eat All Week,* a paleo meal planning program that helps busy professionals save time and add deliciousness to their paleo and Whole30 cooking.

Facebook: iheartumami

Instagram: @iheartumami.ny

YouTube: iheartumami

Pinterest: iheartumami

Savor & Fancy: Sarah Steffens

savorandfancy.com

Sarah Steffens is a Los Angeles-based personal chef who cooks meals that support her clients' intention to physically and mentally thrive.

Instagram: @sarahsteffens_personalchef

The Sophisticated Caveman:
Brian Kavanagh

thesophisticatedcaveman.com

Brian Kavanagh is an outdoor enthusiast who creates and shares simple recipes featuring real food with an added "touch of class."

Facebook: socaveman

Instagram: @sophisticatedcaveman

Twitter: @socaveman

Pinterest: socaveman

Cook at Home Mom: Laura Miner

cookathomemom.com

Laura Miner is a home cook who loves to help families prepare and enjoy simple, delicious meals together.

Instagram: @cookathomemom

Pinterest: cookathomemom

Primal Gourmet: Ronny Joseph

cookprimalgourmet.com

Ronny Joseph is a self-taught cook, food photographer, and coffee enthusiast who shares real-food recipes that are easy and healthy but don't sacrifice flavor.

Facebook: cookprimalgourmet

Instagram: @primal_gourmet

YouTube: PrimalGourmet

Meal Planning

Real Plans

w30.co/w30realplans

Delicious, totally compliant Whole30 meals in a weekly plan to fit your taste and schedule. Fully customizable; choose which days of the week and meals to plan, exclude ingredients to which you are allergic or just don't like, and generate an automated shopping list and meal prep instructions for each week. Features more than 1,000 Whole30-compliant recipes to build into your family's perfect weekly meal plan.

Whole30 Certified Coaches

Work with a Coach

whole30.com/coaches

Our Whole30 Certified Coaching program allows those with the education, experience, and passion for the Whole30 to lead others through the program in a group (or in some cases, one-on-one) coaching environment. Our coaches lead Whole30 group resets, teach seminars, hold cooking and meal prep events, and provide other Whole30 and food freedom services to their local communities. To work with a coach in your area, visit our website and search by state or zip code.

Whole30 Approved

This is a list of our official Whole30 Approved partners, with the addition of some Whole30-friendly products from companies we love. These companies make a variety of products to support your Whole30 journey, but in many cases, not *every* product they make fits our guidelines. Read your labels, or look for the official Whole30 Approved logo on their website or packaging. We add to our list of official Whole30 Approved partners every week, so visit whole30.com/whole30-approved for the full roster.

Whole30 Curated Kits

THRIVE MARKET WHOLE30 CURATED KITS (THRV.ME/ WHOLE30FBLIVE): Whole30 Approved curated kits, "Melissa's Picks" featuring her favorite Whole30 products, and more than 100+ compliant pantry staples delivered to your door. New members save 25 percent and free shipping on their first order.

BAREFOOT PROVISIONS WHOLE30 KITS (W30.CO/ W30BAREFOOT): Whole30 Approved curated kits for emergency foods, healthy fats, and pregnancy nutrition, shipped throughout the world, no membership required.

On-the-Go and Travel Food

RXBAR (RXBAR.COM): Egg white protein–based bars. Most flavors are Whole30 compliant; read your labels. Don't use these as treats, please. Use the discount code "whole30" online to save 10 percent.

EPIC (EPICBAR.COM): Grass-fed/pastured jerky bars, bits, and strips, and bacon bites for salads and soups. Most varieties are Whole30 compliant (read your labels).

CHOMPS SNACK STICKS (GOCHOMPS.COM): Grass-fed and free range beef, venison, and chicken snack sticks.

WILD ZORA (WILDZORA.COM): Natural and grass-fed meat and veggie bars.

BROOKLYN BILTONG (BROOKLYNBILTONG.COM): Seasoned, all-natural dried beef snacks.

SOPHIA'S SURVIVAL JERKY (GRASSFEDJERKYCHEWS. COM): Grass-fed beef jerky in multiple flavors.

SEASNAX (SEASNAX.COM): Nutrient-packed roasted seaweed sheets in a variety of flavors.

Fresh Foods (Meat and Produce)

BUTCHERBOX (BUTCHERBOX.COM/WHOLE30): 100-percent grass-fed, grass-finished beef, organic chicken, and heritage breed pork, delivered to your door CSA-style for less than $6.50 per meal.

HUNGRY HARVEST (HUNGRYHARVEST.NET): Recovered farm-fresh produce and organic produce, delivered to your door CSA-style in the mid-Atlantic (and rapidly growing).

U.S. WELLNESS MEATS (GRASSLANDBEEF.COM): Grass-fed and free-range meats from family farmers, including the first-ever Whole30 Approved sugar-free bacon.

VITAL FARMS (VITALFARMS.COM): Eggs from certified humane, certified organic, pasture-raised hens raised on land without pesticides, herbicides, or harmful chemicals.

PANORAMA (PANORAMAMEATS.COM): Grass-fed beef from certified organic family farmers.

VERDE FARMS (VERDEFARMS.COM): Pasture-raised grass-fed beef raised according to strict animal welfare protocols.

THE HONEST BISON (HONESTBISON.COM): Grass-fed and humanely raised bison offerings, including soup bones.

PEDERSON'S NATURAL FARMS (PEDERSONSNATURAL-FARMS.COM): Certified humane and sugar-free bacon, sausages, hot dogs, and ham.

NAKED BACON (NAKEDBACONCO.COM): Sugar-free, nitrite-/nitrate-free, all-natural bacon and breakfast sausage.

LOKI FISH CO. (LOKIFISH.COM): Sustainably harvested and direct-marketed wild fish, free of added sugars, additives, or preservatives.

VEGGIE NOODLE CO. (VEGGIENOODLECO.COM): Fresh, raw spiralized veggie noodles made from zucchini, butternut squash, sweet potatoes, and beets.

Healthy Fats

PRIMAL KITCHEN AVOCADO OIL AND MAYO (PRIMALKITCHEN.COM): Heart-healthy avocado oil and avocado oil–based sugar-free mayonnaise, in original and chipotle flavors.

EPIC ANIMAL OILS (EPICBAR.COM): Beef tallow, pork lard, and duck fat from their Whole Animal Project.

FATWORKS (FATWORKSFOODS.COM): Traditional handcrafted cooking fats, including tallow (beef, buffalo, and lamb), lard, leaf lard, duck fat, goose fat, and chicken schmaltz.

TIN STAR GHEE (TINSTARFOODS.COM): Cultured, handmade pastured ghee and brown butter ghee made from the milk of grass-fed cows.

PURE INDIAN FOODS GHEE (PUREINDIANFOODS.COM): Grass-fed, organic, non-GMO ghee and cooking oils.

OMGHEE (OMGHEE.COM): Small-batch, grass-fed, organic, non-GMO ghee.

MEENUT BUTTER (MEEEATPALEO.COM): Handmade, small-batch sugar- and peanut-free nut butter blends.

Pantry Staples

SAFE CATCH (SAFECATCH.COM): Wild-caught tuna in cans and pouches, featuring the lowest mercury content of any brand-safe even for pregnant women.

NEW PRIMAL MARINADES AND COOKING SAUCES (NEWPRIMAL.COM): Classic, citrus herb, and spicy marinades and cooking sauces for meat and veggies.

BIG TREE FARMS COCONUT AMINOS (BIGTREEFARMS. COM): A soy sauce substitute made from brewed and naturally-fermented coconut blossom nectar and sea salt.

RED BOAT FISH SAUCE (REDBOATFISHSAUCE.COM): All-natural, first-press, "extra-virgin" Vietnamese fish sauce made without MSG, added water, or preservatives using a 200-year-old artisanal process.

YAI'S THAI SAUCES (YAISTHAI.COM): Thai-inspired, hand-crafted salsas, sauces, almond sauce, and curry sauces.

HORSETOOTH HOT SAUCE (HORSETOOTHHOTSAUCE. COM): Family-owned Colorado-based company specializing in delectable hot sauces from mild to ultra-spicy.

PRIMAL PALATE ORGANIC SPICES (PRIMALPALATE.COM): Organic, gluten-free, non-GMO, non-irradiated high-quality spices and spice blends, including an AIP-friendly spice pack.

SPICE CAVE ORGANIC SPICE BLENDS (THESPICECAVE. COM): All-natural spice blends to pair with your protein choices: Land, Sea, and Wind. (Save the lightly sweetened Fire for life after your Whole30.)

SPICE HOUND (SPICEHOUND.COM): More than 100 high-quality, freshly ground, and custom-blended spices, herbs, salts, and spice accessories.

PALEO POWDER SEASONINGS (PALEOPOWDERSEASON-ING.COM): All-purpose paleo, MSG-free, and gluten-free seasonings.

Fridge and Freezer Staples

PRE-MADE PALEO MEALS (PREMADEPALEO.COM): Chef-prepared, seasonal, and organic breakfasts, lunches, dinners, and snacks shipped frozen across the United States.

GRANDCESTORS MEALS (GRANDCESTORS.COM): Individual serving sizes of prepared frozen meals with hearty portions.

TESSEMAE'S ALL NATURAL (TESSEMAES.COM): All-natural and certified organic dressings, sauces, condiments, and marinades from their family to yours.

PRIMAL KITCHEN DRESSINGS (PRIMALKITCHEN.COM): Avocado oil–based, sugar-free Greek, ranch, Caesar, and green goddess dressings.

FARMHOUSE CULTURE (FARMHOUSECULTURE.COM): Organic, probiotic-rich krauts, Gut Shots, and vegetables with zingy, zesty flavors.

ZÜPA NOMA SOUPS (DRINKZUPA.COM): Ready-to-sip nutrient-dense soups containing over four servings of whole, organic vegetables per bottle.

BROTHS AND COLLAGEN

VITAL PROTEINS (VITALPROTEINS.COM): Pasture-raised collagen, gelatin, bone broth, and more, for healthier skin, nails, and hair; to promote joint and bone health; and aid in athletic performance.

EPIC (EPICBAR.COM): The first-ever ready-to-heat pasture-raised and grass-fed beef, chicken, and turkey broth, from their Whole Animal Project.

BARE BONES (BAREBONESBROTH.COM): Nutritious, pasture-raised and grass-fed, organic chicken and beef bone broths.

BONAFIDE PROVISIONS (BONAFIDEPROVISIONS.COM): Organic, grass-fed, pasture-raised chicken and beef bone broth, and Drinkable Veggie bone broth beverages.

KETTLE & FIRE (KETTLEANDFIRE.COM): Grass-fed, organic beef and chicken bone broth in shelf-stable packaging.

OSSO GOOD (OSSOGOODBONES.COM): Pasture-raised and grass-fed, all-natural chicken and beef sippable, organic bone broths.

Beverages

HINT WATER (DRINKHINT.COM): Pure, unsweetened water infused with truly natural fruit flavors. Available in more than 25 refreshing flavors, in still and sparkling.

LACROIX WATER (LACROIXWATER.COM): Sugar- and calorie-free naturally flavored sparkling waters.

NUTPODS MILK (NUTPODS.COM): Unsweetened, carrageenan-free almond and coconut milk coffee creamers in three delicious varieties.

NEW BARN ALMOND MILK (THENEWBARN.COM): The first Whole30 Approved almond milk, with only four simple, organic ingredients.

CRIO BRU COFFEE ALTERNATIVE (CRIOBRU.COM): All-natural 99-percent caffeine-free coffee alternative made from Fair Trade cocoa beans, roasted, ground, and brewed just like coffee.

CHOFFY BREWED CHOCOLATE (CHOFFY.COM): Artisan quality 100-percent premium ground cacao beans, brews just like coffee.

KLIO HERBAL TEA (KLIOTEA.COM): Unique herbal teas imported from Greece.

Lifestyle

SFH FISH OIL (SFH.COM): All-natural, filler-free omega-3 high-potency fish oil.

ELETE ELECTROLYTES (ELETEWATER.COM): Sugar-free electrolyte concentrates for athletes.

ORA WELLNESS (ORAWELLNESS.COM): Organic, all-natural tooth and gum hygiene products.

Whole30 Support

Resources to give you Whole30 support, motivation, and accountability.

Whole30 Day by Day: Your Daily Guide to Whole30 Success

whole30.com/daybyday

Advice, tips, hacks, and inspiration to guide you through every day of your Whole30, with guided reflections, dedicated space to track your non-scale victories and Whole30 meals, and daily check-ins to keep you motivated.

Wholesome

whole30.com/wholesome

Our free biweekly newsletter filled with Whole30-related advice, tips, recipes, reader stories, discounts, giveaways, and more.

Whole30 Daily

daily.whole30.com

A subscription newsletter delivering a daily dose of Whole30 wisdom, support, and tough love straight to your inbox every morning.

The Whole30 Forum

forum.whole30.com

If you have a question, we can almost guarantee it's been answered. Find those answers, solicit expert advice from our moderators, and get support from fellow Whole30ers on our free forum.

Whole30 Resources

whole30.com/pdf-downloads

Home to a host of helpful PDF downloads (including our shopping list, meal template, label-reading guide, pantry-stocking guide, and more).

Dear Melissa

whole30.com/category/dear-melissa

My own Whole30 (and life after) advice column, where I answer your questions and share from my own experience.

Connect with Melissa

I love hearing your stories, answering your questions, giving you my best Whole30 and food freedom advice... and tough-loving you when you need it.

Facebook: hartwig.melissa

Instagram: @melissa_hartwig

Twitter: @melissahartwig_

Ziing: #melissahartwigwhole30

Cooking Conversions

Metric weights listed here have been slightly rounded to make measuring easier.

Weight

U.S.	METRIC
¼ oz	7 grams
½ oz	15 g
¾ oz	20 g
1 oz	30 g
8 oz (½ lb)	225 g
12 oz (¾ lb)	340 g
16 oz (1 lb)	455 g
2 lb	900 g
2¼ lb	1 kg

Volume

U.S.	METRIC	IMPERIAL
¼ tsp	1.2 ml	
½ tsp	2.5 ml	
1 tsp	5 ml	
½ Tbsp (1½ tsp)	7.5 ml	
1 Tbsp (3 tsp)	15 ml	
¼ cup (4 Tbsp)	60 ml	2 fl oz
⅓ cup (5 Tbsp)	75 ml	2½ fl oz
½ cup (8 Tbsp)	125 ml	4 fl oz
⅔ cup (10 Tbsp)	150 ml	5 fl oz
¾ cup (12 Tbsp)	175 ml	6 fl oz
1 cup (16 Tbsp)	250 ml	8 fl oz
1¼ cups	300 ml	10 fl oz (½ pint)
1½ cups	350 ml	12 fl oz
2 cups (1 pint)	500 ml	16 fl oz
2½ cups	625 ml	20 fl oz (1 pint)
1 quart	1 liter	32 fl oz

Oven Conversions

FAHRENHEIT (degrees F)	CELSIUS (degrees C)	GAS NUMBER	OVEN TERMS
225	110	¼	Very Cool
250	130	½	Very Slow
275	140	1	Very Slow
300	150	2	Slow
325	165	3	Slow
350	177	4	Moderate
375	190	5	Moderate
400	200	6	Moderately Hot
425	220	7	Hot
450	230	8	Hot
475	245	9	Hot
500	260	10	Extremely Hot
550	290	10	Broiling

INDEX

Note: Page references in *italics* indicate photographs.

A

Alcohol, note about, x

Almond(s)

-Crusted Pork Piccata with Zucchini Noodles, *76,* 77

Gazpacho Noodle Soup, *184,* 185

Satay Sauce, 278

Toasted, Blistered Green Beans with, *266,* 267

Apple(s)

–Butternut Squash Soup, 168, *169*

Carrot-Parsnip Soup with Bacon Crumble, *176,* 177

Fennel, and Pork Radicchio Wraps, *12,* 13

and Harvest Vegetables, Roasted Chicken Thighs with, *150,* 151

-Pork Meatball Noodle Bowls, 186, *187*

Apricot-Lamb Loaves with Roasted Cauliflower, *144,* 145

Artichoke Hearts, Slow-Cooker Shakshuka with, *216,* 217

Asparagus

Cream Soup, *200,* 201

Green Curry Pork with, *226,* 227

and Salmon, Lemon-Ginger, *128,* 129

and Shrimp Dinner Omelets, 108, *109*

Avocado(s)

Easy Beef Salad Wraps, *38,* 39

Greek-Style Meatball Salad, *24,* 25

Grilled Steak and Charred Onion Salad, *10,* 11

Hearty Chopped Salad, 37

Mango and Ahi Tuna Poke Salad, 28, *29*

Mango Salsa, *106,* 107

No-Rice Spicy Tuna Rolls, *4,* 5

Quick Blender Green Goddess Dressing, 275

Shrimp and Mango Salad, 32, *33*

B

Bacon

and Eggs with Sweet Potato Noodles, 84

and Pearl Onions, Bolognese Sauce with, 245

-Wrapped Cabbage, Rosemary-Garlic Chicken with, 118, *119*

Baked goods, note about, x

Basil

Pesto, 170

Roasted Garlic Chimichurri, 274

-Zucchini Chicken Hash, 80, *81*

Beef

and Bell Pepper Stir-Fry, Indian, *66,* 67

Bolognese Sauce with Bacon and Pearl Onions, 245

Bone Broth, 280

and Broccoli Salad, Hot, 6, *7*

and Broccoli Stir-Fry, *68,* 69

Chili Con Carne, 253

Coffee au Poivre Steaks with Spiral Potatoes, *142, 143*

Cuban, with Peppers and Onions, 230, *231*

Fajita, Skillet, *96,* 97

Flank Steak with Zucchini Noodle Ramen, *194,* 195

Garlicky Pepper, with Crunchy Cabbage, *228,* 229

Grilled Steak and Charred Onion Salad, *10,* 11

Mongolian, 64, *65*

One-Pan Meatballs with Potatoes and Broccoli, 147

Pan-Seared Steaks with Chimichurri Brussels Slaw, 52, *53*

Roast, Balsamic, and Root Vegetables, *250,* 251

Salad Wraps, Easy, *38,* 39

Salisbury Steak Meatball and Noodle Bowls, 196, *197*

Skillet Grass-Fed Burgers with Roasted-Red-Pepper Ketchup, *90,* 91

Soup, Italian, *192,* 193

Steak and Portobello Rutabaga-Noodle Bowls, *162,* 163

Veggie Wraps with Lemon-Zucchini Dressing, 36

Beet(s)

and Cabbage Salad, Quick, 261

Six-Ingredient Chicken Salad, 22, *23*

Bok Choy and Spicy Lemongrass Chicken Stir-Fry, *54,* 55

Bowls, xv–xvi

Broccoli

and Beef Salad, Hot, 6, *7*

and Beef Stir-Fry, *68,* 69

Coconut-Curry Chicken Drumsticks, 254, *255*

-Kale Soup, Creamy, 204, *205*

Orange Chicken with Cauliflower Rice, 102, *103*

and Potatoes, One-Pan Meatballs with, 147

Sesame, Sheet Pan Shrimp with, 132, *133*

Tuna, and Snow Pea Salad, Asian, with Sesame Dressing, *30,* 31

Broth

Beef Bone, 280

Chicken Bone, 280

Brussels Sprout(s)

Baked, with Tahini, 258

and Chicken Skillet, Thai, 50, *51*

Pan-Seared Steaks with Chimichurri Brussels Slaw, 52, *53*

Roasted, Zucchini-Wrapped Cod with, *134, 135*

Roasted Chicken Thighs with Harvest Vegetables and Apples, *150,* 151

Burgers, Skillet Grass-Fed, with Roasted-Red-Pepper Ketchup, *90,* 91

Butter, Clarified, 283

C

Cabbage

Bacon-Wrapped, Rosemary-Garlic Chicken with, 118, *119*

Banh Mi Pork Salad, 2, *3*

Beef and Broccoli Stir-Fry, *68,* 69

and Beet Salad, Quick, 261

Crunchy, Garlicky Pepper Beef with, *228,* 229

and Potatoes, Roasted Sausages with, *138,* 139

Red, Cups, Shrimp-Prosciutto, 40, *41*

Simple Greek Slaw, *60,* 61

Carrageenan, note about, x

Carrot(s)

Balsamic Beef Roast and Root Vegetables, *250,* 251

BBQ-Pulled-Chicken Lettuce Wraps, *14,* 15

Chicken Sauté with Ginger and Basil, 70, *71*

Grilled Chicken Satay Salad, *20,* 21

Carrot(s) (*continued*)
-Noodle and Pork Bowls, Asian, 182, *183*
-Parsnip Soup with Bacon Crumble, *176,* 177
Rosemary Baby, Mustard-Rubbed Pork Tenderloin with, *140,* 141
Skillet Turkey and Squash Chili, 94, *95*
Veggie Hash with Eggs, *122,* 123
Veggie Noodle Soup with Basil Pesto, 170

Cashew
-Cauliflower Alfredo Sauce, 276
-Coconut Cream, 160, *161*
-Crusted Chicken and Wilted Kale Salad, 8, *9*

Cauliflower
-Cashew Alfredo Sauce, 276
and Chicken Skillet, Spanish, *56,* 57
Coconut-Curry Chicken Drumsticks, 254, *255*
Crumbles, Homemade, 75
Fajita Beef Skillet, *96,* 97
Fennel Soup with Spinach and Spicy Sausage, 180, *181*
Grits, Shrimp Stir-Fry over, 74, *75*
Italian Roasted Whole, 269
Lemon-Garlic Shrimp and Veggies, *98,* 99
Red Curry Shrimp Skillet, 92, *93*
Rice, Chicken Tikka Masala with, *232,* 233
Rice, Homemade, 75
Rice, Orange Chicken with, 102, *103*
Rice, Simple, 284
Roasted, Apricot-Lamb Loaves with, *144,* 145
Sheet Pan Buffalo Chicken with, *152,* 153
Skillet Butter Chicken, *82,* 83
Slow-Cooker Moroccan Chicken, 212, *213*
Southwest "Breakfast for Dinner" Bowls, 202, *203*
-Sweet Potato Mash, 270, *271*
Veggie Confetti Cauli-Rice, 260

Celery Root Fries, Herbed, with Lemon Aioli, 264, *265*

Chicken
Adobo with Mashed Sweet Potatoes, *242,* 243
Balsamic, 244
BBQ-Pulled-, Lettuce Wraps, *14,* 15
Bone Broth, 280

and Brussels Sprout Skillet, Thai, 50, *51*
Buffalo, Dip, 248, *249*
Cashew-Crusted, and Wilted Kale Salad, 8, *9*
and Cauliflower Skillet, Spanish, *56,* 57
Chile Verde, Slow-Cooker, 222, *223*
Chopped Salad, Fruity, 26, *27*
Cilantro-Lime, 236, *237*
Drumsticks, Coconut-Curry, 254, *255*
Grilled, Satay Salad, *20,* 21
Hash, Zucchini-Basil, 80, *81*
Hearty Chinese Egg Drop Soup, 165
Hearty Chopped Salad, 37
Kalamata Olives, and Tomatoes, Spaghetti Squash with, *240,* 241
Legs, Cajun-Style, with Roasted Okra and Peppers, 124, *125*
and Mushroom Soup, *188,* 189
Noodle Bowl, Southwest, 199
Orange, with Cauliflower Rice, 102, *103*
Red Pepper Skillet, Spicy, *110,* 111
Roasted Sausages with Potatoes and Cabbage, *138,* 139
Rosemary-Garlic, with Bacon-Wrapped Cabbage, 118, *119*
Salad, Curry, 18, *19*
Salad, Six-Ingredient, 22, *23*
Sauté with Ginger and Basil, 70, *71*
Sheet Pan Buffalo, with Cauliflower, *152,* 153
Shredded Barbecue, on Sweet Potato "Buns," 238, *239*
and Shrimp with Peppers, Fajita, 136, *137*
Skillet, North African, with Sweet Potato Noodles, 100, *101*
Skillet Butter, *82,* 83
Slow-Cooker Moroccan, 212, *213*
Soup, Mexican, 172, *173*
Spicy Lemongrass, and Bok Choy Stir-Fry, *54,* 55
Spicy Seared, with Watermelon-Spinach Salad, *42,* 43
Thai, Sweet-Potato-Noodle Bowls, 160, *161*
Thighs, Roasted, with Harvest Vegetables and Apples, *150,* 151
Thighs with Stuffed Mushrooms, 154, *155*
Tikka Masala with Cauliflower Rice, *232,* 233
Veggie Wraps with Lemon-Zucchini Dressing, 36
Zoodle Pho, *206,* 207

Chili
Con Carne, 253
Skillet Turkey and Squash, 94, *95*
Slow-Cooker Chicken Chile Verde, 222, *223*
Slow-Cooker Pork, 234, *235*
Chimichurri, Roasted Garlic, 274
Cilantro-Lime Chicken, 236, *237*
Citrus juicer, xvi
Clarified Butter, 283
Clementine-Ancho Salmon with Herbed Sweet Potato Fries, 126, *127*
Coconut aminos, note about, xi
Coconut-Curry Chicken Drumsticks, 254, *255*

Cod
Citrusy Fish Stew, 190, *191*
Steamed, with Spicy Roasted Tomato-Fennel Sauce, 214, *215*
Zucchini-Wrapped, with Roasted Brussels Sprouts, 134, *135*
Coffee au Poivre Steaks with Spiral Potatoes, 142, *143*

Cucumbers
Grilled Chicken Satay Salad, *20,* 21
No-Rice Spicy Tuna Rolls, 4, *5*
Sizzling Pork Greek Salad, *34,* 35
Curried Butternut Squash–Shrimp Soup, Creamy, 246, *247*
Curried Sunflower Seed Sauce, 276
Curry, Green, Pork with Asparagus, *226,* 227
Curry, Red, Shrimp Skillet, 92, *93*
Curry Chicken Salad, 18, *19*
Curry-Coconut Chicken Drumsticks, 254, *255*
Cutting boards, xv

D

Dairy, note about, x
Dip, Buffalo Chicken, 248, *249*
Dressings (Salad)
Apple-Mustard Vinaigrette, 277
Asian Citrus, 277
Everyday Whole30, 278
Green Goddess, Quick Blender, 275
Whole30 Ranch, 282

E

Egg(s)
and Bacon with Sweet Potato Noodles, 84
Drop Soup, Hearty Chinese, 165
Flank Steak with Zucchini Noodle Ramen, *194,* 195

Hearty Chopped Salad, 37
Poached, Winter Greens and Potato
Soup with, 178, *179*
Roasted Potato and Kale Hash with,
120, 121
Shrimp and Asparagus Dinner
Omelets, 108, *109*
Slow-Cooker Shakshuka with Artichoke
Hearts, 216, 217
Southwest "Breakfast for Dinner"
Bowls, 202, *203*
Veggie Hash with, *122,* 123

F

Fajita Beef Skillet, *96, 97*
Fajita Chicken and Shrimp with Peppers,
136, *137*
Fennel
Apple, and Pork Radicchio Wraps, *12,*
13
Citrusy Fish Stew, 190, *191*
Soup with Spinach and Spicy Sausage,
180, *181*
–Spicy Roasted Tomato Sauce, Steamed
Cod with, 214, *215*
and Tomatoes, Roasted Salmon with,
116, *117*
Fish. *See* Cod; Salmon; Tuna
Food processor, xvi–xvii
Fruit. *See specific fruits*
Fruit juice, note about, xi
Fruity Chicken Chopped Salad, 26, *27*

G

Garlic, Roasted, Chimichurri, 274
Garlic peeler and press, xvi
Ghee, note about, xi
Grains, note about, x
Green Beans
Blistered, with Toasted Almonds, *266,*
267
note about, xi
Six-Ingredient Chicken Salad, 22, *23*
Veggie Noodle Soup with Basil Pesto,
170
Green Curry Pork with Asparagus, *226,*
227
Green Onions, Pork Chops and Squash
over, *130,* 131
Greens. *See also* Kale; Lettuce; Radicchio;
Spinach
Hot Beef and Broccoli Salad, 6, *7*
Mongolian Beef, 64, *65*
Winter, and Potato Soup with Poached
Eggs, 178, *179*

H

Herbs. *See also specific herbs*
Pan-Seared Steaks with Chimichurri
Brussels Slaw, 52, *53*
Quick Blender Green Goddess
Dressing, 275
Roasted Garlic Chimichurri, 274
Whole30 Ranch Dressing, 282

I

Immersion blender, xvii
Instant Pot, xvii

J

Junk food, note about, x

K

Kale
-Broccoli Soup, Creamy, 204, *205*
Chicken Thighs with Stuffed
Mushrooms, 154, *155*
and Potato, Roasted, Hash with Eggs,
120, 121
Wilted, and Cashew-Crusted Chicken
Salad, 8, *9*
Winter Greens and Potato Soup with
Poached Eggs, 178, *179*
Ketchup
Roasted-Red-Pepper, *90,* 91
Whole30, 282
Kitchen tools, xv–xvii
Knives and sharpeners, xv

L

Lamb-Apricot Loaves with Roasted
Cauliflower, *144,* 145
Leek and Turnip Soup, Creamy, *174,* 175
Legumes, note about, x
Lemon
Aioli, Herbed Celery Root Fries with,
264, *265*
-Ginger Salmon and Asparagus, *128,*
129
Lettuce
Easy Beef Salad Wraps, 38, *39*
Fruity Chicken Chopped Salad, 26, *27*
Greek-Style Meatball Salad, 24, *25*
Grilled Chicken Satay Salad, *20,* 21
Grilled Steak and Charred Onion
Salad, *10,* 11
Hearty Chopped Salad, 37
Shrimp and Mango Salad, 32, *33*
Sizzling Pork Greek Salad, 34, *35*
Veggie Wraps with Lemon-Zucchini
Dressing, 36

Wraps, BBQ-Pulled-Chicken, *14,* 15
Lime-Cilantro Chicken, 236, *237*

M

Mango
and Ahi Tuna Poke Salad, 28, *29*
Avocado Salsa, *106, 107*
and Shrimp Salad, 32, *33*
Mayonnaise
Basic, 281
Egg-Free, 281
Meat. *See* Beef; Lamb; Pork
Meatball(s)
Big Turkey, with Roasted Cherry
Tomatoes, *114,* 115
One-Pan, with Potatoes and Broccoli,
147
Pork-Apple, Noodle Bowls, 186, *187*
Salad, Greek-Style, 24, *25*
Salisbury Steak, and Noodle Bowls,
196, *197*
Microplane, xvi
MSG, note about, x
Mushroom(s)
and Chicken Soup, *188,* 189
Hearty Chinese Egg Drop Soup, 165
Steak and Portobello Rutabaga-Noodle
Bowls, *162,* 163
Stuffed, Chicken Thighs with, 154, *155*
-Tarragon Cream Sauce, Pork
Scaloppini with, 78, *79*
Veggie Hash with Eggs, *122,* 123
Mussels in Spicy Tomato Sauce with
Squash Ribbons, 85

N

Nuts. *See* Almond(s); Cashew

O

Okra and Peppers, Roasted, Cajun-Style
Chicken Legs with, 124, *125*
Olives
Kalamata, Chicken, and Tomatoes,
Spaghetti Squash with, *240,* 241
Sizzling Pork Greek Salad, 34, *35*
Spanish Chicken and Cauliflower
Skillet, *56, 57*
Omelets, Shrimp and Asparagus Dinner,
108, *109*
Onion(s)
Charred, and Grilled Steak Salad, *10,* 11
Pearl, and Bacon, Bolognese Sauce
with, 245
and Peppers, Cuban Beef with, 230, *231*

Orange(s)
Asian Citrus Dressing, 277
Chicken with Cauliflower Rice, 102, *103*
Fruity Chicken Chopped Salad, 26, *27*

P

Parchment paper, xvi
Parsnip(s)
Balsamic Beef Roast and Root Vegetables, *250*, 251
-Carrot Soup with Bacon Crumble, *176*, 177
Lemon-Dill, 262
Veggie Hash with Eggs, *122*, 123
Pea(s)
Chicken Sauté with Ginger and Basil, 70, *71*
Pork and Pepper Stir-Fry, 72, *73*
Snow, Tuna, and Broccoli Salad, Asian, with Sesame Dressing, *30*, 31
snow/snap, note about, xi
Sugar Snap, Sautéed, 268
Pepper(s)
Bell, and Beef Stir-Fry, Indian, *66*, 67
Chile-Lime Roasted Sweet Potatoes, 259
Chili Con Carne, 253
Fajita Beef Skillet, *96*, 97
Fajita Chicken and Shrimp with, 136, *137*
Ginger Shrimp and Zucchini-Noodle Stir-Fry, *46*, 47
Green Chile Pork Stew, 171
Green Curry Pork with Asparagus, *226*, 227
Italian Beef Soup, *192*, 193
Lemon-Garlic Shrimp and Veggies, *98*, 99
Mexican Chicken Soup, 172, *173*
and Okra, Roasted, Cajun-Style Chicken Legs with, 124, *125*
and Onions, Cuban Beef with, 230, *231*
and Pork Paprikash, Quick, *166*, 167
and Pork Stir-Fry, 72, *73*
Ratatouille Stew with Seared Scallops, 208, *209*
Red, Chicken Skillet, Spicy, *110*, 111
Roasted-Red- , Ketchup, *90*, 91
Slow-Cooker Chicken Chile Verde, 222, *223*
Southwest "Breakfast for Dinner" Bowls, 202, *203*
Southwest Chicken Noodle Bowl, 199

Turkey Tenderloins with Cherry Tomato–Serrano Peperonata, 48, *49*
Whole30 Sriracha, 274
Pesto, Basil, 170
Pineapple
Ginger-Caramelized, Seared Salmon Fillets with, 88, *89*
and Quick-Toasted Cumin Taco Sauce, 275
Pork. *See also* Bacon; Sausage(s) (pork)
Apple, and Fennel Radicchio Wraps, *12*, 13
Apple-Cider, Slow-Cooker, 218, *219*
-Apple Meatball Noodle Bowls, 186, *187*
and Carrot-Noodle Bowls, Asian, 182, *183*
Chili, Slow-Cooker, 234, *235*
Chops, Sheet Pan Barbecue, with Potatoes, 148, *149*
Chops, Skillet, with Sweet Potatoes, *60*, 61
Chops, Skillet Rosemary, with Potatoes and Onions, *104*, 105
Chops and Squash over Green Onions, *130*, 131
Chops with Sweet Potato Colcannon, *62*, 63
Green Curry, with Asparagus, *226*, 227
and Pepper Paprikash, Quick, *166*, 167
and Pepper Stir-Fry, 72, *73*
Piccata, Almond-Crusted, with Zucchini Noodles, *76*, 77
Salad, Banh Mi, 2, *3*
Scaloppini with Mushroom-Tarragon Cream Sauce, 78, *79*
Shrimp-Prosciutto Red Cabbage Cups, 40, *41*
Sizzling, Greek Salad, *34*, 35
Spaghetti Squash with Sausage Arrabbiata Sauce, 58, *59*
Stew, Green Chile, 171
Tacos with Sweet Potato Mash, 224, *225*
Tenderloin, Mustard-Rubbed, with Rosemary Baby Carrots, *140*, 141
-Vegetable Stew, Sweet and Spicy, 252
Potato(es). *See also* Sweet Potato(es)
Balsamic Beef Roast and Root Vegetables, *250*, 251
and Broccoli, One-Pan Meatballs with, 147
and Cabbage, Roasted Sausages with, *138*, 139
Green Chile Pork Stew, 171

and Kale, Roasted, Hash with Eggs, *120*, 121
and Onions, Skillet Rosemary Pork Chops with, *104*, 105
and Salmon Salad, Warm, 16, *17*
Sheet Pan Barbecue Pork Chops with, 148, *149*
Southwest Chicken Noodle Bowl, 199
Spiral, Coffee au Poivre Steaks with, *142*, 143
and Winter Greens Soup with Poached Eggs, 178, *179*
Poultry. *See* Chicken; Turkey
Prosciutto-Shrimp Red Cabbage Cups, 40, *41*

R

Radicchio Wraps, Apple, Fennel, and Pork, *12*, 13
Ratatouille Stew with Seared Scallops, 208, *209*
Red Curry Shrimp Skillet, 92, *93*
Rosemary-Garlic Chicken with Bacon-Wrapped Cabbage, 118, *119*
Rutabaga
-Noodle Bowls, Steak and Portobello, *162*, 163
Sweet and Spicy Vegetable-Pork Stew, 252

S

Salads
Banh Mi Pork, 2, *3*
Beet and Cabbage, Quick, 261
Cashew-Crusted Chicken and Wilted Kale, 8, *9*
Chicken, Six-Ingredient, 22, *23*
Curry Chicken, 18, *19*
Fruity Chicken Chopped, 26, *27*
Grilled Chicken Satay, *20*, 21
Grilled Steak and Charred Onion, *10*, 11
Hearty Chopped, 37
Hot Beef and Broccoli, 6, *7*
Mango and Ahi Tuna Poke, 28, *29*
Meatball, Greek-Style, 24, *25*
Salmon and Potato, Warm, 16, *17*
Shrimp and Mango, 32, *33*
Sizzling Pork Greek, *34*, 35
Tuna, Snow Pea, and Broccoli, Asian, with Sesame Dressing, *30*, 31
Watermelon-Spinach, Spicy Seared Chicken with, *42*, 43
Salmon
Ancho-Clementine, with Herbed Sweet Potato Fries, 126, *127*

and Asparagus, Lemon-Ginger, *128,*
129
Fillets, Seared, with Ginger-
Caramelized Pineapple, 88, *89*
and Potato Salad, Warm, 16, *17*
Roasted, with Tomatoes and Fennel,
116, *117*
Salsa, Mango Avocado, *106,* 107
Salsa Verde
–Shrimp Soup, *220,* 221
Slow-Cooker Chicken Chile Verde,
222, *223*
Salt, iodized, note about, xi
Sauces. *See also* Ketchup; Mayonnaise
Almond Satay, 278
Basic Mayonnaise, 281
Basil Pesto, 170
Bolognese, with Bacon and Pearl
Onions, 245
Cashew-Coconut Cream, 160, *161*
Cauliflower-Cashew Alfredo, 276
Curried Sunflower Seed, 276
Egg-Free Mayonnaise, 281
Quick-Toasted Cumin and Pineapple
Taco, 275
Roasted Garlic Chimichurri, 274
Roasted-Red-Pepper Ketchup, *90,* 91
Whole30 Sriracha, 274
Sausage, Turkey, and Sweet Potato Soup,
Quick, 198
Sausages, Roasted, with Potatoes and
Cabbage, *138,* 139
Sausage(s) (pork)
Chicken Thighs with Stuffed
Mushrooms, 154, *155*
Chorizo and Sweet Potato Skillet, *86,*
87
Southwest "Breakfast for Dinner"
Bowls, 202, *203*
Spicy, and Spinach, Fennel Soup with,
180, *181*
Scallop(s)
Seared, Ratatouille Stew with, 208, *209*
Smoky, Noodle Bowls, 164
Sesame Broccoli, Sheet Pan Shrimp with,
132, *133*
Shears, kitchen, xv
Sheet pans, xvi
Shellfish. *See also* Shrimp
Mussels in Spicy Tomato Sauce with
Squash Ribbons, 85
Ratatouille Stew with Seared Scallops,
208, *209*

Smoky Scallop Noodle Bowls, 164
Shrimp
and Asparagus Dinner Omelets, 108,
109
–Butternut Squash Soup, Creamy
Curried, 246, *247*
and Chicken with Peppers, Fajita, 136,
137
Gazpacho Noodle Soup, *184,* 185
Ginger, and Zucchini-Noodle Stir-Fry,
46, 47
Lemon-Garlic, and Veggies, *98,* 99
and Mango Salad, 32, *33*
-Prosciutto Red Cabbage Cups, 40, *41*
Red Curry, Skillet, 92, *93*
–Salsa Verde Soup, *220,* 221
Sheet Pan, with Sesame Broccoli, 132,
133
Stir-Fry over Cauliflower Grits, 74, *75*
Veggie Noodle Soup with Basil Pesto,
170
Veggie Wraps with Lemon-Zucchini
Dressing, 36
and Zoodle Soup, Mexican, 158, *159*
Slow cooker, xvii
Soups
Apple–Butternut Squash, 168, *169*
Asparagus Cream, *200,* 201
Beef, Italian, *192,* 193
Broccoli-Kale, Creamy, 204, *205*
Carrot-Parsnip, with Bacon Crumble,
176, 177
Chicken, Mexican, 172, *173*
Chicken and Mushroom, *188,* 189
Chicken Zoodle Pho, *206,* 207
Curried Butternut Squash–Shrimp,
Creamy, 246, *247*
Egg Drop, Hearty Chinese, 165
Fennel, with Spinach and Spicy
Sausage, 180, *181*
Flank Steak with Zucchini Noodle
Ramen, *194,* 195
Gazpacho Noodle, *184,* 185
Quick Pork and Pepper Paprikash,
166, 167
Shrimp and Zoodle, Mexican, 158, *159*
Shrimp–Salsa Verde, *220,* 221
Southwest Chicken Noodle Bowl, 199
Steak and Portobello Rutabaga-Noodle
Bowls, *162,* 163
Thai Chicken Sweet-Potato-Noodle
Bowls, 160, *161*

Turkey Sausage and Sweet Potato,
Quick, 198
Turnip and Leek, Creamy, *174,* 175
Veggie Noodle, with Basil Pesto, 170
Winter Greens and Potato, with
Poached Eggs, 178, *179*
Spinach
Chorizo and Sweet Potato Skillet, *86,*
87
Mango and Ahi Tuna Poke Salad, 28,
29
Red Curry Shrimp Skillet, 92, *93*
and Spicy Sausage, Fennel Soup with,
180, *181*
-Watermelon Salad, Spicy Seared
Chicken with, *42,* 43
Spiral slicer, xvi
Squash. *See also* Zucchini
Butternut, –Apple Soup, 168, *169*
Butternut, –Shrimp Soup, Creamy
Curried, 246, *247*
Pork-Apple Meatball Noodle Bowls,
186, *187*
and Pork Chops over Green Onions,
130, 131
Ribbons, Mussels in Spicy Tomato
Sauce with, 85
Spaghetti, with Chicken, Kalamata
Olives, and Tomatoes, *240,* 241
Spaghetti, with Sausage Arrabbiata
Sauce, 58, *59*
Sweet and Spicy Vegetable-Pork Stew,
252
and Turkey Chili, Skillet, 94, *95*
Sriracha, Whole30, 274
Stews. *See also* Chili
Fish, Citrusy, 190, *191*
Green Chile Pork, 171
Ratatouille, with Seared Scallops, 208,
209
Vegetable-Pork, Sweet and Spicy, 252
Sugar, note about, x
Sulfites, note about, x
Sunflower Seed Sauce, Curried, 276
Sweet Potato(es)
"Buns," Shredded Barbecue Chicken
on, 238, *239*
–Cauliflower Mash, 270, *271*
Chicken and Mushroom Soup, *188,* 189
Chile-Lime Roasted, 259
and Chorizo Skillet, *86,* 87
Colcannon, Pork Chops with, 62, *63*

Sweet Potato(es) (continued)
  Fries, Herbed, Ancho-Clementine
    Salmon with, 126, 127
  Mash, Pork Tacos with, 224, 225
  Mashed, Chicken Adobo with, 242, 243
  -Noodle Bowls, Thai Chicken, 160, 161
  Noodles, Bacon and Eggs with, 84
  Noodles, North African Chicken Skillet
    with, 100, 101
  Roasted Chicken Thighs with Harvest
    Vegetables and Apples, 150, 151
  Salisbury Steak Meatball and Noodle
    Bowls, 196, 197
  Skillet Butter Chicken, 82, 83
  Skillet Pork Chops with, 60, 61
  Slow-Cooker Moroccan Chicken, 212,
    213
  Southwest "Breakfast for Dinner"
    Bowls, 202, 203
  and Turkey Sausage Soup, Quick, 198

T
Tacos, Pork, with Sweet Potato Mash, 224,
  225
Taco Sauce, Quick-Toasted Cumin and
  Pineapple, 275
Tahini, Baked Brussels Sprouts with, 258
Tomatillos
  Shrimp–Salsa Verde Soup, 220, 221
Tomato(es)
  Bolognese Sauce with Bacon and Pearl
    Onions, 245
  Cherry, Roasted, Big Turkey Meatballs
    with, 114, 115
  Cherry, –Serrano Peperonata, Turkey
    Tenderloins with, 48, 49
  Chicken, and Kalamata Olives,
    Spaghetti Squash with, 240, 241
  Chili Con Carne, 253
  Easy Beef Salad Wraps, 38, 39
  and Fennel, Roasted Salmon with, 116,
    117
  Gazpacho Noodle Soup, 184, 185
  Hearty Chopped Salad, 37
  Quick-Toasted Cumin and Pineapple
    Taco Sauce, 275
  Ratatouille Stew with Seared Scallops,
    208, 209
  Sauce, Spicy, Mussels in, with Squash
    Ribbons, 85
  Six-Ingredient Chicken Salad, 22, 23
  Skillet Butter Chicken, 82, 83

Skillet Turkey and Squash Chili, 94, 95
Slow-Cooker Pork Chili, 234, 235
Slow-Cooker Shakshuka with Artichoke
  Hearts, 216, 217
Smoky Scallop Noodle Bowls, 164
Spaghetti Squash with Sausage
  Arrabbiata Sauce, 58, 59
Spanish Chicken and Cauliflower
  Skillet, 56, 57
Spicy Roasted, –Fennel Sauce, Steamed
  Cod with, 214, 215
Whole30 Ketchup, 282
Tuna
  Ahi, and Mango Poke Salad, 28, 29
  Ahi, Seared, with Mango Avocado
    Salsa, 106, 107
  Rolls, No-Rice Spicy, 4, 5
  Snow Pea, and Broccoli Salad, Asian,
    with Sesame Dressing, 30, 31
Turkey
  Greek-Style Meatball Salad, 24, 25
  Meatballs, Big, with Roasted Cherry
    Tomatoes, 114, 115
  Sausage and Sweet Potato Soup, Quick,
    198
  and Squash Chili, Skillet, 94, 95
  Tenderloins with Cherry Tomato–
    Serrano Peperonata, 48, 49
Turnip and Leek Soup, Creamy, 174, 175

V
Vegetable chopper, xvi
Vegetables. See also specific vegetables
  Veggie Confetti Cauli-Rice, 260
Vinegar, note about, xi

W
Watermelon-Spinach Salad, Spicy Seared
  Chicken with, 42, 43
Weighing yourself, xi, xiv
Whole30
  approved partners and products,
    290–293
  Certified Coaches, 290
  committing to, xi–xii
  cookbooks, 287–288
  fast and easy kitchen hacks, xvii–xix
  getting started with, xiii–xiv
  how it works, viii
  kitchen essentials, xv–xvii
  meal planning, 290
  off-limits food exceptions, xi

off-limits foods, x–xi
the results, viii–ix
rules for, x–xii
social media feeds, 288–289
support, 294
websites, 285–286
Whole30 guest chefs
  Anya Kaats, 5
  Brian Kavanagh, 16
  ChihYu Smith, 65
  Dana Monsees, 213
  Jessica Beacom and Stacie Hassing, 19
  Kelly Smith, 219
  Laura Miner, 135
  Ronny Joseph, 79
  Sarah Steffens, 81
  Scott Gooding, 63
Wraps
  Apple, Fennel, and Pork Radicchio,
    12, 13
  BBQ-Pulled-Chicken Lettuce, 14, 15
  Beef Salad, Easy, 38, 39
  Veggie, with Lemon-Zucchini Dressing,
    36

Z
Zucchini
  -Basil Chicken Hash, 80, 81
  Chicken Zoodle Pho, 206, 207
  Creamy Turnip and Leek Soup, 174, 175
  Gazpacho Noodle Soup, 184, 185
  Hasselback, with Gremolata, 263
  Italian Beef Soup, 192, 193
  -Lemon Dressing, Veggie Wraps with,
    36
  Lemon-Garlic Shrimp and Veggies,
    98, 99
  Mexican Shrimp and Zoodle Soup,
    158, 159
  -Noodle and Ginger Shrimp Stir-Fry,
    46, 47
  Noodle Ramen, Flank Steak with, 194,
    195
  Noodles, Almond-Crusted Pork Piccata
    with, 76, 77
  Ratatouille Stew with Seared Scallops,
    208, 209
  Smoky Scallop Noodle Bowls, 164
  Veggie Noodle Soup with Basil Pesto,
    170
  -Wrapped Cod with Roasted Brussels
    Sprouts, 134, 135